Modern Dermatologic Radiation Therapy

Herbert Goldschmidt
Renato G. Panizzon

Modern Dermatologic Radiation Therapy

With special contributions by John C. Breneman, Robert O. Gorson, and Bernt Lindelöf

With 99 illustrations in 105 parts, 22 tables, and 510 references

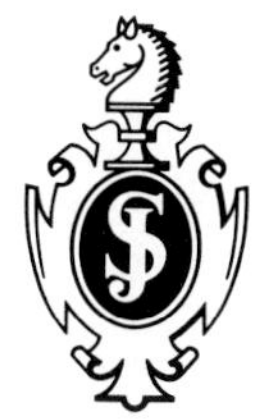

Springer-Verlag New York Berlin Heidelberg
London Paris Tokyo Hong Kong Barcelona

Herbert Goldschmidt, M.D.,
F.A.C.P.
Clinical Professor of Dermatology
University of Pennsylvania
Philadelphia, PA, USA

Renato G. Panizzon, Dr. med.
Privatdozent
Universität Zürich
Zürich, Switzerland

Library of Congress Cataloging-in-Publication Data
Goldschmidt, Herbert, 1923–
    Modern dermatologic radiation therapy / Herbert Goldschmidt,
Renato G. Panizzon ; special contributions by J.C. Breneman, R.O.
Gorson, B. Lindelöf.
        p. cm.
    Includes bibliographical references.
    Includes index.
    ISBN 0-387-97328-1 (alk. paper).–ISBN 3-540-97328-1 (alk.
paper)
        1. Skin–Diseases–Radiotherapy. 2. Skin–Cancer–Radiotherapy.
I. Panizzon, Renato G. II. Title.
        [DNLM: 1. Skin Diseases–radiotherapy. 2. Skin Neoplasms–
radiotherapy. WR 660 G623m]
RL113.G65 1990
616.5'0642–dc20
DNLM/DLC
for Library of Congress   90-9894

Printed on acid-free paper

Typeset by Publishers Service of Montana, Bozeman, MT.
Printed and bound by Edwards Brothers, Ann Arbor, MI.
Printed in the United States of America.

9 8 7 6 5 4 3 2 1

ISBN 0-387-97328-1 Springer-Verlag New York Berlin Heidelberg
ISBN 3-540-97328-1 Springer-Verlag Berlin Heidelberg New York

Preface

Radiation therapy of cutaneous cancers and other dermatologic disorders is not covered adequately in many current textbooks of dermatology and radiation oncology. This book is intended to fill that gap.

Both text and illustrations are oriented toward the practical aspects of radiation therapy. The beginner will find a concise introduction to physical and biological principles, selection of radiation factors, dose definitions, indications for treatment, and radiation sequelae. The experienced dermatologist and radiation oncologist will find a detailed discussion of specific indications for various radiation techniques in different body regions. A special effort was made to add pertinent references to the world literature for those who wish to pursue particular topics still further. We have tried to include all major American and European publications of the last 20 years in our bibliography of more than 500 references, and we also have attempted to review the most important scientific papers on principles and practice of ionizing radiation therapy in a constructive way.

We are grateful to Professor Gorson, Dr. Breneman, and Professor Lindelöf, who generously contributed chapters in their areas of expertise despite their many other commitments.

Herbert Goldschmidt
Philadelphia, Pennsylvania
Renato G. Panizzon
Zürich, Switzerland

Acknowledgments

This book would not have been possible without the generous assistance of others. Most of all, we want to express our gratitude to our wives, Wiltrud and Nicole, for their active editorial help and their patient support during the preparation of the manuscripts. We owe special thanks to our secretaries, Mrs. Susan McKown and Mrs. Cordula Cohen for their excellent work in preparing the typescripts. Prof. Schnyder and Dr. Sherwin gave valuable advice on theoretical and clinical problems. We wish also to thank the staff at Springer-Verlag for their assistance in this project.

In the preparation of this text we have used illustrations, tables, and excerpts of our previous publications in the field of dermatologic radiation therapy, especially the following books and papers:

Goldschmidt H, Sherwin WK. Reactions to ionizing radiation. *J Am Acad Dermatol.* 1980;3:551–579.

Goldschmidt H, Sherwin WK. Office radiotherapy of cutaneous carcinomas. *J Dermatol Surg Oncol.* 1983;9:31–76.

Goldschmidt H, Sherwin WK. Dermatologic radiation therapy. In: Moschella SC, Hurley HJ, eds. *Dermatology.* 2nd ed. Philadelphia, Penn: WB Saunders; 1985.

Goldschmidt H. Treatment planning. In: Goldschmidt H, ed. *Physical Modalities in Dermatologic Therapy.* New York, NY: Springer-Verlag; 1978.

Goldschmidt H. Radiodermatitis and other sequelae of ionizing radiation. In: Demis J, ed. *Dermatology, Vol. IV.* Philadelphia, Penn: JB Lippincott; 1986.

Gorson RO. Physical aspects of dermatologic radiotherapy. In: Goldschmidt H, ed. *Physical Modalities in Dermatologic Therapy.* New York, NY: Springer-Verlag; 1978.

Panizzon RG. Die Strahlentherapie des Basalioms. In: Eichmann E, Schnyder UW, eds. *Das Basaliom.* Heidelberg: Springer-Verlag; 1980.

Panizzon RG, Hanson WR, Schwartz D, et al. Ionizing radiation induces early, sustained increases in collagen biosynthesis: a 48 week study in mouse skin and skin fibroblasts cultures. *Radiat Res.* 1988;116:145–156.

Herbert Goldschmidt
Renato G. Panizzon

Contents

Contributors

John C. Breneman, M.D.   Assistant Professor of Radiology, University of Cincinnati, Cincinnati, Ohio, USA

Herbert Goldschmidt, M.D.   Clinical Professor of Dermatology, University of Pennsylvania, Philadelphia, Pennsylvania, USA

Robert O. Gorson   Professor of Medical Physics, Jefferson University, Philadelphia, Pennsylvania, USA

Bernt Lindelöf, M.D.   Associate Professor, Department of Dermatology, Karolinska Hospital, Karolinska Institute, Stockholm, Sweden

Renato G. Panizzon, Dr. med.   Privatdozent, Universität Zürich, Zürich, Switzerland

1

Physical Aspects of Dermatologic Radiotherapy

Robert O. Gorson

X-Ray Phenomena

X rays are electromagnetic radiations of high energy.[1] Figure 1.1 shows the relative position of x rays in the electromagnetic spectrum. γ rays also cover the same energy range as do x rays and are indistinguishable from them. γ rays originate from within the atomic nucleus, whereas x rays are generated outside the nucleus. As do all other electromagnetic radiations, x and γ rays consist of oscillating electric and magnetic fields characterized by the following parameters:

Velocity c (2.997925 × 10^8 m/sec)
Wavelength λ
Frequency ν
Period T
Energy E

The velocity of all electromagnetic radiation is the same in a vacuum, that is, approximately 3 × 10^8 m/sec. The wavelength (λ) is the distance between any two corresponding points on two adjacent waves, which is the same as the distance traveled during the time for one cycle. The time for one cycle is the period (T). The frequency (ν) is the number of cycles per second and is expressed in hertz (Hz), which is a special unit of frequency equal to one cycle per second. The period and frequency are inversely related, so that $T = 1/\nu$. By definition of velocity,

$$c = \lambda T = \lambda \nu \tag{1}$$

In addition to their wave-like characteristics, electromagnetic radiations exhibit particle-like qualities in their interactions (transfers of energy) with matter. Each x ray is characterized by a definite amount of energy that is directly proportional to its frequency and inversely proportional to its wavelength. These "packets" of energy are called "photons" or "quanta." The relationship between the energy of a photon and its frequency is

$$E = h\nu \tag{2}$$

where h = 6.625 × 10^{-34} joule-seconds (Planck's constant) and E is expressed in joules (J). By combining equations (1) and (2) the following relationship between photon energy and wavelength is obtained:

$$E = hc/\lambda \tag{3}$$

The joule is a relatively large unit of energy for use in radiation physics. A more convenient unit is the electron volt (eV). An electron volt is the amount of energy that an electron acquires when it is accelerated through a difference of potential of one volt. Multiple units are 1000 eV (1 keV) and 1,000,000 eV (1 MeV). One eV equals 1.6 × 10^{-19} J.

When values for the velocity of light and Planck's constant are substituted into equation (3), and when the wavelength is expressed in angstroms (1 Å = 10^{-10} m) and the energy in keV, the following useful relationship can be derived:

$$E = 12.4/\lambda \tag{4}$$

Table 1.1 lists various photon energies and their corresponding frequencies and wavelengths derived from equations (1) and (4).

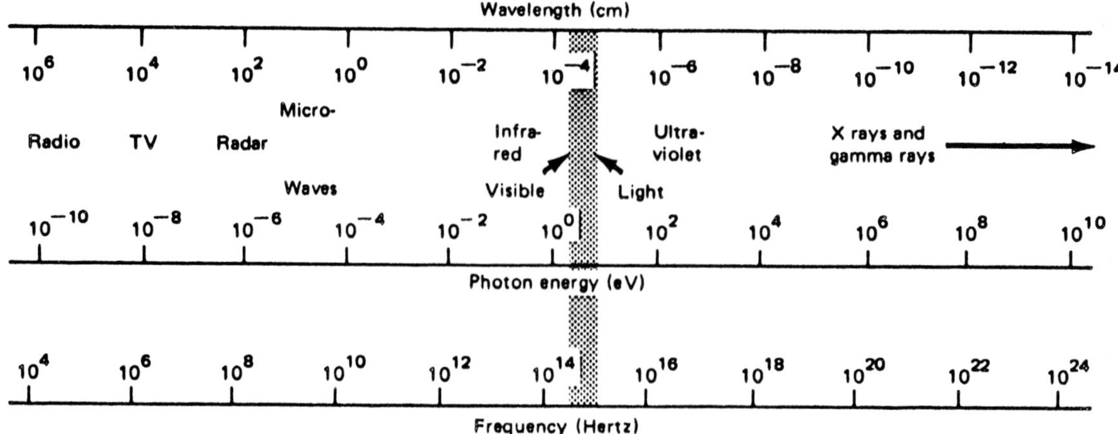

FIGURE 1.1. Diagram of the electromagnetic spectrum indicating the relative position of different parts of the spectrum in terms of wavelength, photon energy, and frequency (From ref. 1, with permission.)

Production of X Rays

X rays are produced by two processes involving the deceleration of high-energy electrons in matter. High-energy electrons are readily obtained by accelerating electrons boiled off a heated filament (thermionic emission) through a high electric potential in an evacuated tube (x-ray tube). Figure 1.2 diagrams the principal parts of an x-ray tube. By varying the electric potential between the filament (cathode) and the anode, the kinetic energy of the electrons striking the target in the anode may also be varied. Most of the electrons striking the target lose their energy by "colliding" with orbital electrons of the atoms of the target material (usually tungsten). Many of the orbital electrons are knocked out of the atoms or into higher energy levels within the atoms. As the target atoms return to the ground state, electromagnetic photons are released. Some of the photons may have sufficient energy to be categorized within the x-ray region of the electromagnetic spectrum. Most of the photons have energies in the ultraviolet, visible light, or infrared regions. In any case, radiation produced by excited atoms returning to the ground state is called "characteristic" radiation because the energies of the released photons correspond to differences in the energy levels of the orbital electrons of the target atoms, and the energy differences depend on the atomic number of the atoms comprising the target. Characteristic (or fluorescent) radiation consists of a line spectrum of energies

TABLE 1.1. Photon energy wavelength and frequency.[a]

Energy (keV)	Wavelength (Å)	Frequency (Hz × 10¹⁸)
0.5	24.8	0.12
1.0	12.4	0.24
6.2	2.0	1.5
12.4	1.0	3.0
24.8	0.5	6.0
49.6	0.25	12

[a] From ref. 1, with permission.

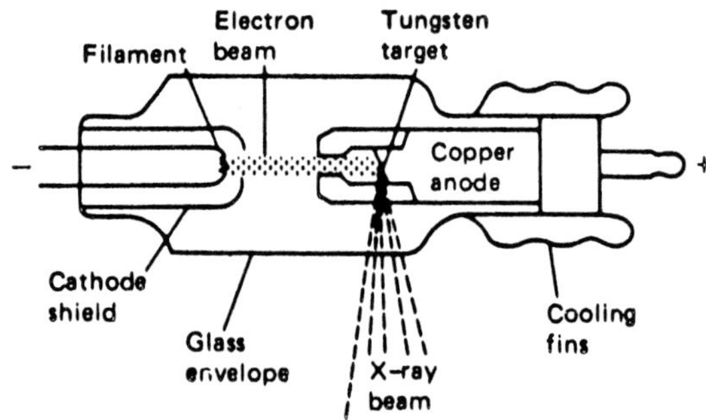

FIGURE 1.2. The principal parts of an x-ray therapy tube. Electrons emitted by the heated filament are accelerated to the copper anode where they strike the tungsten target from which the resultant x rays are emitted (From ref. 1, with permission.)

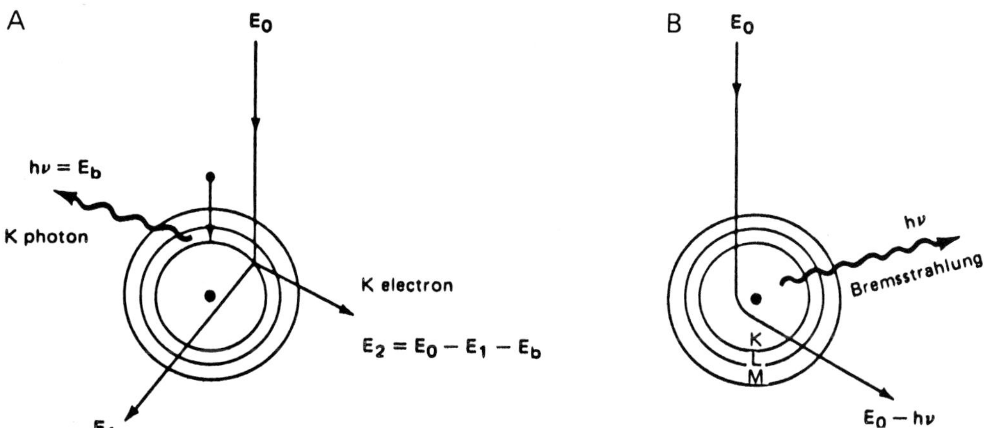

FIGURE 1.3. Electron interactions. A, Collision loss. The incident electron with energy E_0 collides with a K electron, knocking it out of the atom. This is followed by the emission of the K-characteristic x-ray photon when the vacancy in the K shell is filled by another electron. E_b is the binding energy of the K electron. B, Radiation loss. The incident electron loses energy as it is decelerated by the atomic nucleus, producing an x-ray photon (bremsstrahlung) (From ref. 1, with permission.)

corresponding to the energy differences of the electron levels in the excited and ground states.

X rays are also produced when high-energy electrons are decelerated by the nuclei of the target atoms. This radiation is called "bremsstrahlung" or braking radiation. Usually only part of the kinetic energy of a decelerating electron is converted into an x-ray photon; hence, most of the x rays generated have energies less than the kinetic energies of the striking electrons. On rare occasions, all of the energy of an electron is converted into an x ray. Thus, the maximum energy of x rays generated in an x-ray tube, when expressed in electron volts, is numerically equal to the accelerating voltage across the x-ray tube. Figure 1.3 illustrates two kinds of electron interaction. Figure 1.3A (collision loss) shows the ejection of a K electron followed by the emission of a K-characteristic x ray when the vacancy in the K shell is filled. Figure 1.3B (radiation loss) shows the emission of a bremsstrahlung x ray when the striking electron is deflected from its path by the atomic nucleus. The relative intensities of x rays generated by 50- and 100-keV bombarding electrons are shown in Figure 1.4 by dashed lines. The solid lines show the relative intensity distribution of the x rays transmitted through the x-ray tube. The difference between the two curves is the intensity of the x rays absorbed in the target material and the glass envelope of the x-ray tube. Note that all of the x rays below a certain energy level are absorbed within the x-ray tube. If more filtration is added to the x-ray tube, an even greater proportion of lower energy photons will be removed and the peak of the curve will shift to higher energies and the effective energy of the transmitted x-ray beam will increase. Increasing the accelerating voltage of the x-ray tube, and hence the kinetic energy of the bombarding electrons, will produce a similar shift.

Superimposed on the bremsstrahlung intensity spectrum is the line spectrum of the characteristic x rays. The characteristic x-ray spectrum constitutes a small fraction of the total x-ray intensity and can usually be disregarded. This is particularly the case for x-ray tubes operated at tube potentials below 69 kV because the binding energy of the tungsten K electrons is about 69 keV.

Because most of the electrons striking the target suffer collision losses with orbital electrons and only a small portion undergo bremsstrahlung-producing interactions with atomic nuclei, the efficiency of x-ray production is low. For x-ray tubes operating at potentials below 100 kV, less than 1% of the total energy of the electron beam striking the target appears in the emerging x-ray beam.

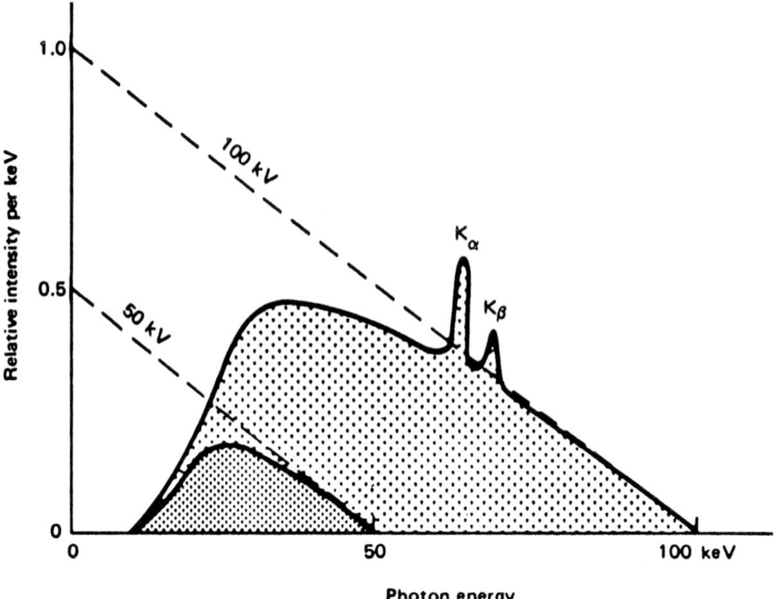

FIGURE 1.4. Energy distribution of x rays generated by x-ray tubes operated at 50 and 100 kV. The dashed curves show the theoretical distribution of bremsstrahlung generated within a thick tungsten target. The solid curves show the energy distribution of the x rays that escape from the target and penetrate the x-ray tube. In both cases, the maximum energy of the x rays expressed in electron volts is numerically equal to the voltage across the x-ray tube. Also shown are the K$_\alpha$- and K$_\beta$-characteristic x rays for tungsten, which are produced by electrons having energies above approximately 69 keV (From ref. 1, with permission.)

X-Ray Absorption

In general, when an x-ray beam is directed at a human body, some x rays will be absorbed or scattered and some will pass through as though the body were not present. The probability that a given x-ray photon will be absorbed depends on the energy of the photon, the atomic number of the constituent atoms of the body, and the density and thickness of the part of the body through which the photon passes. When x rays are used to treat superficial lesions, the energy spectrum of the x-ray beam is adjusted (by selecting an appropriate combination of x-ray tube voltage and filtration) so that most of the energy is absorbed within the tissue volume to be treated. The absorption process involves the interaction of photons with orbital electrons producing ionization and excitation of the affected atoms. There are two such processes that are of importance in the energy range of x rays used in superficial radiation therapy. These are illustrated in Figure 1.5. The first process, called the "photoelectric" effect, occurs whenever a photon transfers all of its energy to an orbital electron. The photon disappears and the electron is ejected from the atom with a kinetic energy equal to the photon energy minus the binding energy of the electron. The second process, called the "Compton" effect, occurs whenever a photon interacting with an orbital electron transfers only part of its energy to the electron. The electron, called a "Compton electron," leaves the atom with a kinetic energy equal to the transferred energy minus the electron-binding energy. The remaining energy appears in the form of another photon of lower energy than that of the original (longer wavelength), emitted in a different direction. The Compton scattered photon will either pass out of the body or will interact with another atom in the body by either the Compton or photoelectric process. In any case, the energies of the photoelectric and Compton electrons are dissipated by subsequent interactions with other electrons (collision losses) producing further ionization and excitation or,

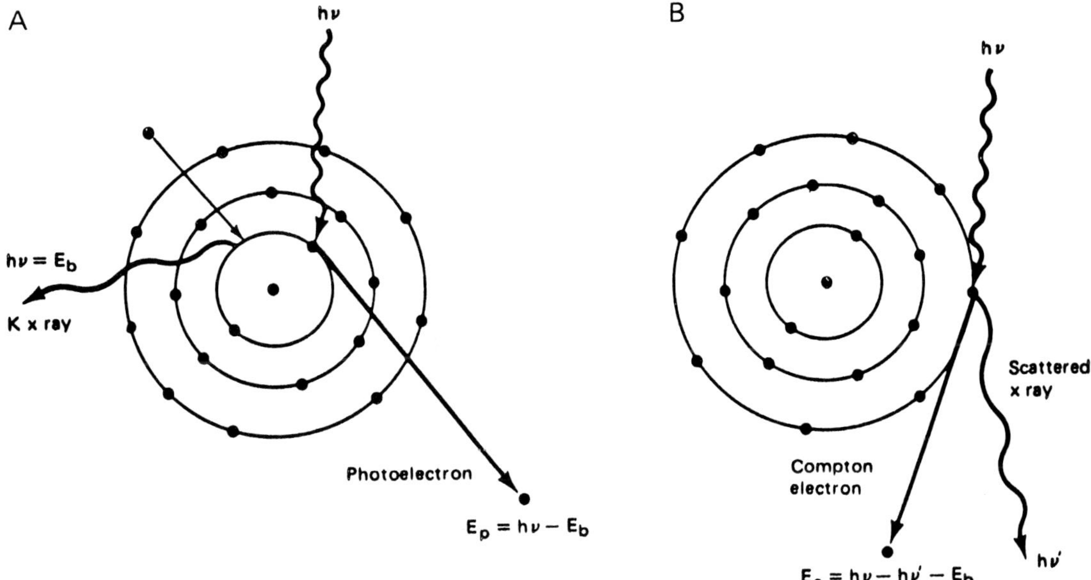

FIGURE 1.5. X-ray interactions with electrons. A, An x-ray photon transfers all of its energy to a K electron, which is ejected from the atom with a kinetic energy equal to the photon energy minus the electron-binding energy. A K x ray is emitted when the vacancy in the K shell is filled by another electron. B, An x-ray photon interacts with one of the outer orbital electrons transferring only part of its energy to the electron. The remaining energy appears in the form of a scattered x-ray photon of longer wavelength (From ref. 1, with permission.)

very infrequently, by bremsstrahlung production (radiation losses). Since it takes approximately 34 eV of energy (on the average) to produce an ion pair, the complete absorption of a 34-keV photon will result in the production of about 1000 ion pairs. Some of the ions recombine and some initiate chemical changes and the production of free radicals, leading to further chemical reactions. The energy not used in chemical changes is degraded into heat. The increase in temperature, however, is negligible.

X-Ray Quality

X-ray quality is a term loosely used to denote the relative penetrating characteristics of an x-ray beam. If the photons were monoenergetic, as, for example, γ rays emitted by certain radioisotopes, they would all have the same probability of being absorbed per unit thickness of an absorbing material, and each additional unit thickness of the same material would remove the same fraction of the incident photons. Suppose 1 mm of aluminum absorbs $\frac{2}{3}$ and transmits $\frac{1}{3}$ of the incident monoener-

getic photons comprising a narrow x- or γ-ray beam. Then, 2 mm of aluminum would transmit $\frac{1}{3}$ × $\frac{1}{3}$ or $\frac{1}{9}$ and 3 mm would transmit $(\frac{1}{3})^3$ or $\frac{1}{27}$ of the incident photons. Hence, the transmission of monoenergetic photons decreases exponentially with increasing thickness of absorbing material and can be expressed as follows:

$$N = N_0 e^{-\mu} \tag{5}$$

where N is the number of photons remaining in the transmitted beam after passing through an absorbing material of thickness t, N_0 is the original number of photons in the incident beam (the number of photons removed from the beam by the photoelectric and Compton processes is $N_0 − N$), and μ is the probability of absorption per unit thickness and is called the attenuation co-efficient. The value of μ depends on the energy of the photons and the atomic number of the absorbing material. Hence, one index of radiation quality is the value of the attenuation co-efficient for a given material. Another index is the half-value layer (HVL): that is, the thickness of a given material that will attenuate a narrow beam of photons to 50% of its

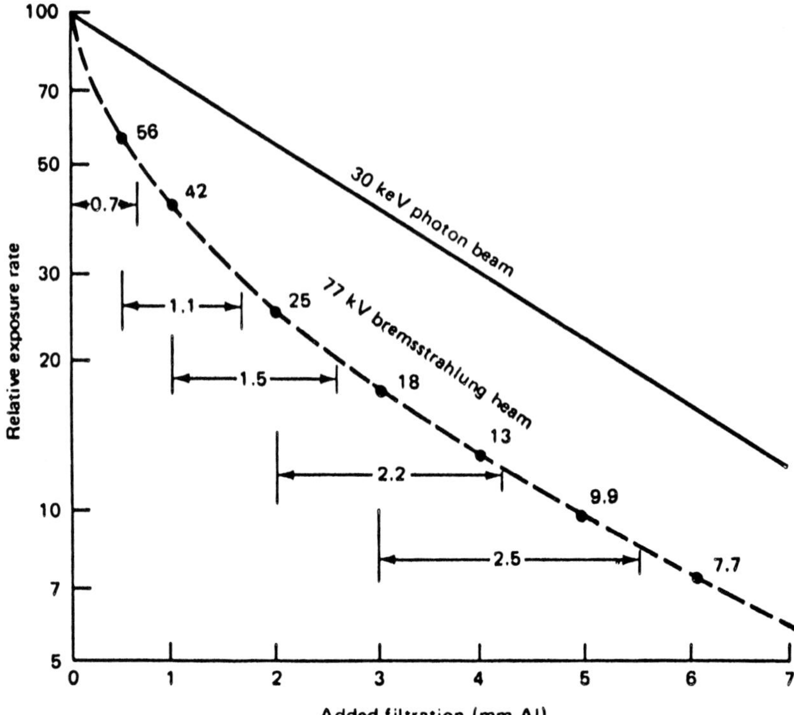

FIGURE 1.6. X-ray attenuation curves. The upper curves illustrates the attenuation of a narrow 30-keV monoenergetic x- or γ-ray beam in aluminum. The curve is a straight line on semilog paper showing that the HVL and the energy of the beam remain constant with added filtration. The lower curve illustrates the attenuation of a 77-kV bremsstrahlung beam emitted by an x-ray tube. Since the beam contains a wide spectrum of energy, the attenuation curve is not a straight line and the average energy and the HVL, shown below the curve, increase with increased filtration (From ref. 1, with permission.)

original intensity. Thus, $N/N_0 = \frac{1}{2}$ when $t = T\frac{1}{2}$ or 1 HVL. When these values are substituted into equation (5) and natural logarithms of both sides are taken, the following relationship is derived:

$$T\frac{1}{2} = \ln 2/\mu = 0.693/\mu \qquad (6)$$

When attenuation data for a monoenergetic photon beam are plotted on semilog paper, the points fall along a straight line, as is expected for an exponential function. However, when attenuation data for a heterogeneous photon beam, such as the bremsstrahlung produced by an x-ray tube, are plotted on semilog paper, a curve is obtained that asymptotically approaches a straight line as the absorber thickness increases. Such a beam has a wide spectrum of energies, each with its own attenuation coefficient, so that the resulting attenuation curve is the sum of a large number of exponential curves.

Figure 1.6 shows attenuation curves for two photon beams: a monoenergetic beam of γ rays and a heterogeneous beam of x rays. For the monoenergetic beam, all the HVLs are equivalent. For the bremsstrahlung beam, the slope of the curve decreases with absorber thickness and the HVLs increase. For x-ray machines, it is customary to use the first HVL as an index of x-ray beam quality. Sometimes, the ratio of the first to the second HVL, called the "homogeneity factor," is used to denote the degree of energy homogeneity. The homogeneity factor is equal to one for monoenergetic beam. It is less than one for a bremsstrahlung beam, but it approaches unity as greater thicknesses of absorbing material (filters) are placed in the beam.

Other indices of radiation quality are the equivalent energy, equivalent kilovoltage, and equivalent wavelength. The equivalent energy of a heterogeneous beam of x rays is defined as the energy of a monoenergetic beam that would have the same HVL as the first HVL of the heterogeneous beam. The effective attenuation co-efficient can be derived from the first HVL using equation (6), and the corresponding energy can be obtained from a table of attenuation co-efficients. The equivalent kilovoltage is numerically equal to the equivalent energy in keV. The equivalent wavelength can then be calculated from equation (4). The effective energy, HLV, and effective attenuation co-efficient of an x-ray beam are functions of the magnitude and waveshape of the x-ray tube potential and the total filtration of the x-ray beam. The x-ray tube potential in kV and the added equivalent filtration in mm of aluminum are sometimes specified together as an index of x-ray quality. The index most commonly used, however, is the HVL (or thickness) of aluminum (Al) (for x-ray machines operating below 120 kV) or copper (above 120 kV). The HVL increases with increasing tube potential and increasing added filtration.

Dosimetry

To treat tumors with x rays, there must be some method for specifying not only the quality of the beam of radiation used, but also the quantity of radiation absorbed at various points in the tissue volume.[2,3] It is not practical to measure the amount of radiation absorbed directly. This must be calculated from measurements made on the x-ray beam in air prior to tissue penetration. These measurements are made during the calibration of the x-ray machine. One of the calibration parameters is the exposure rate measured under specified conditions of distance, x-ray tube potential, tube current, and collimation (x-ray beam size).

Exposure

One of the oldest concepts in radiation dosimetry is that of "radiation dose," or "dosage," which later became "exposure dose" and now is called "exposure." It refers to the amount of ionization produced in a small volume of air around a point of interest under certain defined conditions of measurement. Figure 1.7 illustrates the concept of exposure. As the x-ray beam passes through the

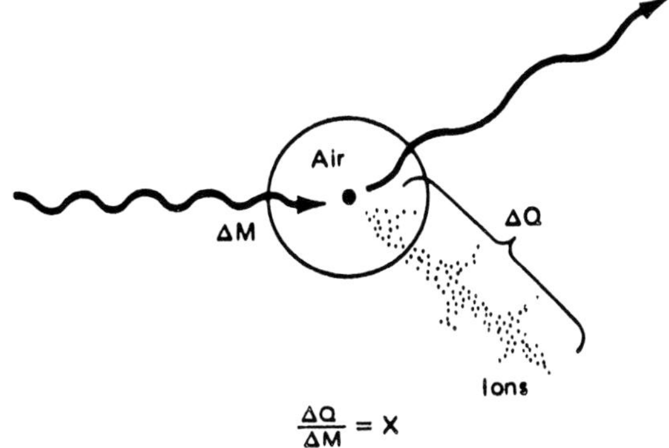

FIGURE 1.7. The concept of exposure. ΔM is an incremental mass of air surrounding the point of interest. ΔQ is the sum of the electric charges of all the ions, of either sign, produced by primary electrons released by the interaction of x rays within the air mass (From ref. 1, with permission.)

incremental air volume surrounding the point of interest, a very small fraction of the photons interact with the air atoms within the volume, releasing primary (photoelectric and Compton) electrons that produce additional ionization, thereby releasing secondary electrons within and outside the incremental air volume. The total absolute charge produced is the charge of one electron multiplied by the sum of all of the primary electrons released within the air volume plus all of the secondary electrons. The total charge is divided by the mass of the incremental volume. The exposure is the limiting value of this ratio as the volume becomes infinitely small.

In 1971 the International Commission on Radiation Units and Measurements (ICRU) adopted the following formal definition[3]:

The *exposure*, X, is the quotient $dQ/$ by dm, where dQ is the absolute value of the total charge of the ions of one sign produced in air when all of the electrons liberated by photons in a volume element of air having a mass dm are completely stopped in air:

$$X = dQ/dm \qquad (7)$$

In the International System (SI) of Units, the unit of exposure is the coulomb per kilogram. Historically, the special unit of exposure has been the

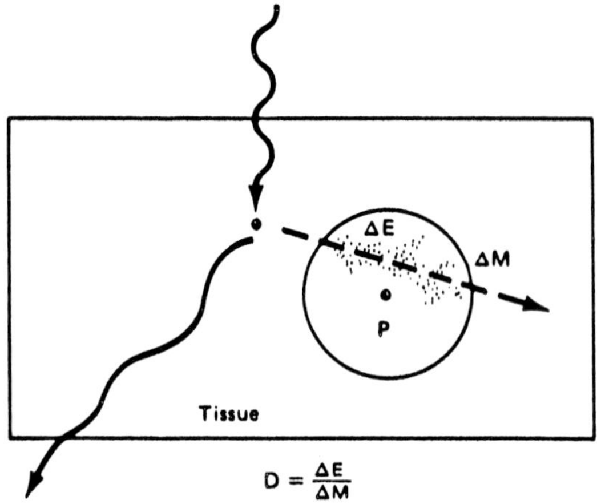

FIGURE 1.8. The concept of absorbed dose. ΔM is an incremental mass (of tissue) surrounding the point of interest, P. ΔE is the total energy dissipated by the primary (photo- or Compton) electron *within* the incremental mass. The absorbed dose at P is the ratio $\Delta E/\Delta M$ as ΔM surrounding P becomes vanishingly small.[3] (From ref. 1, with permission.)

roentgen (R).* The roentgen was originally defined as the exposure required to produce one electrostatic unit of charge (of either sign) per cubic centimeter of air at standard temperature and pressure (0°C, 760 mmHg). The new equivalent definition in terms of SI units is:

$$1 \text{ R} = 2.58 \times 10^{-4} \text{ C/kg (exactly)}$$

At present, exposure and exposure rate, which describe the ability of an x-ray beam to ionize air, are generally used for x-ray machine calibration purposes as the first step in determining the amount of radiation energy absorbed by the patient. This is done by taking ionization measurements in air at the position where the surface to be treated subsequently will be placed. However, one can refer to the exposure at some locus within the patient. In such a case, the exposure value would be determined for a small quantity of air inserted at the point of interest in the patient.

It is not easy to measure exposure rates directly, even in free air. In practice, appropriately designed

---

*In 1975, the ICRU recommended that the special units roentgen and rad (and curie) be gradually abandoned over a period of not less than 10 years and be replaced by the SI units coulomb per kilogram (C/kg) and the gray (Gy) (and the becquerel (Bq), respectively.[4]

ionization chambers are used, which have been compared directly or indirectly with standard ionization chambers at the National Bureau of Standards or with secondary chambers maintained by regional calibration centers approved by the American Association of Physicists in Medicine (AAPM). The chambers must be calibrated for the same quality of x rays as those that will be used for irradiation. The concept of exposure is limited only to ionization in air and only to x and γ rays.

In recent years, the concept of exposure has gradually been replaced in many countries by the concept of Kerma (*k*inetic *e*nergy *r*eleased in *mat*ter) in air, which is the energy equivalent of exposure. However, for the low x-ray energies used in dermatology, there is no practical difference between Kerma-in-air and absorbed dose (discussed next) in air.

Absorbed Dose

An easier concept to understand than that of exposure and a more relevant one for biologic purposes is that of "absorbed dose." This is simply the energy absorbed per unit mass at the point of interest. According to the 1971 formal definition of the ICRU,[4]

The absorbed dose, D, is the quotient of $d\bar{e}$ by dm, where $d\bar{e}$ is the mean energy imparted by ionizing radiation to the matter in a volume element and dm is the mass of the matter in that volume element.

$$D = d\bar{e}/dm \qquad (8)$$

In SI units, the unit for absorbed dose is the joule per kilogram. In 1974 the ICRU recommended and in 1975 the International Committee of Weights and Measures (CIPM) adopted the following new special unit:[5]

the gray, symbol Gy, equal to the joule per kilogram (J/kg). Historically, the special unit of absorbed dose has been the rad.* The rad was defined as the absorbed dose equal to 100 ergs of energy per gram of absorbing material. Since one joule equals 10^7 ergs, and one kilogram equals 10^3 gm,

$$1 \text{ Gy} = 10^7 \text{ ergs}/10^3 \text{ gm} = 10^4 \text{ ergs per gm} = 100 \text{ rads}.$$

The concept of absorbed dose is illustrated in Figure 1.8. Note that the concept of absorbed dose is not restricted to x and γ rays, but also applies to all other ionizing radiations and to any absorbing medium.

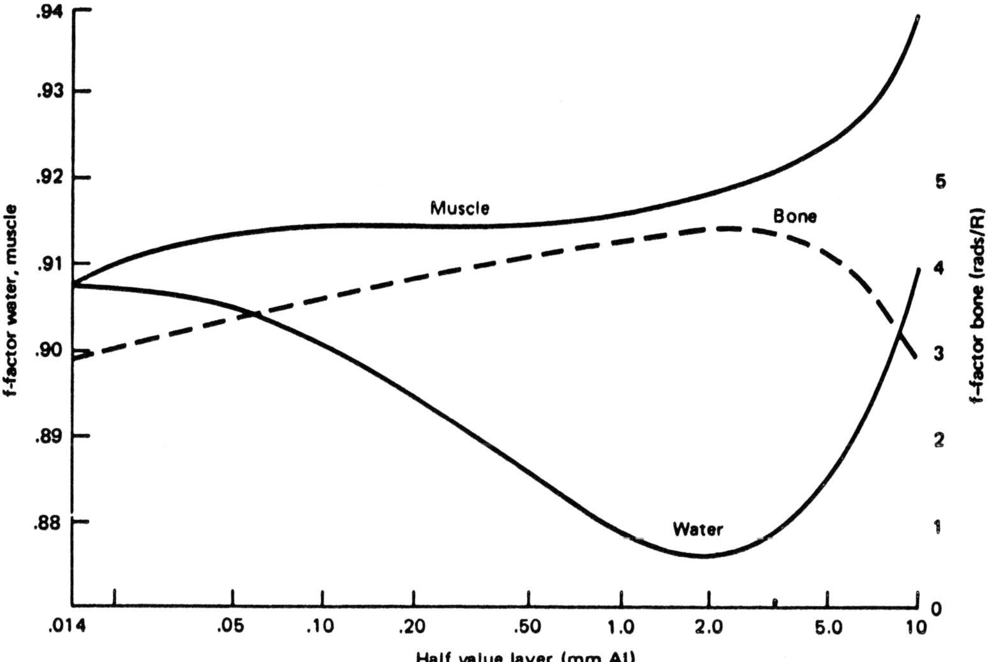

FIGURE 1.9. The R-to-rad conversion factor is shown as a function of HVLs of Al for bone, muscle, and water (soft tissue.) (From ref. 1, with permission.)

In general, one cannot readily measure absorbed dose directly. However, in the case of x and γ rays, the absorbed dose at any point is proportional to the exposure at that point; if the exposure is known, the absorbed dose can be calculated taking into account the differences between the x-ray absorption co-efficients of air and the absorbing medium. The first step is to determine the energy equivalence of a roentgen (R) in order to evaluate the absorbed dose in air.

The charge of an electron is equal to 1.6×10^{-19} coulombs (C). If we divide 2.54×10^{-4} C/kg used in the definition of a roentgen by the electronic charge, we obtain 1.61×10^{15} electrons/kg. Each electron represents one ionization or the release of one ion pair (i.e., electron and positive ion). Therefore, an exposure of 1 R produces 1.61×10^{12} ion pairs/gm of air. The average amount of energy required to produce an ion pair is 33.7 eV (to convert to ergs, multiply by 1.6×10^{-12} ergs/eV). The result is that an exposure of 1 R produces an absorbed dose of 86.9 ergs/gm in air, or 0.869 rads. Thus,

$$D_{\text{air}} = 0.869 \, \frac{\text{rads}}{\text{R}} \times X \, \text{R} = 0.869 \, X \, \text{rads} \quad (9)$$

If after measuring the exposure at some point of interest we wish to determine the absorbed dose in a tiny mass of some other medium at that point, we can do so by taking into account the difference in the mass energy absorption co-efficients for the medium and for air.

$$D_{\text{med}} = \left(0.869 \, \frac{\mu_{\text{med}}}{\mu_{\text{air}}}\right) \times X = f \times X \quad (10)$$

The quantity in parentheses is of such importance in absorbed dose calculations that it is often referred to as the R-to-rad conversion factor, or f-factor. The value of the mass energy absorption co-efficient (μ) depends on the energy of the photon beam and the effective atomic number of the absorbing material. It is less than the attenuation co-efficient used in equation (5) because it refers only to that part of the energy removed from the beam by the incremental mass, which is also absorbed by the mass. The radiation scattered from the beam at the point of interest does not contribute to the absorbed dose at that point.

The f-factor has been calculated for a number of photon energies and HVLs for bone, muscle, and water (soft tissue). These are plotted in Figure 1.9.

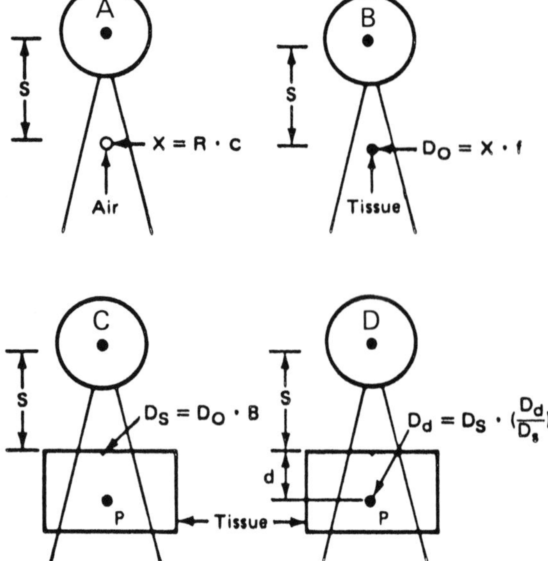

FIGURE 1.10. A–D, The steps necessary to determine the absorbed dose at some point P on the central axis of the x-ray beam located d cm below the skin surface (From ref. 1, with permission.)

Depth Dose Calculations

Exposure measurements are not normally made in the patient because it is not practical to insert calibrated air ionization chambers at all points of interest. Instead, exposure measurements are made in "phantom patients" composed of tissue-equivalent material or in tanks of water for a wide range of exposure conditions. Readings below the surface are usually normalized in terms of a percentage of the maximum readings that occur at the surface for x-ray energies used in dermatology. These depth dose data have been collected and published by others.[6] In order to apply this information to dose calculations in radiation therapy, we need to introduce the concepts of *backscatter factor, skin dose*, and *percentage depth dose*.

Backscatter Factor and Skin Dose

Figure 1.10 illustrates the steps necessary to determine the absorbed dose at some point P on the central axis of the x-ray beam located d cm below the skin surface (Fig. 1.10D). S represents the target-skin distance (TSD); that is, the distance from the target in the anode of the x-ray tube to the surface of the patient when in position for treatment. The first step (Fig. 1.10A) is to take ionization readings for a given exposure time with a calibrated ionization chamber in air, with the TSD, added filtration, kVp, mA, and collimation values that will be used for treatment. The exposure X, in R, is obtained by multiplying the average reading R by the calibration factor C, and making any necessary corrections for air temperature and pressure. These data are obtained at the time the x-ray machine is calibrated and are part of the calibration report. Figure 1.10B shows an imaginary tiny spherical mass of tissue (radius equal to the maximum range of the photoelectric and Compton electrons) located at the position of the ionization chamber. The absorbed dose, D_o, of this incremental mass of tissue suspended in air is $f \times X$ rads, according to equation (10). Figure 1.10C shows the same mass element as part of the skin at the surface of the area to be treated. The absorbed dose, D_s, at the skin (skin dose) will be greater than D_o because of the additional contribution from x rays scattered back from tissue below the skin. This scattered radiation is often called *backscatter*, and the ratio D_s/D_o is called the *backscatter factor, B*.[7]

The magnitude of the backscatter depends on the radiation quality (HVL) and the area and geometric shape of the x-ray beam at the skin. Backscatter factors have been measured for a wide range of HVLs and areas, and some of the data of interest for superficial radiation therapy are plotted in Figure 1.11. Note that the backscatter factor increases with x-ray beam size and increases with HVL over the range shown. It reaches a maximum at about an HVL of 10 mm Al, much beyond the range of interest in dermatology.

Percentage Depth Dose

In Fig. 1.10D, the absorbed dose at P is D_d. The ratio D_d/D_s is known as the *"fractional depth dose."* When multiplied by 100, the ratio is called the *"percentage depth dose."* The percentage depth dose is a complicated function of the depth d, HVL, area A, shape of the field, and TSD. Depth dose data have been obtained in water phantoms over a wide range of these parameters. Some data are plotted in Figure 1.12 for a 30-cm TSD and a 4.4-cm diameter beam size over the HVL range of interest in dermatologic radiation therapy.

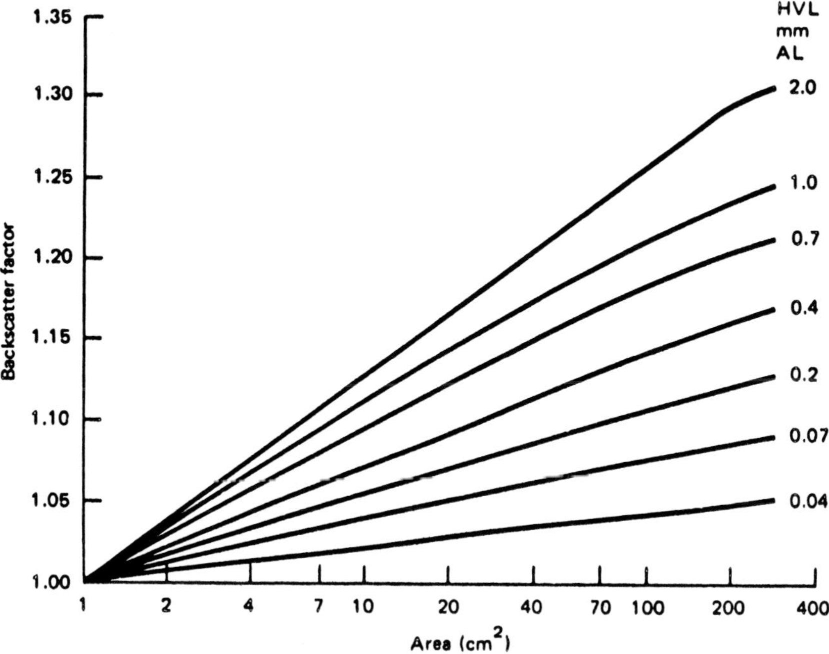

FIGURE 1.11. The backscatter factor plotted as a function of circular area of x-ray beams for different HVLs of Al (From ref. 1, with permission.)

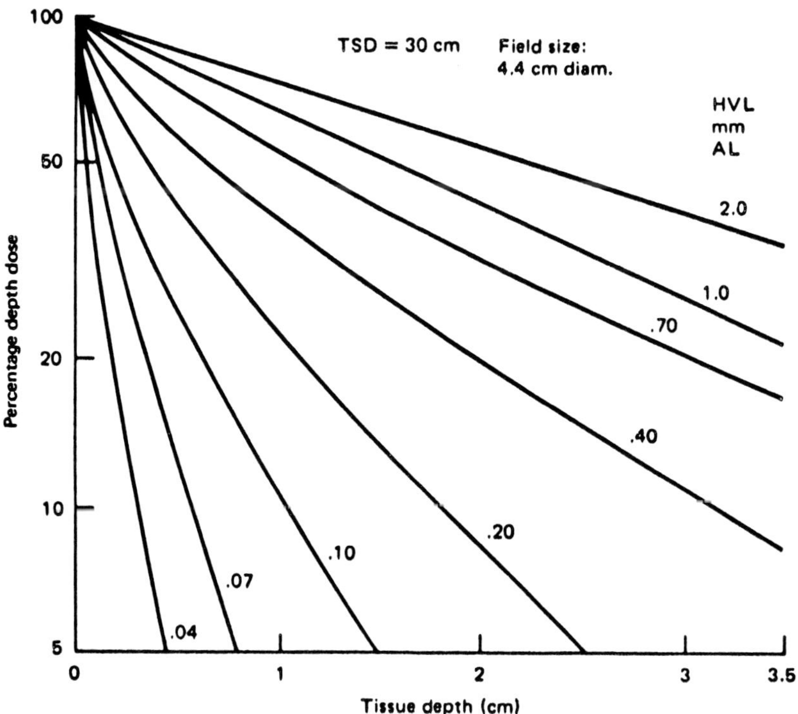

FIGURE 1.12. Percentage depth dose plotted for various HVLs as a function of tissue depth (From ref. 1, with permission.)

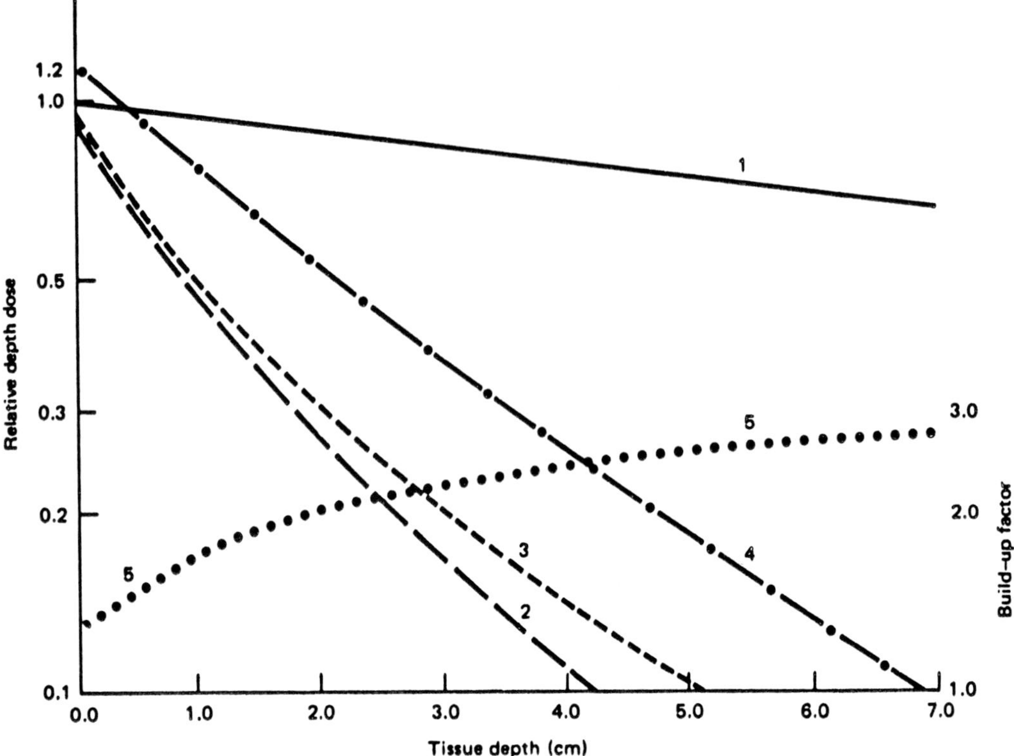

FIGURE 1.13. The component parts of a depth dose curve. Curve 4 is a depth dose curve for a 1-mm Al HVL x-ray beam, with a 30-cm TSD and a circular area of 100 cm². Curve 1 is the component part due only to the inverse square factor. Curve 2 is a plot of depth dose data for the same x-ray beam as in Curve 4, except that the cross-sectional area has been reduced to essentially zero, thus eliminating scattered radiation. Curve 3 is Curve 2 divided by Curve 1, eliminating the inverse square factor. Hence, it is a plot of the tissue attenuation of the x-ray beam. Curve 5 is the result of dividing Curve 4 by Curves 1 and 3 to eliminate both the tissue attenuation and inverse square factors, leaving only the build-up factor due to scattered radiation (From ref. 1, with permission.)

The following example will illustrate further the calculation of absorbed dose at a given depth below the skin. Suppose we wish to treat a superficial lesion so that the base of the tumor 5 mm below the skin surface receives 200 rads per treatment and we need to determine the treatment time. We decide to operate the beryllium-window x-ray tube at 29 kV, 25 mA, with a 0.3 mm Al filter and a 30-cm TSD, 4-cm diameter cone. Under these conditions, according to the calibration of the machine, the exposure rate is 115 R/min and the HVL is 0.17 mm Al. According to Figure 1.9, the R-to-rad conversion factor f is about 0.88 for water (soft tissue) at this HVL. The backscatter factor B is about 1.05 for an x-ray beam size of 12.6 cm², as obtained by interpolation in Figure 1.11. Hence, the absorbed dose rate at the skin is:

$$D_s = 115 \text{ R/min} \times 0.88 \text{ rads/R} \times 1.05$$

$$= 106.3 \text{ rads/min}$$

By interpolation of the depth dose data in Figure 1.12, we find that the percentage depth dose at 5 mm is approximately 37% for a 4.4-cm diameter field, 30-cm TSD, and a 0.17-mm HVL of Al. Therefore, the absorbed dose rate at the base of the lesion is:

$$D_p = 106.3 \text{ rads/min} \times 0.37 = 39.3 \text{ rads/min}$$

The treatment time (T) to deliver 200 rads is:

$$T = \frac{200 \text{ rads}}{39.3 \text{ rads/min}} = 5.09 \text{ min} = 5 \text{ min} + 5 \text{ sec}$$

Factors Affecting Percentage Depth Dose

Three factors are involved in determining the percentage depth dose at some reference point below the skin on the central axis. These are: (1) the geometric divergence of the x-ray beam, (2) the attenuation of the primary beam by the tissue between the surface and the point of reference, and (3) the contribution of radiation scattered from the surrounding tissue to the point of reference. The geometric divergence of the x-ray beam is described by the inverse square law. If there were no tissue attenuation of the primary beam and if there were no scattered radiation, the dose at depth d in Figure 1.10 would be related to the dose at the surface as follows:

$$D_\mathrm{d} = D_\mathrm{s} \times \left(\frac{S}{S + d}\right)^2$$

For example, if the TSD were 30 cm, the percentage depth dose at a depth of 4 cm due to divergence alone would be the following:

$$\frac{D_\mathrm{d}}{D_\mathrm{s}} \times 100 = \left(\frac{30}{30 + 4}\right)^2 \times 100 = 78\%$$

Hence, the divergence of the beam from a distance of 30 to 34 cm decreases the x-ray intensity, exposure rate, and absorbed dose rate by 22%. At a distance of 60 cm, the beam intensity would drop to $(30/60)^2$, or 25%. The effect of beam divergence on percentage depth dose is illustrated by curve 1 in Figure 1.13, which is a plot of the inverse square factor for a TSD of 30 cm. Curve 2 in Figure 1.13 is a plot of the depth dose data for a narrow beam of x rays with essentially zero cross-sectional area, a 1-mm HVL of Al, and a 30-cm TSD. Since the beam is so narrow, there is virtually no contribution from scattered radiation at the surface (backscatter) or below the surface (build-up factor). Hence, curve 2 is the result of attenuation of the primary beam by tissue and the inverse square law divergence. If the ordinate values of curve 2 are divided by the corresponding ordinate values of curve 1, the beam divergence is factored out, producing curve 3. Curve 3 shows the contribution of tissue attenuation of the x-ray beam on the depth dose curve, $e^{-\mu d}$, where μ is the effective attenuation co-efficient for a 1-mm HVL beam in tissue. Curve 4 is a plot of the depth dose data for a circular beam of 100-cm² area, with the same HVL and TSD as above. This curve has been normalized to 100% of the skin dose for zero area. Hence, the skin dose for 100-cm² area is 1.2 times the zero-area skin dose because of the backscatter

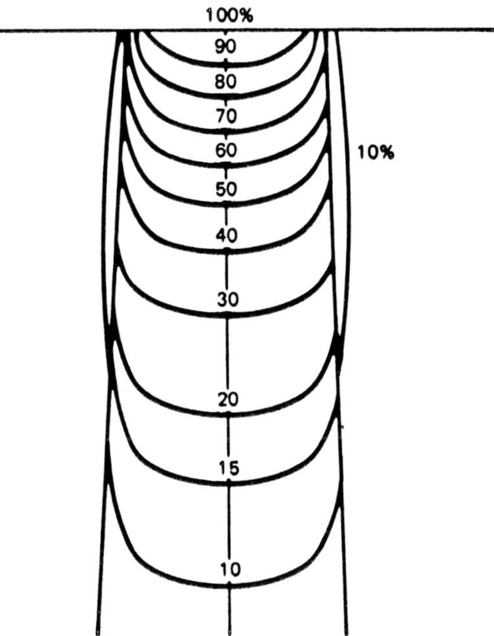

FIGURE 1.14. A set of isodose curves indicating dose distribution normalized to 100% of the skin for a given HVL, TSD, and beam size (From ref. 1, with permission.)

factor. Curve 4 includes the effects of tissue attenuation, inverse square divergence, and scattered radiation (build-up factor). If curve 4 is divided by curves 3 and 1 to factor out tissue attenuation and inverse square factors, only the build-up factor due to scattered radiation is left. The result is plotted in curve 5. The build-up factor increases rapidly with depth, so that at 5 cm the scattered radiation contributes considerably more to the dose than does the energy absorbed from the primary beam.

Isodose Distributions

The central axis depth dose tables or graphs are of limited value for describing the absorbed dose distribution throughout the treatment volume. The dose drops off rapidly toward the edge of the x-ray field. To take this effect into account, one must either treat an area considerably larger than the tumor or refer to 2-dimensional depth dose distributions usually presented graphically as families of isodose curves. An isodose curve is the locus of points along which the percentage depth dose is constant. A set of isodose curves for a particular combination of HVL, TSD, and beam size is shown in Figure 1.14. Isodose curves usually are drawn

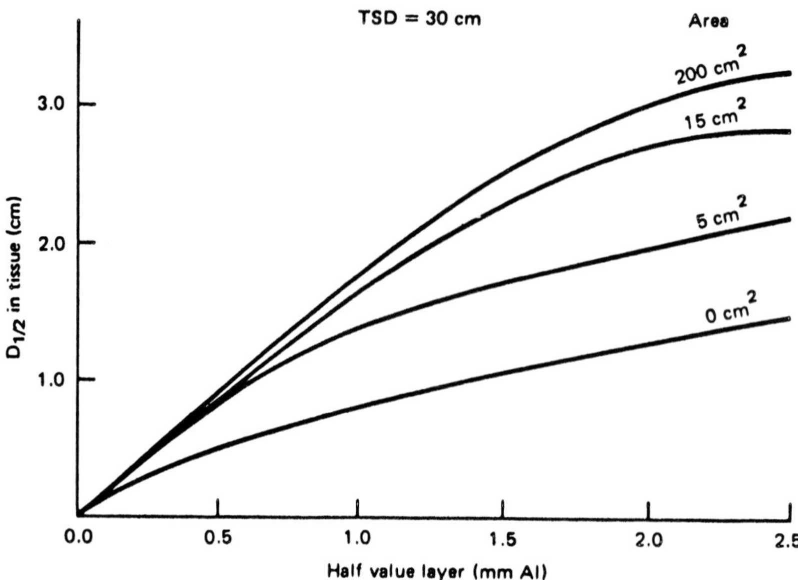

FIGURE 1.15. $D_{\frac{1}{2}}$ in tissue as a function of HVL and beam size (From ref. 1, with permission.)

full scale on transparent sheets, which can be overlaid on an outline of the area to be treated in order to select an x-ray field size that will adequately treat the entire tumor volume. Although the central axis depth dose data measured in a tissue-equivalent phantom for one x-ray therapy machine is reasonably reliable for use with other x-ray machines operated under the same conditions of HVL, TSD, and x-ray beam size, isodose curves should be generated with the same type of machine as the one to be used.

Half-Value Depth and Fall-Off Ratio

The half-value depth, or $D_{\frac{1}{2}}$, is the tissue depth at which the dose drops to 50% of the surface dose. In like manner, D_{10}^{9} is the tissue depth at which the dose falls to 10% of the surface dose. The fall-off ratio for a given set of treatment parameters is defined as D_{10}^{9} divided by $D_{\frac{1}{2}}$. The fall-off ratio is a clinical index of the rate the dose decreases with increasing tissue depth. The $D_{\frac{1}{2}}$ and fall-off ratio depend, of course, on all of the parameters that determine percentage depth dose. Figure 1.15 shows how the $D_{\frac{1}{2}}$ varies with HVL for various field sizes at a TSD of 30 cm. Additional data for a wide range of parameters have been published by Tuddenham.[8]

Summary

In radiotherapy, one major objective is to maximize the amount of absorbed dose in the region occupied by the lesion and to minimize the dose to other adjacent tissues. In deep therapy, where the lesion to be treated is some distance below the surface, multiple fields intersecting at some internal point are often used or sometimes the primary beam (or patient) is rotated, with the axis of rotation in the vicinity of the tumor. In superficial therapy, however, the tumor volume is at or near the surface and it generally is not advisable to treat with more than one field. The problem then is to select the treatment parameters (kV potential, added filtration, TSD, and field size) so as to deliver an adequate dose to the base and edges of the lesion while sparing the underlying structures as much as possible. If isodose curves are available, one can readily visualize the expected dose distribution for the given treatment conditions and select the combination of parameters that provides a reasonable compromise. When isodose curves are not available, as is often the case, one must consult central axis percentage depth dose tables or $D_{\frac{1}{2}}$ tables or graphs to estimate the percentage dose reaching the base of the tumor and underlying

TABLE 1.2. Qualitative effect of increasing physical parameters used in dermatologic x-ray therapy.[a]

Related parameters	Physical parameters					
	X-ray tube potential (kV)	X-ray tube current (mA)	Added filter (mm Al)	Target-to-skin distance (TSD)	Collimator or cone size	Exposure time (T)
Exposure rate (R/min) in air[b]	↑[j]	↑	↓	↓	—	—
Absorbed dose rate (rads/min) at the skin[c]	↑	↑	↓	↓	↑	—
Total skin dose (rads)[d]	↑	↑	↓	↓	↑	↑
Effective energy (HVL) of the x-ray beam[e]	↑	—	↑	—	—	—
Maximum photon energy[f]	↑	—	—	—	—	—
Minimum photon wavelength[f]	↓[k]	—	—	—	—	—
Backscatter factor[g]	↑	—	↑	—	↑	—
Percentage depth dose[h]	↑	—	↑	↑	↑	—
$D_{\frac{1}{2}}$ values[h]	↑	—	↑	↑	↑	—
Surface area in the primary beam[i]	—[l]	—	—	↑	↑	—

[a] From ref. 1, with permission.

[b] The exposure rate increases with increased production of x rays. The number of x rays produced per second depends on the number of electrons striking the target per second (i.e., the tube current). X-ray production also depends on the energy of the electrons striking the target. The electron energy increases with tube potential (kV). Exposure rate decreases with added filter, which absorbs the weaker x rays. Exposure rate also decreases with increasing TSD because of the inverse square divergence.

[c] The absorbed dose rate is directly proportional to the exposure rate. At the skin surface it also increases with the beam size because of increased scatter.

[d] The total skin dose depends on the absorbed dose rate and the exposure time.

[e] As the tube potential (kV) is increased, the energy of the electrons striking the tube target increases, thus increasing the average energy of the emitted x rays. Increasing the aluminum filtration selectively absorbs the lower energy (weaker) x rays, thus effectively increasing the energy of the transmitted x-ray beam.

[f] The maximum photon energy and minimum photon wavelength depend only on the energy of the striking electrons, and hence only on the tube potential.

[g] The backscatter factor increases with photon energy and reaches a maximum at about an HVL of 10 mm of Al (0.6 mm Cu), depending on field size. Hence, the backscatter radiation increases with tube potential and with added filtration for the ranges of interest in dermatologic radiation therapy. The backscatter factor also increases with field size.

[h] The percentage depth dose and $D_{\frac{1}{2}}$ value increase with photon energy (hence, with tube potential and added filtration) because of the greater penetrating ability of higher energy x rays. They also increase with TSD because of the reduced effectiveness of the inverse square law factor at increasing distances.

[i] The surface area in the primary beam increases, of course, with field size or cone size and increases with TSD because of the inverse square divergence of the beam.

[j] ↑ = increases.

[k] ↓ = decreases.

[l] — = no change.

tissues. One must also keep in mind that the dose rate falls off sharply near the edge of the field. This must be considered when choosing the size of the primary beam to adequately treat the entire tumor volume.

Table 1.2 summarizes qualitatively the effects of varying the physical parameters used in radiologic treatment of superficial lesions.

References

1. Gorson RD, Lassen M: Physical aspects of dermatologic radiotherapy. In: Goldschmidt H, ed. *Physical Modalities in Dermatologic Therapy: Radiotherapy Electrosurgery, Phototherapy, Cryosurgery.* New York, NY: Springer-Verlag, 1978.

2. International Commission on Radiation Units and Measurements. ICRU Report No. 17. *Radiation Dosi-*

metry: x rays Generated at Potentials of 5 to 150 kV. Washington, DC: 1970.

3. International Commission on Radiation Units and Measurements. ICRU Report No. 33. *Radiation Quantities and Units*. Bethesda, Md: 1980.

4. International Commission on Radiation Units and Measurements. ICRU Report No. 19. *Radiation Quantities and Units*. Washington, DC: 1971.

5. Wyckoff HO (chairman). Statement by the ICRU. *Med Phys*. 1976; 3:52.

6. British Institute of Radiology. Central axis depth dose data for use in radiotherapy. *Radiology*. 1972; 11 (Suppl).

7. Johns HE, Cunningham JR. *The Physics of Radiology*, 4th ed. Springfield, Ill: Charles C Thomas: 1983.

8. Tuddenham WJ. Half-value depth and fall-off ratio as functions of portal area, target-skin-distance and half-value layer. *Radiology*. 1957; 69:79.

2

Radiobiology

Renato G. Panizzon

Radiobiology, the study of the interaction of ionizing radiation with living matter, began about the turn of the century with the discovery of x rays by Roentgen in 1895. Within months, Becquerel discovered natural radiation from the nuclear disintegration of uranium atoms. The process by which an x-ray image of Roentgen's hand could be produced was quickly recognized as a potential technique for the diagnosis of diseases, but it also became rapidly apparent that cells could be injured or killed by radiation. Although radiobiology is the study of the interaction of any radiant energy (including microwaves and radiowaves) with living matter, this chapter will discuss only ionizing radiation used as a therapeutic tool. Photons of x rays or γ rays are forms of electromagnetic radiation, whereas electrons, protons, and neutrons are forms of particulate radiation. The interaction of radiation with matter will be used to illustrate the events that culminate in a biological effect.

Interaction of Radiation with Matter

Photons of x rays or γ rays can interact with atoms in different ways:

1. Absorption: The photon is absorbed by the atom and possesses enough energy to dislodge an electron
2. Scattering: low-energy photons are deflected by an outer electron
3. Recoil interaction: the incoming high energy photon interacts with an outer electron imparting only part of the photon's energy to the recoiling electron (Compton). This is the dominant type of interaction over 100 keV

4. Nuclear interaction: the photon of very high energy ($>$ 1,02 MeV) interacts with the atomic nucleus. This process is also known as "pair production"
5. If photon energies greater than 10 MeV collide with the nucleus, an ejection of a proton or a neutron may result

Units of Exposure/Absorbed Dose

All radiations may be completely absorbed in a particular volume, pass through unaffected, or pass with reduced energy. Since only the absorbed radiation is biologically effective, we are primarily dealing with absorbed energy. The absorbed dose of ionizing radiation has in the past been expressed in units called "rad" (*r*adiation *a*bsorbed *d*ose), which is equal to 100 ergs per gram of matter (10^{-2} J/kg in SI units). The SI unit of absorbed dose is the gray (Gy), which is defined as 1 J/kg and equals 100 centigrays (cGy) or 100 rads (Table 2.1).[1]

The kinetic energy released in matter (kerma) is the total kinetic energy transferred by the incoming radiation to the ionizing particles that it generates. For photons of energy less than 1 MeV, the absorbed dose and kerma are quite identical. The kerma dose is expressed in Gy or cGy.

Linear Energy Transfer

The amount of energy deposited by a particle or photon as it passes through a material will be deposited as energy linearly along the track of the radiation. This transfer of energy along the track is referred to as the linear energy transfer (LET). Linear energy transfer is expressed in keV/μm.

TABLE 2.1. Dose units (gray, kerma, sievert).

Use	Dose	SI units
Radiation therapy	Absorbed dose	$1\ Gy^a = 100\ cGy = 1\ J/kg$ $= 100\ rad$
Radiation research	Activity	$1\ Bq^b = 1/s$
Radiation physics	Absorbed dose	See above
	Secondary radiation (>1 MeV): *kinetic energy released in matter* = kerma	K (in Gy or cGy)
Radiation protection	Energy dose $\times$ factor q q = 1 for photons/electrons/beta rays 3–10 for neutrons 20 for alpha particles	$1\ Sv^c = 1\ J/kg$ $= 100\ rem$

[a] Gy = Gray.
[b] Bq = Becquerel.
[c] Sv = Sievert.

Different types of radiation have characteristic LET values according to their incident radiation energy. X rays of high energy tend to have low LET values. On the other hand, LET increases with decreasing particle energy, and the number of ionizations per unit length increases as the particle slows down (Table 2.2).[1,2]

Biologic Effects

The ions formed as electrons that are set in motion occur mostly in water, which is about 70% of most tissues; this is called the "indirect effect." From ions, free radicals are formed; these are atoms or molecules that have unpaired valence electrons and are associated with a high degree of chemical reactivity. These active radicals function primarily as potent oxidizing agents. In water the radicals H·, OH·, and solvated electrons (e^-) are formed, affecting biomolecules by H abstraction (RH +

TABLE 2.2. Examples of LET values.

Radiation	Energy (MeV)	LET (keV/μm)
x rays	0.25	1.5
γ rays (^{60}Co)	1.25	0.3
Electrons	1.00	0.25
	0.01	2.30
Protons	10	4
	5	8
Neutrons (recoil protons)	20	7
Alpha particles	5	100

OH· → R· + HOH) or by OH addition (R^- + OH· → R^- OH·). In the presence of oxygens, these radicals can be transformed into peroxyradicals: R· + O_2 → ROO·. This reaction prevents the recombination to the original biomolecule, R· + H· → RH, and therefore increases the radical yield in the medium in the presence of oxygen. In addition, O_2 reacts quickly with the solvated electron and, thus, recombination of the biomolecules with the electron, RH· + e^- → RH, is prevented. These potent active radicals produce biochemical injury in all molecules, which is distributed randomly throughout the cell. Therefore, one can measure ionizing radiation effects on any measurable cell function such as enzyme activity, cell membrane permeability, protein synthesis, or ion transport rates. Radiation effects might be considered to be those of localized intracellular chemotherapy, the process being the conversion of normal body water molecules into potent intracellular chemicals. These same processes can occur in complex biological molecules such as deoxyribonucleic acid (DNA). This process is then referred to as a "direct effect." The absorption of ionizing radiation in biological matter occurs in the following order: formation of ions, production of free radicals, and atomic bond alterations that lead to chemical changes, which in turn can lead to a biological effect of the radiation (Fig. 2.1).[3]

In the treatment of malignant disease, tumor cell death is the biological effect of greatest interest. Cell death in the treatment of cancer is actually the

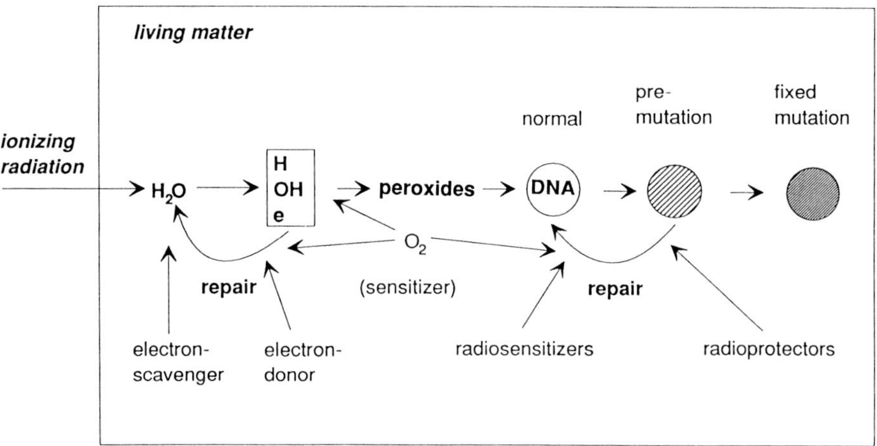

FIGURE 2.1. Biologic effects of radiation, factors of modification. (Modified from Fritz-Niggli,[3] with permission.)

loss of the cell's ability to divide in an unlimited manner or the loss of reproductive integrity. Although most cells will actually lyse and disappear when they attempt to divide after lethal radiation injury, some lethally irradiated cells may exist for some time and carry on respiratory and enzymatic functions. However, if they can no longer divide, these cells pose no threat and they can be considered dead tumor cells. Although radiation affects all cellular molecular structures, DNA is the most sensitive molecule, the injury of which causes the loss of reproductive integrity. All the methods used to understand the relationship of dose of irradiation to magnitude of cell kill utilize the capability of cells to undergo unlimited division. In vitro techniques of growing cells in Petri dishes or culture flasks have been used extensively in these experiments. The ability of a single cell to grow into a large colony that can easily be seen with the naked eye (clonogenicity) is a convenient proof of its reproductive integrity. The loss of this ability as a function of the dose of irradiation can be expressed in a cell survival curve, where the reproductive capability can be calculated and plotted. Figure 2.2 shows a curve plotted on a log-linear graph.[4] The shape of the curve in Figure 2.2 demonstrates the loss of cell viability as an exponential function of the dose; that is, a specified radiation dose kills a constant fraction of irradiated cells. The fraction of the cells killed is independent of the number of cells irradiated. The absolute number of cells killed by this dose depends on the absolute number of cells irradiated. This process is similar to the decay of a radioactive isotope. Basic parameters used to describe the curve are:

1. Do: the dose required to reduce the number of cells to 37% of the initial value on the exponential portion of the curve
2. n: extrapolation number, which is found by extrapolating the straight-line portion of the curve until it cuts the surviving fraction axis
3. Dq: the dose at which the straight-line portion of the curve extrapolated backward intersects with the dose axis

In other words, Do is the measure of sensitivity of cells to each increment of dose of radiation, and Dq and n are measures of the "shoulder" effects denoting the magnitude of radiation-damaged cells accumulated before lethality is expressed as an exponential function of dose. This relationship of cell lethality to the radiation dose has been the basis of understanding various factors that influence the efficacy of radiation for cancer treatment. Cell survival curves obtained on various cell lines in vitro and various in vivo systems are similar because they both have a "shoulder portion" and an "exponential portion" (curve B). This is true of cells from animals or humans, tumors or normal tissues.[5]

The cell survival curve described above, whether determined in tissue cultures in vitro or proliferating cells in vivo, shows the effect on the clonogenic cells of a single exposure to radiation. Single doses of radiation are rarely used in the clinical setting.

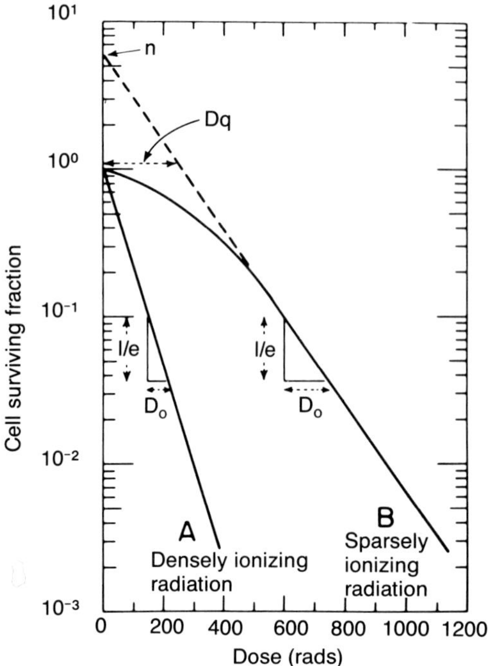

FIGURE 2.2. Cell survival curve. (From Hall EJ. *Radiobiology for the Radiologist*, 2nd ed. Philadelphia, Penn: J.B. Lippincott Company, 1978.)

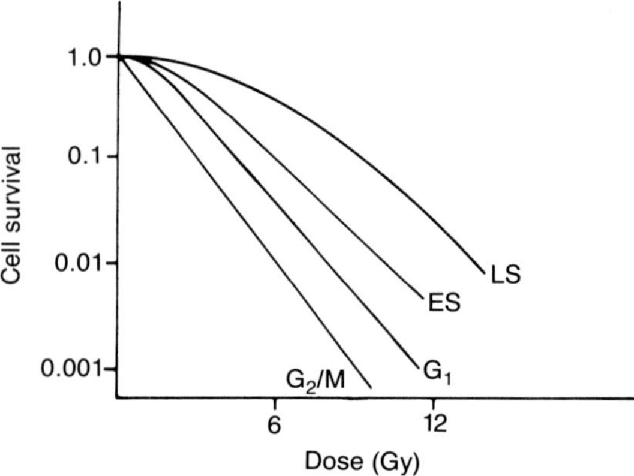

FIGURE 2.3. Cell survival curve for cultured Chinese hamster cells. (Sinclair 1968. From Potten CS. *Radiation and Skin*. London: Taylor and Francis; 1985.)

When a dose of radiation is fractionated, the partially injured cells undergo a repair process. There are two types of repair; sublethal and potentially lethal repair. Repair of sublethal damage is the process whereby surviving cells undergo complete repair of the accumulated radiation damage. If these cells are subjected to another dose of irradiation after a length of time, they can tolerate the same amount of damage as if they had never been irradiated. Potentially lethal damage repair appears to be a separate process from sublethal repair, and can be observed when irradiated cells are grown in suboptimal conditions, such as in a balanced solution rather than in full growth media. Potentially lethal damage and its repair have been observed in animal tumors; however, the potential clinical significance of this observation is not clear.[2,4,5]

Cell Kinetics

The radiosensitivity of the cell depends on its position in the cell cycle. This has been shown with cells grown in culture where the cell cycle can be synchronized. Cells tend to be most sensitive in G_2/M or G_1 phase and are most resistant in late S-phase (LS) (Fig. 2.3).[1,4,6,7] The time of maximum radioresistance varies from one cell line to another. Generally it occurs during the S-phase when enzymes involved in DNA duplication are most abundant.

Cells that have been irradiated show a delay in their progression down the cell cycle. The cells in the premitotic G_2 phase show a maximum delay. Another factor that influences the sensitivity of cells to radiation injury is the presence or absence of oxygen. Radiation damage is caused by production of highly reactive "free radicals," which can combine with oxygen to produce powerful oxidizing agents. Without oxygen, the damaged site of the molecule would have a higher probability of being repaired; that is, oxygen appears to increase the probability of a permanent radiation lesion. Hypoxic cells are about 3 times more resistant to radiation damage (Fig. 2.4) than oxygenated cells.[4,7] This factor is called the "oxygen enhancement ratio" (OER), which means that oxygen enhances the radiosensitivity of anoxic cells. The difference is reduced when high LET radiation is used. Tumors have areas of frank necrosis, areas with viable but hypoxic cells, and areas of well-oxygenated dividing cells. The concentration of oxygen at a particular point in a tumor depends on the distance from the nearest capillary and the rate of O_2 consumption from the capillary to that point.[4,6,8] The cell becomes severely hypoxic when it is more

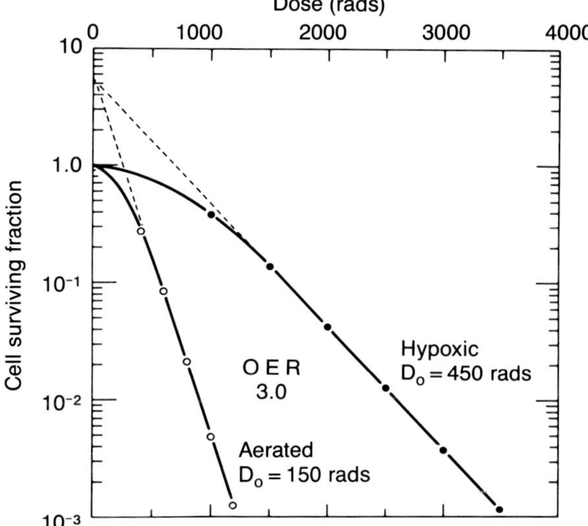

FIGURE 2.4. Survival curves for cultured hamster cells exposed to x rays under aerated conditions and under hypoxic conditions. (From Hall EJ. *Radiobiology for the Radiologist*, 2nd ed. Philadelphia, Penn: J.B. Lippincott Company; 1978.)

than about 100 to 150 μm from a blood capillary (Fig. 2.5). In a course of fractionated radiation therapy during the interval between fractions, hypoxic cells receive more oxygen because of the death of sensitive oxygenated cells, and they become reoxygenated and sensitive to subsequent radiation injury.

In a heterogeneous population of cells, whether in tumor or normal tissue, there are subpopulations of cells with varied reproductive potential. In general they can be grouped into:

1. Clonogenic cells in proliferative phase: cells that are capable of unlimited division and are actively proliferating
2. Clonogenic cells in quiescent phase: cells that are capable of unlimited division but not proliferating at the particular moment (G_0 cells or prolonged G_1 cells)
3. Proliferating cells committed to becoming mature cells after a limited number of divisions or amplifications
4. Mature or functioning cells incapable of division, i.e., cells in normal tissues or tumor cells on their way to cell death

The preceding discussion dealt with basic concepts of radiation biology at the cellular level. When a tissue is irradiated, the expression of damage depends on many factors. Clinical observations of radiation injury depend on the dose of radiation, the time interval between the delivery of radiation to the manifestation of cell death, the volume of tissue that is irradiated, and the type of tissue irradiated.

We distinguish three groups of tissues: rapid cell renewal systems (mucosa of the gut or the bone marrow), slowly proliferating cell renewal systems (epithelial cells, endothelial cells of blood vessels, and connective tissue cells of the stroma), and nonproliferating systems (nerve cells and muscle cells). Radiation effects on tissues, whether seen

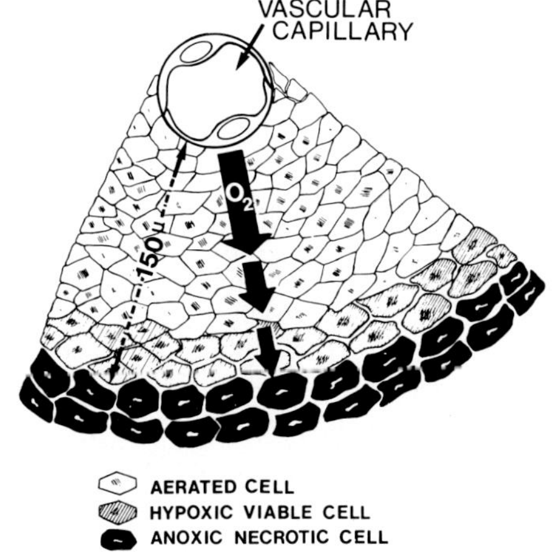

FIGURE 2.5. Diffusion of oxygen from a capillary through tumor tissue. (From Hall EJ. *Radiobiology for the Radiologist*, 2nd ed. Philadelphia, Penn: J.B. Lippincott Company; 1978.)

acutely or after several months, depend on total dose, volume of tissue irradiated, total time over which the treatment was protracted, and dose fraction used or the number of fractions. For example, the effect of 2000 cGy delivered in five fractions in 5 days is approximately equal biologically to 3000 cGy delivered in 3 weeks in 15 fractions. Rapidly growing tumors that have high growth fractions and high cell loss factors will seem to regress rapidly with radiation, yet may regrow because the last tumor cell might not have been lethally injured. In contrast, the tumor that seemingly does not respond eventually might be cured because expression of cellular lethality could be slow owing to the lower growth fraction and lower cell loss factor. It is the reduction of the tumor stem cell population that is of greatest importance, not the rapidity of cell death.

Therapeutic regimens using radiation in the treatment of malignant neoplasms are designed to reduce the clonogenic tumor cells to zero and to preserve the normal tissue within the fields of radiation. Withers outlined the four R's of radiobiology that determine the therapeutic ratio: repair, re-distribution around the cell cycle, re-oxygenation, and re-population in tumors and normal tissues.[6] The therapeutic ratio is the key to the successful treatment of cancer; most research in the field of therapeutic radiology involves attempts to modify the radiation effects on tumor or normal tissue. One such attempt involves radiosensitivity modifiers.

Radiosensitivity Modifiers

Radiosensitivity modifiers have been developed because of the interest in sensitizing tumor cells and protecting normal cells.[8] We distinguish four different groups: physiological modifiers affect cell cycle proliferation rate, oxygen availability, and change of blood flow; physical modifiers are represented by fractionation and dose rate; chemical modifiers work on sensitizers or protectors; biochemical modifiers repair enzyme inhibitors.

The most widely investigated chemical sensitizer is a compound called misonidazol, which in many ways mimics oxygen, the most potent radiation sensitizer. Misonidazol is electron-affinic like O_2 and is lipid soluble, allowing it to diffuse into poorly vascularized areas. This compound should sensitize tumor tissue to radiation without affecting normal tissue. However, misonidazol causes neurotoxic side effects that limit the dose to a level where its efficacy as a clinically effective hypoxic cell sensitizer has not been proven. Other compounds that mimic O_2 but have fewer side effects are being investigated.[7,8]

Another approach to modify the effects of radiation by drug treatment is to protect normal tissue through the use of sulphydryl compounds. The thiol groups within these compounds act as free radical scavengers and reduce the degree of injury at the given radiation dose. This approach attempts to take advantage of poor tumor vascularization that would delay the time of tumor uptake of the radioprotector. Normal tissues rapidly take up the protective compounds. The result could be an increase in the therapeutic ratio, which is the major aim of radiation effect modification.

Several clinical trials are underway that use various chemotherapeutic agents or drugs in combination with radiation; however, little is known about the proper timing of the two modalities or about the general biological principles involved in the use of combined treatment.

Another promising modality of cancer therapy is hyperthermia, alone or in combination with radiation. Temperatures higher than 40°C are cytotoxic. The higher the temperature and the longer the exposure to hyperthermia, the greater the cytotoxicity. It has been shown that heat is more toxic to radioresistant S-phase cells. When combined with radiation heat is a potentiator of radiation effects on all cells, and especially hypoxic cells.[2,7,8] In some studies, the OER at 42°C has been shown to be about 1.6. Methods of delivery of heat have been developed and are showing clinical promise.

References

1. Potten CS. *Radiation and Skin*. London and Philadelphia, Penn: Taylor and Francis; 1985.
2. Berry RJ. Basic concepts in radiobiology. A review. In: Mansfield CM, ed. *Therapeutic Radiology*. New York, NY: Medical Examination Publishing Co; 1983:1–15.
3. Fritz-Niggli H. Klinische Strahlenbiologie. *Schweiz Med Wschr*. 1988;118(suppl 25):76–84.
4. Hall EJ. *Radiobiology for the Radiologist*, 3rd ed. Philadelphia: Penn: JB Lippincott; 1987.

5. Suit HD. Radiation biology: the conceptual and practical impact on radiation therapy. *Radiat Res.* 1983; 94:10–40.
6. Withers HR, Peters LJ. Biological aspects of radiation therapy. In: Fletcher GH, ed. *Textbook of Radiotherapy*, 3rd ed. Philadelphia, Penn: Lea & Febiger; 1980:103–180.
7. Malkinson FD. Some principles of radiobiology: a selective review. *J Invest Dermatol.* 1981;76:32–38.
8. Steel GG, Adams GE, Peckham MJ, eds. *The Biological Basis of Radiotherapy.* Amsterdam: Elsevier; 1983.

3

Radiation Reactions and Sequelae

Renato G. Panizzon and Herbert Goldschmidt

The first reports on therapeutic and damaging effects of x rays were published within a year of Roentgen's discovery. Reversible and irreversible effects were soon distinguished, and the first cases of radiogenic carcinomas were reported at the turn of the century. Comprehensive reviews on this subject were published by Ellinger,[1] Epstein,[2] Goldschmidt and Sherwin,[3] and Goldschmidt.[4]

Radiation reactions can be divided into two groups: nonstochastic and stochastic effects. Nonstochastic effects (for details see Chapter 4) occur only after a substantial threshold has been exceeded; among these are acute and chronic radiodermatitis, radiogenic cancer, and cataracts. Stochastic effects may occur in large populations even after very small radiation doses; typical examples are genetic changes and radiogenic internal neoplasms (Fig. 3.1).

The nonstochastic manifestations of ionizing radiation on the skin may be classified as (1) reversible changes, such as roentgen erythema, reversible epilation of hair, and temporary suppression of sebaceous gland function, (2) conditional reversible changes, such as pigmentation of irradiated skin, and (3) irreversible changes, usually secondary to acute radiodermatitis and potential causes of chronic radiodermatitis and radiation cancer.

Reversible Radiation Effects

Roentgen Erythema—Erythema Dose

The first visible response of the skin to a single dose of ionizing radiation is the appearance of an erythematous reaction in the exposed field. The "erythema dose" was used for quantitative purposes before reliable physical measurements of radiation doses became available.[2] The threshold erythema dose for superficial x rays [half-value layer (HVL) 1 mm aluminum (Al)] ranges from 300 to 400 cGy; for higher energies it can be as high as 800 cGy. Because of their limited penetration, the erythema dose of grenz rays is also higher than that for superficial x rays.

Reaction Pattern

After exposure to a single dose of conventional x irradiation, the skin responds with a reaction pattern in three phases[3] (Fig. 3.2). The first phase consists of an erythema that may occur within minutes or up to 24 hours following the exposure and may last 2 to 3 days. This erythema is attributed to vascular dilatation caused by a release of histamine or serotonin. The second phase (delayed erythema) usually begins about 7 days after irradiation and continues to deepen in color for 7 to 8 days. This type of erythema is thought to be secondary to the release of proteolytic enzymes, such as lysozymes, from damaged epithelial cells. Occasionally, a very delayed erythema appears 6 to 7 weeks after the initial treatment. The cause of this erythema is uncertain.

Experimental Aspects

The erythema, a first wave of reaction, is associated with an inflammatory response resulting from the death of epithelial cells. In animal experiments, the severity of this reaction can be assessed with a scoring system. The assessment of erythema is

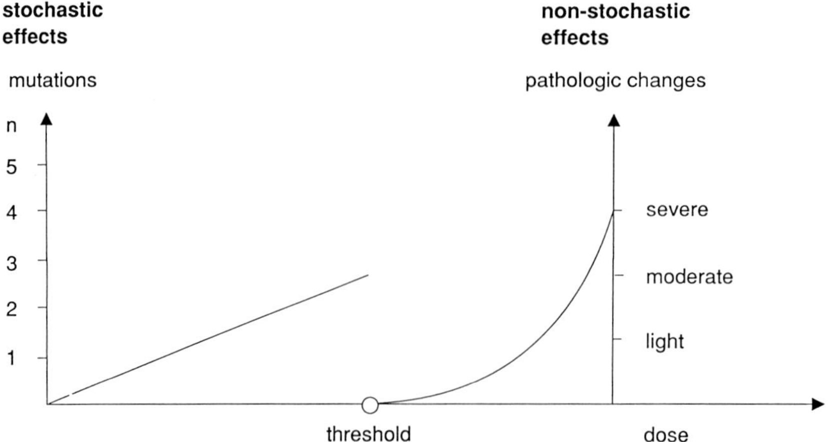

FIGURE 3.1. Stochastic and nonstochastic effects.

subjective and varies with individual observers. It can be influenced by factors such as oxygen tension and the temperature of the environment. Therefore, erythema dose-response relationships are not well defined and sometimes are difficult to interpret. The presence of moist desquamation is a non-subjective assessment that reaches a peak at 4 to 6 weeks after irradiation; this is in keeping with cell kinetic data. Using the incidence of moist desquamation as an end-point to establish quantitative data, reproducible dose-effect curves can be obtained and the dose associated with a 50% incidence of the effect can be determined.[5]

A second wave of reaction, of dermal origin, may begin about 10 weeks after irradiation, reaching a peak after 12 to 14 weeks. These dermal changes are believed to be caused by the impairment of dermal blood flow due to structural and morphological changes in the blood vessels. After irradiation there is a slow depletion of endothelial cells as damaged cells attempt to divide. In response to this cell loss, the few remaining viable endothelial cells start to proliferate, resulting in the development of irregularly spaced cell colonies along the blood vessel wall. These colonies will partially or totally occlude the lumen of the vessels, resulting in a reduction of the blood flow. This in turn will lead to a reduction in the availability of oxygen and nutrients to surrounding tissues, eventually leading to tissue breakdown and necrosis.[6] The severity of acute effects does not necessarily predict the severity of late effects.[7]

Pigment Changes

Following the erythematous reaction, a progressively darkening pigmentation may appear in the treated area, usually 3 weeks after the erythema dose. This pigment commonly disappears after several weeks but, in exceptional cases, may last several months. Histologically, there is storage of melanin in macrophages in the corium.

In most instances, roentgen erythema and radiation pigmentation following small single doses of x rays are temporary and reversible reactions. However, when the skin has been subjected to large single (or multiple fractionated) doses of x irradiation, whether during a therapeutic procedure or through accidental overexposure, inflammation of the skin, adnexal structures, and subcutaneous tissue may occur. These stronger and usually irreversible reactions are discussed later in this chapter.

Effects on Cutaneous Appendages

The germinal layers of anagen hair follicles are highly sensitive to ionizing radiation. Single doses of 300 to 400 cGy (HVL 0.8 mm Al) cause anagen hairs of the scalp to revert to the telogen stage; this is followed by temporary loss of hair. Telogen hairs are less affected by radiation. Re-growth of new hairs can usually be observed after 2 to 3 months. In the past, temporary epilation methods were used in the treatment of tinea capitis and other

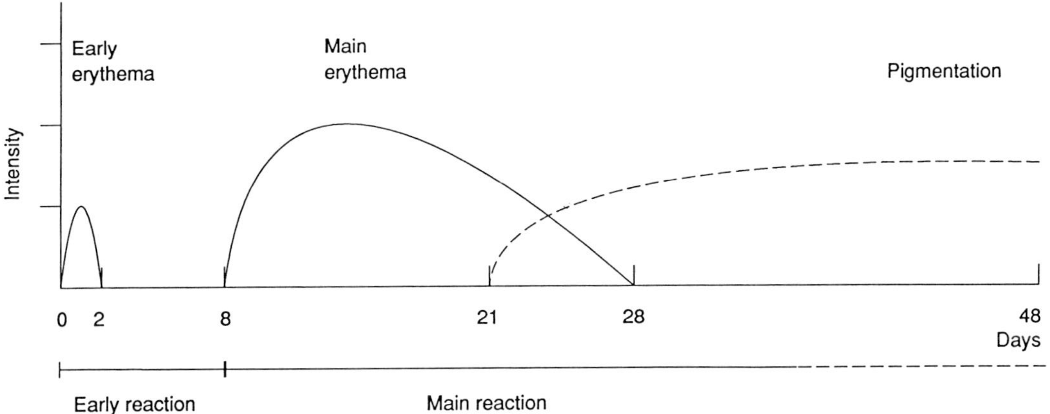

FIGURE 3.2. The phases of skin erythema after exposure to x rays.

scalp conditions.[8] Much larger doses are required for temporary epilation of beard and vellus hairs.

Permanent epilation occurs after single doses above 1200 cGy (HVL 1.0 mm Al). Therapeutic attempts to remove hairs permanently for cosmetic purposes have often resulted in chronic radiodermatitis and radiation cancer.

The sebaceous glands are as sensitive to radiation as the hair follicles. A temporary reduction in sebaceous gland size can be achieved through the use of ionizing radiation.[9] This action is the basis for radiotherapy of acne.[10,11] Older methods of radiotherapy for hyperhidrosis with relatively high cumulative doses have often resulted in chronic radiodermatitis many years after treatment.[11]

Irreversible Radiation Effects

Acute Radiodermatitis

Clinical Symptoms

After exposure to a single dose of ionizing radiation exceeding 10 Gy (1000 cGy), or after equivalent multiple radiation doses, the exposed skin area develops an early response to radiation that has been compared to that of a thermal burn and is frequently referred to as a radiation burn. The main characteristic of acute radiodermatitis is intense local inflammation at the radiation site. This reaction is an unavoidable consequence of radiation designed to destroy cutaneous neoplasms. An accidental overdose (due to inadvertent overlapping of radiation fields, improper shielding, or the use of the wrong filter, kilovoltage, or target-skin distance) may cause similar changes. The clinical signs and symptoms of acute radiodermatitis include erythema, edema, vesiculation, erosion, ulceration, pain, and pruritus. Acute radiodermatitis may be classified as being of first, second, or third degree.[12] The degree of damage depends on the total dose delivered, the quality (penetration) of the radiation, and the size of the exposed area.

First-Degree Acute Radiodermatitis

First-degree acute radiodermatitis is manifested by erythema with some accompanying edema. This reaction is usually more pronounced than the reversible roentgen erythema. There may be slight burning, tingling, or a pruritic sensation, beginning 2 to 7 days after radiation and attaining its maximum sensation at 10 to 14 days. The color of the affected skin may gradually change from a bright erythema to a dull brown-red and then disappear. This process generally takes about 4 weeks, although pigmentation may remain for weeks or months. Temporary or permanent epilation may occur depending on the dose and penetration of the x rays.

Second-Degree Acute Radiodermatitis

In second-degree acute radiodermatitis the reaction is more intense. The main features of second-degree reaction are intense erythema, edema, vesiculation, erosion, and superficial ulceration.

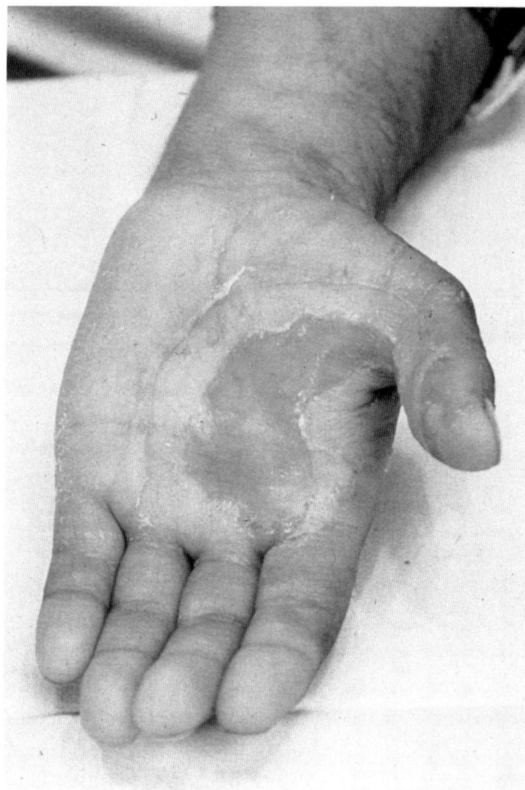

FIGURE 3.3. Third-degree acute radiodermatitis (accidental). Left palm of a 31-year-old patient.

The skin color is often scarlet or violaceous. About 10 days after irradiation, vesiculation develops, which may progress over the next week to leave an oozing eroded surface. Burning, tingling, and pruritus are usually experienced by the patient. A moderate second-degree acute radiodermatitis usually occurs following radiotherapy of skin cancers with multiple fractionated doses. The inflammation ceases 4 or 5 weeks after irradiation, and then repair begins. Depending on the delivered dosage the affected area may become atrophic, with irregular changes of pigmentation and telangiectasia. Alopecia is usually permanent.

Third-Degree Acute Radiodermatitis

Although there is no clear-cut line separating second- and third-degree acute radiodermatitis, a reaction is said to be third degree if more than superficial ulceration and necrosis occur following accidentally administered massive doses of x rays (Fig. 3.3). In this type of reaction the epidermis exfoliates, leaving behind a denuded dermis. Intense hyperemia and edema of the deep tissues develop, and secondary pyogenic infection may occur. Depending on the dose and quality of the irradiation received, the inflammation may extend to the subcutaneous tissue and induce sclerotic changes or even affect bone and viscera. The resulting dry, often indolent ulcer usually has a punched-out appearance. Granulation tissue is frequently absent. Small ulcerative lesions eventually heal, but larger ulcers can persist indefinitely or undergo malignant degeneration.

Except for the unavoidable limited damage that occurs during radiotherapy of malignant tumors of the skin, the occurrence of severe acute radiodermatitis has been (and should remain) a phenomenon of the past. Modern radiotherapeutic methods are designed to avoid such reactions.

Histopathology

The histologic picture of acute radiodermatitis consists of marked intracellular and extracellular edema of the epidermis, together with liquefactive degeneration of the basal cell layer.[1,3] Many pyknotic nuclei are evident. Flattening or effacement of the rete ridges sometimes occurs. In the dermis large accumulations of edema fluid develop, sometimes leading to dermal-epidermal separation and the formation of subepidermal bullae. Swelling of the endothelial cells of blood vessels occurs. The blood vessels themselves are often dilated, and thrombosis and extravasation of red blood cells can be seen. As healing progresses, the stratum corneum and granular layer may thicken while the epidermis itself may be somewhat thinned. The dilation of dermal blood vessels may become permanent, giving rise to telangiectasia. Adnexal structures often undergo atrophy (Fig. 3.4). The dermal collagen may show clumping and fragmentation.

Therapy

During the acute phase of radiation dermatitis, treatment should be as gentle as possible. Vigorous or frequent washing is prohibited because these activities may lead to secondary irritation. Lukewarm compresses, followed by topical antibiotics or steroid preparations, are often helpful in reducing inflammation and secondary bacterial infection.

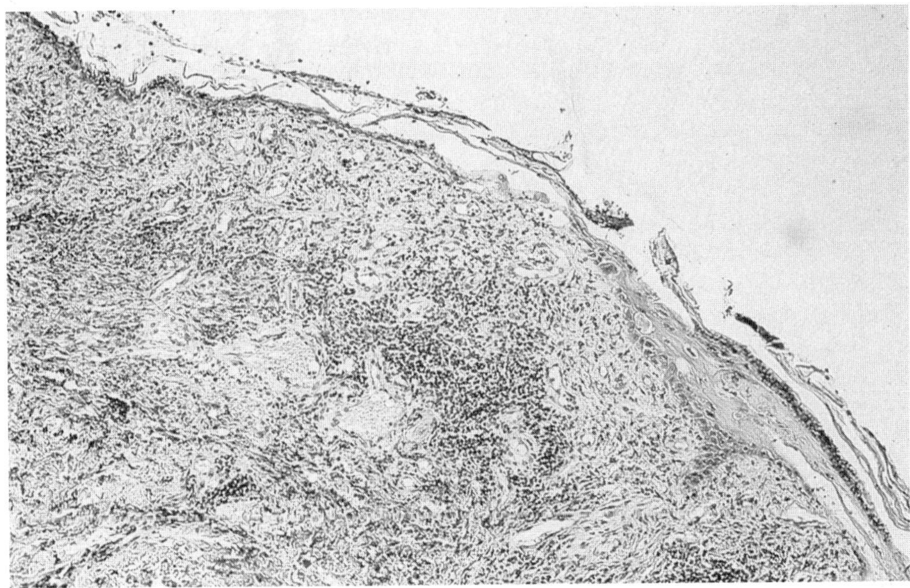

FIGURE 3.4. Histopathology of acute radiodermatitis. For details see text (H & E, × 28).

Some investigators have recommended systemic steroids for severe reactions.

Roentgen Ulcer

As discussed previously, the "roentgen ulcer" (radiation necrosis) is an extremely rare complication that may occur immediately after severe third-degree acute radiodermatitis. It may also develop in chronic radiodermatitis of long duration as a consequence of secondary irritating factors. The most common causes are trauma, thermal injury, excessive cold or ultraviolet exposure, and infection.[14] Most reported cases occurred during the early decades of radiotherapy; common sites were the dorsum of the hand and the facial region, especially over bony prominences. The radionecrosis is characterized by pain, an undermined border, and a beefy base. Radiation ulcers take a long time to heal and in fact may never do so completely, breaking down intermittently instead. When healing does occur, the area may develop marked atrophy, pigment changes, and contractures with deformities. When there is no tendency to healing, the only effective treatment of such ulcerated areas is surgical excision and grafting, with wide and deep margins to ensure that there is relatively healthy tissue on which the graft can take.

Chronic Radiodermatitis

Two clinical types of chronic radiodermatitis (roentgenoderma) can be distinguished; they differ in their tendency to form radiogenic skin cancers. The first type follows fractionated courses of irradiation used in the treatment of cutaneous malignancies in which daily tumor doses are administered over a short period of usually not more than 2 to 6 weeks. The second variety is the result of numerous applications of relatively low doses administered in repeated courses of radiation over longer periods, often several months, leading to large cumulative doses. This type occurred either as the result of occupational exposure or following excessive irradiation of various benign skin conditions; it was more common in the early decades of radiation therapy before the potential radiocarcinogenicity and threshold effects of unlimited courses of small doses of ionizing radiation were recognized.[15]

Chronic Radiodermatitis Following Radiotherapy of Neoplasms

Following the standard treatment for a cutaneous neoplasm with fractionated doses of 4000 to 6000 cGy, sloughing of the irradiated skin occurs, accompanied by an intense erythema but rarely associated with pain. This acute radiodermatitis

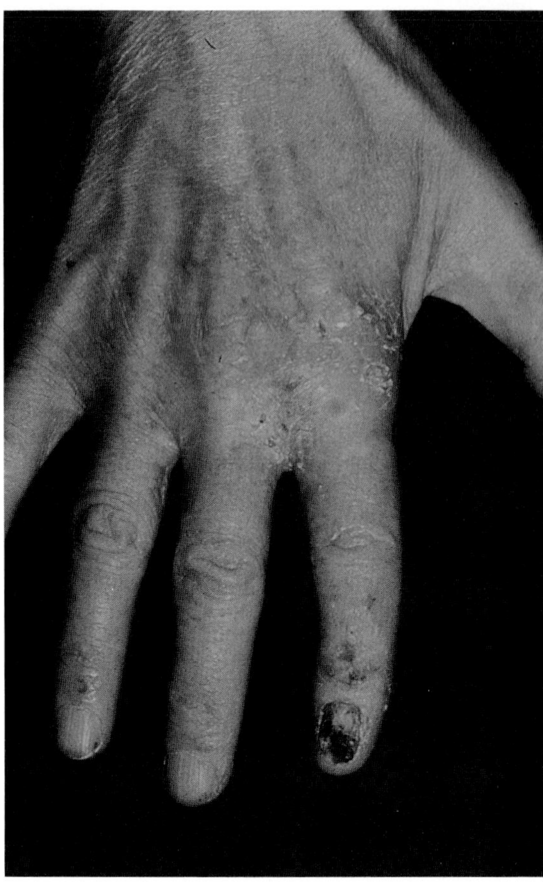

FIGURE 3.5. Chronic radiodermatitis with warty keratoses and superficial squamous cell carcinoma in a 61-year-old dentist (exposed to x rays when holding films).

heals gradually in 3 to 6 weeks. In most cases, the irradiated area looks inconspicuous for many years. However, some patients develop progressive atrophy of the skin after 3 to 24 months, often associated with irregular areas of hypopigmentation or increased pigment formation, telangiectasia (the first evidence usually recognizable after 1 to 2 years), and increased sensitivity to minor trauma. This type of radiodermatitis may also occur after treatment of internal malignancies (e.g., radiotherapy for thyroid, mammary, and prostatic neoplasms) or following treatment of benign skin tumors (e.g., keloids or verrucae). Because of the cell-killing effect, radiation-induced skin carcinomas are rarely seen in radiodermatitis caused by high individual and total doses.

Chronic Radiodermatitis Following Excessive Radiation of Benign Skin Conditions or Occupational Overexposure

Excessive treatment of benign dermatoses with repeated small weekly doses ranging from 50 to 200 cGy with total doses far exceeding 1000 cGy per area may also be followed by chronic radiodermatitis.[12] In the past, this was seen after overdosage of x rays for acne, psoriasis, and eczematous conditions. Although the total doses usually were much smaller than the doses used in cancer therapy, the low individual doses and the relatively long intervals between treatments were more likely to be mutagenic because they did not induce a cell-killing effect. Severe chronic radiodermatitis was also seen many years after permanent x-ray epilation for hirsutism. In these cases, the carcinogenic potential was related to excessive single doses.

In the 1920s, epilation treatments were given at "tricho institutes" where excessive facial hair was irradiated by lay persons.[15] After 10 to 25 years irradiated patients developed x-ray damage in the form of a mask-like face, a thin and pointed nose ("parrot beak"), and furrows radiating from the mouth, along with pigment changes, atrophy, telangiectases, and almost total absence of hair in the affected areas. Similar clinical features are evident in persons with the occupational type of chronic radiodermatitis (Fig. 3.5). This type of radiodermatitis was reported in the early phases of x-ray application and was frequently seen in dentists, veterinarians, workers in industry, and physicians (especially radiotherapists, dermatologists, and internists). The affected skin, often on the hands, turns reddish gray, gradually thickens, and develops premalignant warty keratoses. There is a loss of all hair, and the nails (if included in the irradiated area) become friable and exhibit longitudinal striations. In severe radiation damage sclerotic changes, painful ulcers, and radiogenic neoplasms may develop.

Histopathology

The pathologic changes of chronic radiodermatitis have been studied for many years.[13] The epidermis is often irregular, thickened in some areas, and thinned in others. There is usually marked hyperkeratosis but only few areas of parakeratosis (Fig.

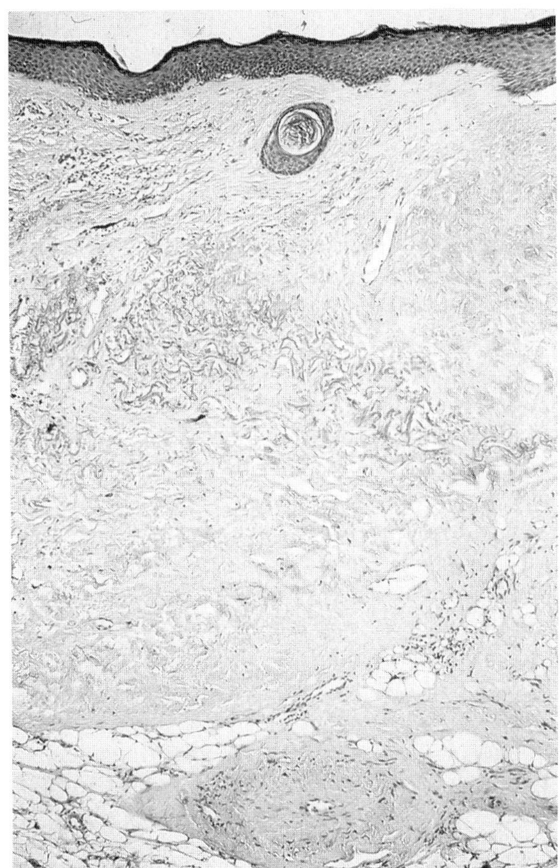

FIGURE 3.6. Histopathology of chronic radiodermatitis. For details see text (H & E, × 23).

3.6). Spongiosis, individual cell keratinization, and nuclear atypia are seen. The epidermis may show a downward proliferation of the rete ridges, which may eventually surround blood vessels in the upper portion of the dermis. The collagen bundles are swollen and often show irregular staining. The changes in the dermal blood vessels comprise the major pathologic findings, with the vessel walls being markedly thickened so that the lumen may be partially or totally occluded. Thromboses are found in many of the larger vessels, and dilated lymphatic channels are frequently seen. The blood vessels lying most superficially in the dermis are widely dilated. The number of normal elastic fibers is markedly diminished, and elastotic fibers predominate. These abnormal fibers have a distinct appearance under the electron microscope. Appendages such as sebaceous glands and hair fol-

licles are entirely absent, but the eccrine sweat glands are usually unaffected, being absent only if the radiation injury was quite severe. Ulceration occurs when there are many vessels that are completely occluded. The pathologic changes may closely resemble those of severe actinic damage, but the basophilic degeneration of the collagen extends much deeper into the dermis in radiodermatitis, and usually the marked parakeratosis of actinically damaged skin is absent.[12]

Experimental Findings

Late radiation effects on animal dermis have been demonstrated histologically; the severity of damage increased with increasing dosage.[16,17] In ^{137}Cs-irradiated DF1 mouse skin the microscopically noticeable fibrosis started 4 weeks after irradiation with 2500 cGy.[17] However, both collagen biosynthesis and collagen content in the skin of the irradiated animals, as well as collagen biosynthesis in cultured fibroblasts explanted from the skin of these mice, showed an increase of newly synthesized collagen as early as 1-week postirradiation, even when only 500 cGy were administered. This increase continued for almost one year (Fig. 3.7). Our results prove that postradiation fibrosis starts much earlier than expected.[18] In pigskin a dose-dependent decrease in dermal thickness was measured 2 years after strontium-90 irradiation with sources 5 to 22.5 mm in diameter. Recent measurements with pulsed ultrasound have demonstrated a 15% reduction in dermal thickness 12 to 18 weeks after strontium-90 irradiation with a single dose of 2700 cGy.[6,16]

Radiogenic Skin Cancer

The main cause of skin cancer in humans is chronic exposure to sunlight; most of the ultraviolet-induced carcinomas occur in exposed areas of the body, particularly the face and arms. Excessive doses of ionizing radiation may also cause cutaneous neoplasms. The cumulative effects of large and small radiation doses on the skin were observed only a few years after Roentgen's discovery. The increasing incidence of radiation sequelae following repeated unlimited courses of x-ray therapy for benign disorders soon made it obvious that, beyond a certain threshold, ionizing radiation could induce chronic radiodermatitis and skin cancer.[3] There are

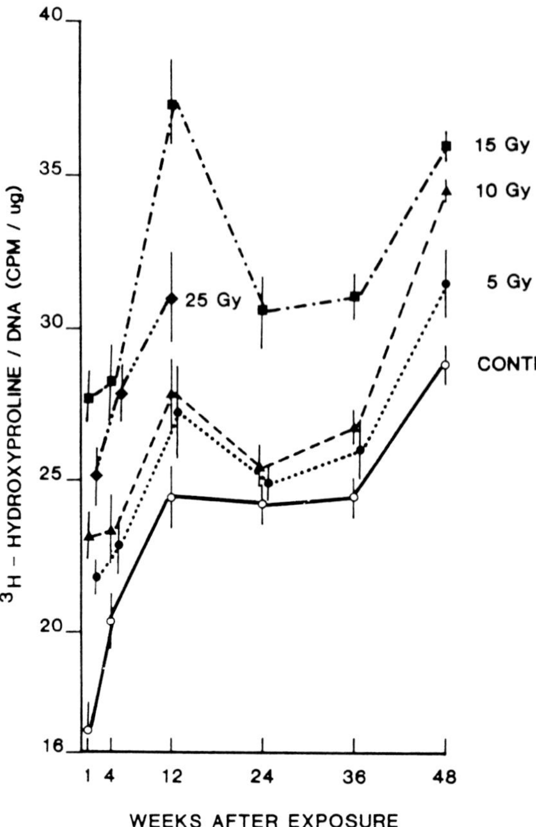

FIGURE 3.7. Effect of single doses of ^{137}Cs on the collagen biosynthesis in skin. The minced tissue was incubated over 22 h with ^{3}H-proline and then the synthesized ^{3}H-hydroxyproline was extracted and measured in counts per minute (CPM). The DNA content was determined (in μg) from the same material and the ratio ^{3}H-hydroxyproline/DNA is expressed as CPM/μg versus time after treatment. The data points represent the mean ± SEM. (From ref. 18, with permission.)

many case reports of skin cancer arising as a consequence of the use and misuse of x rays for a variety of outdated indications, such as ringworm of the scalp, acne of the face, hypertrichosis, hemangioma, lupus vulgaris, toxic goiter, eczema, and multiple fluoroscopies for tuberculosis.

The skin is much less liable to develop potentially fatal cancers after irradiation than other tissues are. The latest recommendations of the International Commission on Radiological Protection[3] mention an absorbed dose of at least 2000 cGy for development of such nonstochastic changes. The macroscopic appearance of radiogenic skin cancers is not substantially different from naturally occurring cutaneous tumors. Most tumors grow rather slowly, but occasionally an aggressive, anaplastic squamous cell cancer or a basal cell cancer may grow with alarming rapidity. The microscopic examination of these tumors reveals a histology nearly identical to that of tumors that may develop in nonirradiated areas, the only difference being the concomitant histologic changes of radiodermatitis in the surrounding tissue.

With few exceptions, radiation cancer does not appear in clinically and/or histologically normal skin; macroscopic and microscopic changes of chronic radiodermatitis are present in the overwhelming majority of radiation-induced skin cancers.

The latent period between irradiation and carcinoma is usually long, varying from 4 to 40 years, with a median of 24.5 years. The tumors are often multiple. Any suspicious lesions that develop in an area that had previously been irradiated must be treated vigorously and as soon as possible in view of the relatively high incidence of metastases in radiogenic squamous cell carcinomas. Lymph node involvement and death secondary to radiogenic squamous cell carcinoma occurred more often during the early years of radiation therapy, especially following occupational exposures with high cumulative doses (e.g., squamous cell carcinomas on the hands of physicians).

A detailed review of the world's literature by Urbach[19] has shown that basal cell carcinomas develop almost exclusively on the head and neck, whereas on all other skin areas squamous cell carcinoma is the predominant type of malignant tumor in chronic radiation dermatitis. He believes that the preponderance of basal cell carcinoma is primarily because patients with occupational radiation dermatitis and secondary squamous cell carcinomas are disappearing by attrition (because few such changes have developed since adequate protective measures became commonplace) and that almost all cases of radiation cancer seen in recent years have been in patients treated for acne, epilation, or benign skin disorders several decades ago. With the general awareness of the potential dangers of repeated low-dose x-ray irradiation during the past three decades, it can be expected that after another 10 to 20 years no new cases of radiogenic skin cancer will be encountered. These cases leave no doubt that ionizing radiation can cause skin cancers. What is not known clearly at this time is the upper limit for x-ray doses (as given for benign disorders) below which the probability of causing cancer is zero or near zero. Many case-control studies provide supporting evidence but do not permit detailed quantitative evaluations.

Quantitative Dose-Effect Data

Radiogenic skin cancers developing many years after irradiation with relatively high total doses for benign skin conditions have been described by a number of authors.[3] Epstein[2] observed malignant changes in 13.9% of 368 patients with chronic radiation dermatitis. Unfortunately, most reports fail to mention the actual doses delivered to the skin.

Once-Weekly Doses Below 100 cGy

Sulzberger and co-workers[20] were the first to investigate the relation between total radiation dose and visible radiation sequelae, such as chronic radiodermatitis and radiogenic skin cancer. They surveyed 1000 patients for the presence of radiation sequelae; 900 of these had been irradiated for various benign skin conditions, such as acne, eczema, psoriasis, and neurodermatitis, and 100 had been treated for skin cancers 5 to 25 years earlier. The results of the survey were compared with an age-matched control group of 1000 patients treated for similar disorders without radiation. Radiogenic sequelae of cosmetic import (atrophy, telangiectasia, depigmentation, hyperpigmentation, keratoses) were seen in only 1.5% of patients who had total doses of more than 1000 cGy in fractional doses up to 2600 cGy. Radiogenic skin cancers were not found in this study. The authors concluded that fractionated doses of 50 to 100 cGy, given in series of three or four treatments at weekly intervals, are not likely to be followed by any visible cutaneous sequelae if the total cumulative dose does not exceed 1000 cGy. (These findings do not apply when 1000 cGy are given in a single dose instead of small fractionated doses.) The validity of these findings has recently been questioned by some authors; Albert and Shore[21] contend that the follow-up period was too short: only 26 irradiated subjects were evaluated more than 15 years after irradiation.

Even though the Sulzberger study may not fulfill epidemiologic and statistical requirements, there is convincing clinical evidence in daily dermatologic practice that small radiation doses below 1200 cGy are not a common cause of skin cancer. One of the few detailed retrospective investigations with reliable dose data was published by Rowell.[22] He examined 100 of 136 patients who had received more than 1500 cGy for benign dermatoses during the years 1930 to 1964 and found a 5% incidence (5 cases) of skin cancer. All patients had been irradiated with measured dosages of superficial x rays with an HVL of 0.75 mm Al. One patient had received 4000 cGy to the hands in 20 years, six patients had more than 3000 cGy to the hands, and 10 had more than 2000 cGy to the face. (A similar number of nonirradiated control subjects matched for age and sex were examined for similar changes.) One of six patients who had more than 3000 cGy to the hands developed squamous cell cancer. Ten patients had received more than 2000 cGy to the facial skin; four of these developed basal cell cancer (the individual doses were 3075 cGy, 2970 cGy, 2450 cGy, and 2090 cGy, respectively). The author ascribes the lower dose for facial cancer to an additive effect of sunlight. He also noted that a high total dose does not necessarily result in visible sequelae; one patient who had 2750 cGy to the face had clinically normal skin (and no skin cancer).

Single or Multiple Doses Greater than 300 cGy

Higher single doses, administered once, twice, or three times at weekly or longer intervals (for now obsolete indications like tinea capitis or hypertrichosis) are more likely to induce skin cancer than individual doses below 100 cGy. Supportive evidence can be demonstrated in animal experiments.[21]

In New York, 2227 patients (average age, 8 years) were treated for tinea capitis. After an average follow-up time of 25 years, 33 skin cancers were found in the irradiated group and only three cases in a control group. Conversely, no increased incidence of skin cancers was seen in Modan and Ron's study of 10,902 x-ray epilated children.[23] A large-scale investigation of atomic bomb survivors[24] also did not show any increased evidence of radiogenic skin cancers.

Types of Radiogenic Cutaneous Neoplasms

The macroscopic appearance of radiogenic skin cancers is not substantially different form naturally occurring cutaneous tumors. In the early years of radiation therapy it was believed that squamous cell carcinoma was virtually the only type of radiation-induced carcinoma occurring on the skin. However, it is now clear that basal cell carcinomas are also common sequelae in radiation-damaged skin. Other, less common tumors encountered as late radiation sequelae include cylindromas and sebaceous and sweat gland carcinomas.[12] Melanomas have been reported as occasional sequelae but there is no credible evidence for an association of melanomas with ionizing radiation.[21] Sarcomas have also been reported following radiation, but many of these actually represent irradiation fibromatosis rather than true sarcomas. In the past, these peculiar growths have been termed "pseudosarcoma" of the skin or "paradoxical fibrosarcoma." The microscopic examination of the various listed tumors reveals a histology nearly identical to that of similar-type tumors that develop in nonirradiated areas, the only difference being the concomitant histologic changes of radiodermatitis in the surrounding tissue.

In most reports, the incidence of basal cell carcinoma in irradiated skin areas was higher than that of squamous cell carcinomas. The incidence of metastases from radiation-induced skin cancers seems to be higher than for ordinary squamous carcinomas arising in actinically damaged glabrous skin. The frequency of metastasis from primary nonradiogenic squamous cell carcinoma is listed as 3% for squamous cell carcinomas arising on nonglabrous skin and 11% for squamous cell carcinomas arising on mucocutaneous junctions. In contrast, some authors report metastases of squamous cell cancers arising in chronic radiodermatitis in 20% to 26% of cases.[19] There is also evidence that the carcinogenic effect of x rays is much greater if obvious radiodermatitis is present.[14,26]

Martin and colleagues[25] described 368 patients with facial or neck skin cancers following irradiation for benign skin conditions (mostly hirsutism and acne). Thirty-five died as a result of radiation-induced cancers. The median interval between exposure and diagnosis was 21 years. No information was available concerning the total dosage and number of treatments. The published photographs strongly suggest radiation effects related to gross overdosage. Allison[27] describes four patients with 129 small, multiple, superficial radiogenic basal cell carcinomas without evidence of radiation damage. Patients had been treated for noncutaneous cancers and one patient had repeated fluoroscopy while receiving pneumothorax therapy for tuberculosis. The author contends that these patients belong to a genetically related subset of the population with an impaired ability to repair radiation damage. Frentz[28] also believes that certain skin cancers following grenz irradiation may occur only in genetically predisposed persons with an abnormal sensitivity to ionizing radiation.

Chronic Radiodermatitis and Radiogenic Skin Cancer

With few exceptions, radiogenic cutaneous neoplasms develop in areas that show clinical and microscopic evidence of chronic radiodermatitis. In some cases, mild atrophy, few telangiectases, and absence of hair are the only clinical symptoms. There are a few reports in the literature indicating that radiodermatitis is not a prerequisite for radiogenic skin cancers. One of these is a study on multiple basal cell epitheliomas following radiotherapy of the spine for spondylitis.[26] Another paper states that 19% of 314 radiogenic skin cancers showed "slight" or no skin changes.[25] As mentioned above, visible changes of chronic radiodermatitis can be subtle; even without macroscopic sequelae there may be clear evidence of microscopic changes.

Van Vloten and colleagues[29] examined 257 patients irradiated with fractions varying from 70 to 400 cGy given at 4-week intervals up to total doses of 5100 cGy (HVL 1 mm Cu) for tuberculous lymphadenitis, hyperthyroidosis, and other benign disorders, mostly in the neck area. They detected 16 skin carcinomas after a median follow-up period of 41 years. The severity of radiodermatitis was associated with a higher prevalence of skin cancer, especially for total doses exceeding 1000 cGy. The number of radiation-induced skin cancers increased with posttreatment time.

Susceptibility Factors

There is increasing evidence that the induction of radiogenic cutaneous neoplasms can be promoted by other carcinogenic factors. One of these is ultraviolet radiation. Investigations of the incidence of skin cancers following psoralen-ultraviolet A (PUVA) therapy for psoriasis showed a statistically significant increase of cancers in patients previously treated with x rays or grenz rays.[30]

In a questionnaire follow-up of 2180 patients who were exposed as children (average age, 9 years) to single doses of 300 to 600 cGy of 120 kV x rays as a treatment for tinea capitis, the number of basal cell carcinomas 25 years after treatment was 5 times higher than normal.[21,31] A greater incidence of cancers per unit area in sun-exposed areas of nonscalp skin suggested the involvement of ultraviolet radiation as a promoter of basal cell cancers initiated by ionizing radiation. Davis and colleagues[32] considered various risk factors in 76 patients with chronic radiation dermatitis and radiogenic carcinomas. They concluded that the sun-reactive skin type, especially type I (always burns, never tans) and type II (always burns, then slightly tans) may be used as a predictor of skin cancer risk when the total dose of ionizing radiation is not known. Increased melanin pigmentation may be directly or indirectly protective against the development of skin cancers in patients who have received low-dose superficial radiation for benign disease. None of the patients had skin types IV to VI. They also mention another explanation for the higher incidence of radiogenic carcinomas in fair-skinned persons, namely, the additive effect of ionizing radiation (as an initiator of malignancy) and ultraviolet radiation acting as a promoter.

The potential influence of genetic predisposing factors was already mentioned.[27,28] Analyses by recombinant DNA technologies have suggested that alterations in the activation of cellular oncogenes may be the genetic basis of the carcinogenic effect of radiation.[31]

Experimental Aspects

Several experiments have been performed on rat skin concerning the location, type, and incidence of tumors after various particulate radiation treatments. Doses in the range of 1000 to 2000 cGy were most effective; many of the tumors were believed to have originated from residual or long-term damage in severely distorted hair follicles. Higher doses (more than 4000 cGy) tended to reduce the number of atrophic follicles. Because all

follicular cells were destroyed, fewer tumors were seen after higher doses. This suggests that a constant fraction of atrophic follicles may develop into tumors. It was also noted that the tumor incidence yield was related to the dose received by cells at the bottom of the resting hair follicle.[33] Although the carcinogenic action of ionizing radiation has been demonstrated for a spectrum of end-points in experimental animals, the peculiarities of each tumor model are such as to preclude generalizations.[34] It is difficult to interpret tumor induction curves on the basis of simple mechanisms of action; physical factors, such as absorbed dose, its temporal distribution, and the linear energy transfer may have an appreciable influence on the carcinogenic action.

References

1. Ellinger F. *Medical Radiation Biology.* Springfield, Il: Charles C Thomas; 1957.
2. Epstein E. *Radiodermatitis.* Springfield, Il: Charles C Thomas; 1962.
3. Goldschmidt H, Sherwin W. Reactions to ionizing radiation. *J Am Acad Dermatol.* 1980;3:551–579.
4. Goldschmidt H. Radiodermatitis and other sequelae of ionizing radiation. In: Demis J, ed. *Dermatology, IV.* Philadelphia, Penn: Harper and Row; 1985.
5. Van den Aardweg GJMJ, Hopewell JW, Simmonds RH. Repair and recovery in the epithelial and vascular connective tissue of pig skin after irradiation. *Radiother Oncol.* 1988;11:73–82.
6. Hopewell JW. Mechanisms of the action of radiation on skin and underlying tissues. *Br J Radiol.* 1986:19(suppl):39–47.
7. Whithers HR. Effects on normal tissues: tolerance. In: Brovsk JJ, Barendsen GW, Kal HB, et al., eds. *Radiation Research.* Amsterdam: Martinus Nijhoff Publishers; 1983:459–466.
8. Wagner G. Die Epilationsbestrahlung. In: Jadassohn J, ed. *Handbuch der Haut und Geschlechtskrankheiten Suppl. V, Vol. 2.* Berlin: Springer Verlag; 1959:655–746.
9. Caccialanza M, Bonelli M, Rivolta M. I lipidi della superficie cutanea in rapporto alla roentgentherapia. *G Ital Dermatol Venereol.* 1980;115:260–262.
10. Strauss JS, Kligman AM. Effect of x rays on sebaceous glands of the human face. *J Invest Dermatol.* 1959;33:347–352.
11. Cipollaro AC, Crossland PM. *X-rays and Radium in the Treatment of Diseases of the Skin.* 5th ed. Philadelphia, Penn: Lea & Febiger; 1967.
12. Rudolph R, Goldschmidt H. Radiodermatitis and

other adverse sequelae of cutaneous irradiation. In: Goldschmidt H, ed. *Physical Modalities in Dermatologic Therapy.* New York, NY: Springer-Verlag; 1978.

13. Montgomery H: Pathologic histology of radiodermatitis. In: Cipollaro AC, Crossland PM, eds. *X-rays and Radium in the Treatment of Diseases of the Skin.* 5th ed. Philadelphia, Penn: Lea & Febiger; 1967.

14. Traenkle HL, Mullay D. Further observations of late radiation necrosis following therapy of skin cancer. *Arch Dermatol.* 1960;81:908–913.

15. Lapidus SM. The Tricho system: hypertrichosis, radiation and cancer. *J Surg Oncol.* 1976;8:267–274.

16. Hamlet R, Rezvani M, Hopewell JW. Ultrasound measurement of atrophy in pig skin following X- or B-irradiation. *Biol Engin Skin.* 1986;2:49–57.

17. Panizzon RG, Malkinson FD, Hanson WR, et al. A one-year comparative study of post-irradiation collagen content and microscopic fibroses in mouse skin. *Br J Radiol.* 1986;32(suppl 19):54–57.

18. Panizzon RG, Hanson WR, Schwartz D, et al. Ionizing radiation induces early, sustained increases in collagen biosynthesis: a 48 week study in mouse skin and skin fibroblasts cultures. *Radiat Res.* 1988;116:145–156.

19. Urbach F. Pathologic effects of ionizing radiation. In: Fitzpatrick TB, Eisen AZ, Wolff K, Freedberg IM, Austen KF, eds. *Dermatology in General Medicine.* New York, NY: McGraw-Hill; 1971:1042–1047.

20. Sulzberger MB, Baer RL, Borota A. Do roentgen ray treatments as given by skin specialists produce cancers or other sequelae? *Arch Dermatol Syphilol.* 1952;65:639–655.

21. Albert RE, Shore RE. Carcinogenic effects of radiation on the human skin. In: Upton AL, Albert RE, Burns FJ, et al., eds. *Radiation Carcinogenesis.* New York, NY: Elsevier; 1986.

22. Rowell NR. A follow-up study of superficial radiotherapy for benign dermatoses: recommendations for the use of x-rays in dermatology. *Br J Dermatol.* 1973;88:583–590.

23. Modan B, Ron E. Thyroid neoplasms in a population irradiated for scalp tinea in childhood. In: Degroot L, Frohmaul, Kaplan E, et al., eds. *Radiation-Associated Thyroid Carcinoma.* New York, NY: Grune and Stratton; 1977.

24. Johnson M, Land L, Gregory P, et al. Effects of ionizing radiation on the skin. Hiroshima and Nagasaki. In: Albert RE, Burns FJ, et al., eds. *Radiation Carcinogenesis.* New York, NY: Elsevier; 1986.

25. Martin H, Strong E, Spiro RH. Radiation induced skin cancers of the head and neck. *Cancer.* 1969;25:61–71.

26. Sarcany I, Fountain RB, Evans CD, et al. Multiple basal cell epitheliomata following radiotherapy of the spine. *Br J Dermatol.* 1968;80:90–96.

27. Allison JR. Radiation-induced basal cell cancer. *J Dermatol Surg Oncol* 1984;10:200–203.

28. Frentz G. Grenz-ray induced nonmelanoma skin cancer. *J Am Acad Dermatol.* 1989;21:475–478.

29. Van Vloten WA, Hermans J, Van Daal WA. Radiation-induced skin cancer and radiodermatitis of the head and neck. *Cancer.* 1987;59:411–414.

30. Stern R, Thibodeau L, Kleinerman R, et al. Risk of cutaneous carcinoma in patients treated with oral methoxsalen photochemotherapy for psoriasis. *N Engl J Med.* 1979;300:809–813.

31. Burns FJ. Cancer risk associated with therapeutic irradiation of the skin. *Arch Dermatol.* 1989;125:979–981.

32. Davis MM, Hauke CW, Zollinger TW, et al. Skin cancer in patients with chronic radiation dermatitis. *J Am Acad Dermatol.* 1989;20:608–616.

33. Albert RE, Burns FJ, Bennett P. Radiation-induced hair-follicle damage and tumor formation in mouse and rat skin. *J Natl Cancer Inst.* 1972;49:1131–1137.

34. UNSCEAR 1986. Genetic and somatic effects of ionizing radiation. United Nations, New York; 1986.

4

Chronic Radiation Effects and Radiation Protection

Herbert Goldschmidt

Late somatic effects of ionizing radiation are classified as either stochastic or nonstochastic (from Greek *stochastikos* = able to hit). Stochastic effects are effects for which the probability of an effect occurring, rather than its severity, is a function of dose without threshold.[1] More generally, stochastic means random in nature. In large irradiated populations even a small radiation dose may induce late effects in a small percentage of exposed individuals; the severity of the effect is dose-dependent. Nonstochastic effects occur only if a substantial threshold dose is exceeded (often several hundred cGy).

Nonstochastic Effects

Nonstochastic effects are those for which the severity of the effect varies with the dose and for which a relatively high threshold dose has been demonstrated. The risk of inducing nonstochastic changes at low doses is minimal.

Cataract

Cataractogenic dose levels range from 200 cGy for a single exposure to 350 to 400 cGy for fractionated doses.[2] In dermatologic therapy, adequate eye protection with lead eyeshields reduces the risk of cataracts to a minimum. Measurements of the effect of various eyeshields were carried out by Kopf and co-workers.[3] During radiotherapy for cancer of the eyelid with a total air dose of 3400 cGy at 0.9 mm Aluminum half-value layer (Al HVL), the shielded cornea received 50 cGy and the lens about 40 cGy when an 0.9-mm thick eye cup was inserted into the conjunctival sac. The routine use of lead eyeshields directly over the closed eyelids during fractionated radiotherapy of the face with 1000 cGy limits the dose to the lens for the same HVL to approximately 12 cGy.

Fertility

Although the sperm count may be depressed temporarily by an absorbed dose of 25 cGy, the absorbed dose required to cause permanent sterility is at least 250 cGy.[4] In contrast to the nonstochastic effect on the sperm count, the genetic effects on the descendants of the irradiated individual are considered stochastic.

Chronic Radiodermatitis and Radiogenic Skin Cancer

The late effects of ionizing radiation on the skin are also nonstochastic and require a substantial threshold dose. These changes are discussed in detail in Chapter 3.

Stochastic Effects

The frequency of stochastic effects is related to the dose without evidence of a threshold. In addition to most hereditary effects, most somatic effects are now regarded as being stochastic. Leukemogenesis and carcinogenesis are the most serious somatic risks of irradiation; other suspected radiation-related injuries are stunted growth, mental retard-

"

ation, and personality disorders. There is an extensive body of knowledge about the effects of ionizing radiation on man[4]; most of it relates to doses of 100 to 1000 cGy or more, delivered at high dose rates in short periods of time.Radiation, from artificial or natural sources, rarely causes unique diseases. Most late radiogenic effects are indistinguishable from those that occur naturally in nonirradiated populations; their relationship to radiation is detectable only in a statistical sense. Thus, in any given individual, a particular effect cannot be attributed conclusively to radiation, as opposed to some other cause. In contrast to the effects of large radiation doses, there is no unequivocal evidence of injury in humans from doses similar to those received during low-dose medical treatments (including properly administered dermatologic radiotherapy), particularly for doses below 50 cGy.[5]

General Considerations

Low-Dose Risk Assessment

Risk assessment for low level exposures to carcinogens is a new branch of mathematical biology. The quantification of risks has been greatly facilitated by the publication of risk co-efficients for various types of radiation-induced cancers in the 1972 report of the Advisory Committee on the Biologic Effects of Ionizing Radiation (BEIR I) of the National Academy of Sciences-National Research Council.[5] The committee has based its recommendations on the "linear hypothesis," which presumes that given effects (such as cancers of various organ systems) observed at relatively high levels of radiation exposure exist proportionately downward toward zero without the presence of any limiting threshold dose.

The 1980 BEIR report assumes a linear-quadratic dose-effect relationship and it eschews extrapolations to single whole-body doses of less than 10 cGy. An updated 1990 version of the BEIR report (the fifth in a series) is now being prepared.[6] New estimates have shown that low levels of ionizing radiation could be 3 to 4 times more harmful than was previously assumed. Since it appears that atomic bomb survivors received smaller doses than originally estimated, high rates of cancer are now attributed to lower exposures. This finding is important for risk estimates for leukemia and may lead to tighter radiation safety rules in hospitals, but it has no consequences for dermatologic radiation therapy.

Radiation Carcinogenicity

An increase in incidence with increasing radiation dose has been documented for several cancers in human populations, as well as for several types of neoplasms in experimental animals.[1] The most frequently reported human radiogenic neoplasms are thyroid cancer, breast cancer, leukemia (in atomic bomb survivors and following treatment of ankylosing spondylitis), bronchial carcinoma (in radon miners), cancer of the skeleton (in radium dial painters and patients treated for ankylosing spondylitis or for tuberculosis of the bone), and cancer of the gastrointestinal tract (in atomic bomb survivors and in patients irradiated for ankylosing spondylitis).

Because of their limited penetration, neither grenz rays nor soft x rays and superficial x rays (as used in dermatology) are likely to induce most of these neoplasms. A recent large-scale study emphasizes the advantages of nonpenetrating x rays in reducing carcinogenicity of other organs that were partially exposed to therapeutic radiation, or to scatter radiation near the treated area. Furst and co-workers[7] investigated the cancer incidence of 18,030 patients irradiated for cutaneous hemangiomas in Sweden between 1920 and 1959. More than 12,000 patients were treated with radium 226, 2500 patients with orthovoltage x rays (HVL 0.1–1.0 mm Cu), and 2500 patients with contact therapy (60 kV); doses ranged from 500 to 1000 cGy. The cancer incidence after nonpenetrating radiation (60 kV contact therapy) was not higher than for the normal population. The other subgroups showed relative risk factors ranging from 0.79 to 1.65 with higher than normal values for breast cancer, thyroid cancer, and soft tissue tumors.

Dermatologic radiotherapy has been suspected as a contributing factor only in patients who developed thyroid cancer, breast cancer, and brain and salivary gland tumors. Almost all of these patients were treated for either acne or tinea capitis; owing to the availability of better treatment methods, neither of these common diseases has been considered an indication for modern dermatologic radiation therapy during the past two decades. (For details on potential risks of dermatologic radiotherapy, the reader is referred to a comprehensive review of the subject by Goldschmidt and Sherwin.[8]) In radiation protection work special units are used. The term "rem" (roentgen equivalent man) is defined as the product of the absorbed dose and quality factor. The new SI unit of dose equivalent is the sievert (Sv): 1 rem = 0.01 Sv. In dermatologic radiotherapy 1 cGy is practically equivalent to 1 rem; the biologic effect of 1 Gy equals 1 Sv (100 rad = 100 rem) because no major adjustment of the quality factor is required.

Thyroid Cancer

Until 1950 most investigations on potential hazards of dermatologic radiotherapy have centered on possible genetic effects and on the definition of a safe cumulative dose below which radiogenic skin cancers would not occur. Now that these problems have been clarified, attention has focused on the possible connection between dermatologic radiotherapy and thyroid cancer. Since this potential side effect has been mentioned in a number of medical publications and in several sensationalized reports in the media, a more detailed review of this problem seems appropriate.

The induction of thyroid cancer by ionizing radiation has been summarized in an authoritative report of the National Council on Radiation Protection and Measurements (NCRP) in 1985.[9] The report provides risk estimates for mean thyroidal doses in the range of 6 to 1500 cGy. Because of their cell-killing effect, higher doses are less likely to induce thyroid cancer.

Thyroid cancer is a relatively rare neoplasm; in the United States there are 8100 new cases per year. The age-adjusted rate is 3.7/100,000. It occurs twice as frequently in women as in men and more frequently in whites than in blacks. The incidence increases with age.[10] Studies have indicated that anywhere from 4% to 13% of thyroid glands in patients dying with no known thyroid disease show foci of malignant cells ("occult tumors"[11,12]). According to the BEIR report,[5] the dose-effect relationship as observed at relatively high doses and high dose rates (like that for leukemia) can be represented by a linear, nonthreshold function, corresponding to a risk of 2.5 cases of fatal thyroid cancer per one million persons exposed per year per rem to the thyroid gland, averaged over the fifth to 25th years after exposure. The average latency period is 15 to 20 years. Susceptibility to induction of these tumors seems to be several times higher in children than in adults. The induction rate is higher in women than in men, just as is the natural

incidence of this form of cancer. The estimated induction rates are high, but the most frequent type of cancer is the rather easily treated papillary tumor, which carries little risk of causing death[13]; only 1% to 3% of the radiogenic tumors have proved fatal in several groups of patients studied[14,15]; the maximum lethal percentage was reported by the NRCP as 10%.[9] The thyroid thus has one of the highest induction rates for cancer but one of the lowest for fatal cancer.[14]

In irradiated populations, particularly in Japanese atomic bomb survivors and residents of the Marshall Islands exposed to radioactive fallout, tumors of the thyroid gland have shown a systematic increase in incidence with increasing dosage. Thyroid cancers were also reported in children after treatment with radioiodine for hyperthyroidism and following therapeutic irradiation of various benign medical conditions, such as enlarged thymus glands or tonsils, or sinusitis. In most of the reported series, thyroid doses varied between 70 and 700 cGy.[1,9]

Thyroid Cancer and Dermatologic Radiotherapy: Controlled Studies

Quantitative risk data can be derived only from rigidly controlled epidemiologic investigations that include a sufficiently large number of exposed persons and cohorts, reliable estimates of the mean thyroid dose, and an adequate follow-up period. Only a few studies fulfill the requirements for estimating the risk of developing thyroid cancer quantitatively.[15] The most frequently quoted controlled investigations include follow-up studies of children irradiated for thymic enlargement in Rochester, N.Y.,[16,17] the study of survivors of the atomic bomb in Hiroshima and Nagasaki,[18] and a follow-up of individuals exposed to radioactive fallout in the Marshall Islands.[19] The mean thyroid doses were high in these studies (143–1225 cGy), and a significant excess of tumors of the thyroid was found. Crile and co-workers[20] reviewed these data and pointed out that the increase in thyroid disease was partially due to an increase in occult cancers and that the mortality was extremely low. No deaths were encountered in the Marshall Island patients, and only one death occurred in 40 Japanese atomic bomb survivors with thyroid cancer.

Of special interest to dermatologists are two controlled studies of x-ray epilation for tinea capitis. Until recently it was assumed that the lowest range of potentially carcinogenic doses varied between 50 and 100 cGy. For this reason it was considered extremely unlikely that the thyroid gland could have been exposed to such high dose levels during properly administered dermatologic radiation therapy with suitable radiation protection measures. These dose estimates have been challenged by Modan and colleagues' study in Israel,[21] where 10,902 children had been treated with the multiple-field Kienböck-Adamson epilation technique for tinea capitis. Single or total doses ranged from 400 to 1200 cGy; the quality of radiation was unusually penetrating (HVL, 3 mm Al). The records of these children were re-examined 12 to 23 years later and compared to an untreated individually matched control group of 5500 children. An increased incidence of various benign and malignant thyroid, parotid, salivary gland, and brain tumors was found in the treated group. There were 12 thyroid cancers in the treated group and two in the untreated group. Dosimetric reconstruction studies on phantom skulls revealed an estimated thyroid dose of only 6.5 cGy. Another group of 2213 patients treated for ringworm of the scalp at the New York University Medical Center was reviewed by Albert and colleagues.[22–24] Comparison with a large clinical control group revealed an increase in the number of benign thyroid tumors but (in contrast to the Modan study) no increased evidence of thyroid cancer.

Since the mean thyroid dose in the previously reported studies amounted to several hundred cGy, the findings of Modan and colleagues' study were unexpected, and serious objections were raised to its procedures and conclusions. The main criticism was the possibility that the treated children moved during treatment and that they received much higher thyroid doses than theoretically established.[25,26] (Five individual exposures ranging from 400 to 1200 cGy were given to different scalp regions of each child in 5 days.) Recent investigations make it clear that low-dose thyroid exposure (as in dermatologic radiotherapy) is unlikely to cause fatal thyroid cancer.[20] This rare possibility is even smaller when proper shielding of the thyroid region and relatively nonpenetrating radiation qualities are used. The importance of these factors was emphasized by thyroid dose measurements during cutaneous radiotherapy.

Thyroid Dose Measurements

In the absence of controlled retrospective studies, the measurement of thyroid doses associated with various obsolete as well as current dermatologic radiation techniques offers the best means of assessing the potential risks to the thyroid gland during properly administered therapy; it also permits evaluation of radiation protection techniques.

Petratos and co-workers[27] reported results of thermoluminescent dosimetry during radiotherapy for skin cancer of the facial area with an HVL of 0.9 mm Al; they measured a thyroid dose of only 0.17 cGy per 1000 cGy dose to the lesion. Cones and overlay lead shielding were used during therapy.

Goldschmidt and co-workers[28] carried out extensive dose measurements with thermoluminescent dosimeters and ionization rate meters. Thyroid doses were measured in an anthropomorphic phantom during simulated treatments of various skin regions. Measurements for a facial exposure of 1000 cGy with an HVL of 0.75 mm Al revealed a thyroid dose of only 0.4 cGy when a lead cone of 12-cm diameter was used and a lead shield of 0.9-mm thickness was applied to the thyroid region.[28] When neither a lead shield nor cone was used, the thyroid dose was markedly increased to 210 cGy. These data emphasize that the use of treatment cones and lead shields over the thyroid region is essential when the facial area is irradiated. Thyroid doses were much lower for less penetrating radiation qualities; for grenz ray qualities thyroid exposure was extremely low.

Determination of thyroid exposure during treatment of other body regions yielded much smaller values than for the facial area. For superficial x-ray qualities (HVL, 0.75 mm Al) with standard cones (thyroid shield omitted, 1000 cGy skin dose), the thyroid dose varied from 0.16 cGy during treatment of the upper arm to 0.008 cGy when the hand was irradiated; 0.0009 cGy was measured when the foot was treated. Soft x rays with an HVL of 0.17 mm Al given to the upper arm yielded a thyroid dose of only 0.007 cGy. Grenz rays (HVL, 0.025 mm Al) showed extremely low values (< 1 microrad).

Comparison of Risks

Because of sensationalized reports in the media, many patients believe that diagnostic and therapeutic x rays are extremely dangerous. They often worry about the risks of radiation suggested for the treatment of skin cancers or other skin conditions even when no other suitable therapeutic methods are available. For these patients a comparison with other risks can be useful. All patients exposed to any form of ionizing radiation should be informed of all potential risks but truly informed consent is possible only when quantitative data can be supplied. Even the results of dose measurements are not directly helpful to the practicing dermatologist, unless they are accompanied by quantitative risk assessments that permit comparisons and predictions of the approximate frequency of cancer and the mortality risk for the affected patients. During properly administered radiotherapy (with cones and thyroid protection) for an HVL of 0.75 mm Al, the measured average thyroid dose was 0.42 cGy when one side of the face was treated. For (now outmoded) acne therapy techniques with a maximum dose of 1000 cGy to both sides of the face, this would amount to 0.84 cGy. For this thyroid dose, the risk of developing a thyroid cancer would be 1:7000 for a child and 1:21,500 for an adult. On the basis of the BEIR data, the mortality risk for a thyroid dose of 0.84 cGy can be calculated as 1:240,000 for a child and 1:700,000 for an adult. Although these risks are by no means negligible (particularly when radiation protection is not used or the neck is irradiated directly), they appear to be small compared with other hazards that most people face and accept every day. During penicillin therapy, the risk of shock is given as 1:25,000 or even 1:6600; the risk of death as 1:50,000.[29] Regarding everyday risks, a one in a million risk of death (reduction of life expectancy by 8 minutes) has been attributed to smoking 1.4 cigarettes, eating 100 charcoal-broiled steaks (benzopyrene) or 40 tablespoons of peanut butter (aflatoxin B), drinking 30 12-oz. cans of diet soda (saccharin), or coloring hair black 5 times (2,4 diaminoanisole). Similar (1:1,000,000) risks are associated with fatal accidents that may occur after spending 3 hours in a coal mine, traveling 6 minutes by canoe, 10 miles by bicycle, 300 miles by car, or 1000 miles by jet.[30–32]

Carcinoma of the Breast

Breast cancer has been observed in atomic bomb survivors[33] who had received more than 90 cGy of radiation, women who received localized x-ray therapy for acute postpartum mastitis,[34] in female patients with tuberculosis of the lung subjected to repeated fluoroscopy (150 cGy cumulative breast dose during pneumotherapy), and in women irradiated during childhood for gynecomastia and hemangioma.[35–38] The current risk-versus-benefit debate over the merits of mammography should also be mentioned[39,40] (skin doses of 0.3–10 cGy and mid-breast doses ranging from 30–1000 mrem per exposure). The risk co-efficient cited in the BEIR report is three deaths per rem per year per one million exposed individuals.

Breast Cancer and Dermatologic Radiotherapy

A possible connection between breast cancer and radiotherapy for acne and hirsutism was postulated in a report about 16 women with breast cancer[41]; 11 of these cases were quoted summarily without any details, and the remaining five cases were anecdotal reports of breast cancer in women who had been irradiated for facial acne in the past. Details of acne treatments, such as dosage, quality of radiation, fractionation, or shielding, were not given. This report has been strongly criticized by epidemiologists[42]; in view of the high incidence of breast cancer in women (7%) and the large number of patients irradiated for acne, the described findings could be completely fortuitous. (The nonirradiated sister of one of the reported patients also developed breast cancer.) Another report described the occurrence of breast cancer in a patient irradiated for hirsutism.[43] The reported severe chronic radiodermatitis with numerous (150) basal cell epitheliomas clearly indicates gross overdosage, having no relationship to proper radiation therapy.

Measurements

During treatments for facial skin cancer with 3400 cGy, Petratos and colleagues measured an average scatter to the breast area of only 200 mR. The calculated breast exposure (50 mrad) for a 1000-cGy skin dose to the facial area is lower than exposures during mammography (200 mrad). Goldschmidt and colleagues[44] reviewed the potential risks of breast cancer; detailed thermoluminescent dose measurements revealed mid-breast doses of 0.1

cGy when one side of the face was exposed to 1000 cGy at a HVL of 0.75 mm Al (0.008 for soft x rays with a HVL of 0.17 mm Al).

Cancer of the Salivary Glands

A possible connection between radiotherapy for various benign disorders and salivary gland neoplasms was recently mentioned.[21] Most of the reported cases had received high doses (several hundred rad) of x rays or showed concomitant chronic radiodermatitis of the overlying skin indicative of gross overdosage.

Review of Recent Literature

Benign and malignant tumors of the salivary glands represent about 6% of all head and neck tumors. Irradiation is an infrequent etiologic factor.[45] Preston-Martin and colleagues[46] reviewed several case reports in the literature and reported responses to interviews of 408 patients with parotid tumors. Patient records were not available. In 139 patients with malignant tumors, a possible relation to prior x-ray exposure was found in 28%, attributable to a combined effect of diagnostic and therapeutic radiation; half of these could have been related to various types of therapeutic irradiation, and 19 of these patients had been irradiated for acne. Sixteen patients (4% of all interviewed patients) had received more than 10 x-ray treatments for acne. The relative risk factor (RR) was higher for patients who had received more than 15 treatments (RR8) than for patients who received only 10 to 14 treatments (RR4). No statistically significant correlation with acne therapy could be established for less frequent exposures or for 269 cases with benign tumors (RR1).

Benninger and co-workers[47] reported multiple parotid gland neoplasms following radiation therapy. Salivary gland neoplasms following atomic radiation were described by Belsky and colleagues[48]; radiation to the tonsils and nasopharynx was mentioned as a possible cause by Schneider and colleagues.[49]

Cancer of the Skeleton

Cancer of the skeleton was seen in radium dial painters and following radiotherapy of ankylosing spondylitis or tuberculosis of the bone.[42] The BEIR risk estimate is two deaths per rem per year per one million exposed persons.

Cancer of the Gastrointestinal Tract

Cancer of the gastrointestinal tract, particularly carcinoma of the stomach, occurred in atomic bomb survivors in Hiroshima and in patients who had received radiation for ankylosing spondylitis.[5] The BEIR risk estimate is one death per rem per year per one million exposed persons. There are no reports relating any of these neoplasms to dermatologic radiotherapy. Such a connection would be highly unlikely in view of the limited penetration of superficial, soft, and grenz ray qualities.

Soft Tissue Neoplasms

Isolated cases of fibrosarcomas, angiosarcomas, chondrosarcomas, mixed mesenchymal sarcomas, malignant fibrous histiocytomas, liposarcomas, and neurogenic sarcomas have been observed in heavily irradiated tissues. In some cases, the diagnoses have been disputed. Alterative diagnoses include spindle-cell epidermoid carcinoma and florid fibromatosis.[50]

Reyes[51] reviewed the literature and reported one case of a radiation-induced soft tissue osteogenic sarcoma of the scalp arising 2 years after excision and radiotherapy of a basosquamous cell carcinoma exposed to 5000 cGy. Similar sarcomatous changes were described following irradiation of breast cancer[52,53] and acne.[50] Postirradiation angiosarcomas were described 20 to 30 years following noncutaneous x-ray therapy by several authors.[54–56]

Leukemia

Leukemia is the best known of the radiation-induced malignancies. In atomic bomb survivors of Hiroshima and Nagasaki,[4,42] in persons exposed to nuclear fallout in the Marshall Islands,[4,42] and in British patients treated with intensive spinal irradiation for ankylosing spondylitis,[57] an increased incidence of all forms of leukemia (except the chronic lymphocytic type) has been observed.[58] Radiation-induced leukemias tend to occur most frequently within a few years after exposure.[59] After 25 years, the frequency tends to return to the levels expected without irradiation. The risk estimate for leukemia is one to six cases of leukemia per one million exposed persons per year per rem.

Because of their limited penetration, grenz rays, soft x rays, and superficial x rays, even in relatively high doses, are not likely to induce leukemia. Almost all radiation is absorbed in the skin and subcutaneous tissue. Dermatologic radiotherapy is not mentioned in any of the major reports dealing with radiogenic leukemia. A slight excess of leukemia in patients treated for tinea capitis was statistically not significant.[21]

Brain Tumors

Ron and co-workers[60] investigated the possible relation between radiotherapy for tinea capitis in childhood and the later development of tumors of the brain and nervous system among 10,834 patients treated in Israel between 1948 and 1960. This form of therapy is now obsolete. A comparison with groups of siblings and untreated patients revealed an increased incidence of meningiomas and gliomas in the irradiated group. The estimated skin dose ranged from 350 to 420 roentgen (R), delivered on 5 consecutive days. Nine percent of patients received more than one course of treatment; the children were not immobilized and overlap of exposure in adjoining fields could not be ruled out. The extrapolated average dose to the brain was 100 to 200 cGy. A possible association between radiation therapy and meningiomas was also reported by Burns[61] and Spallone and colleagues.[62]

Lung Cancer

Lung cancer appears to have been induced at Hiroshima[5] by doses estimated to be equivalent to 50 cGy of external gamma radiation delivered at a high dose rate. Studies of uranium (radon) miners[42] and of patients treated for ankylosing spondylitis[43] also show an excess of lung cancer. The BEIR report gives risk estimates for lung cancer of between two and 10 cases per one million exposed persons per year per rem.

We are not aware of any claimed connection between dermatologic radiotherapy and lung cancer. No significant doses reach lung tissue during dermatologic radiation.

Benign Skin Changes Following Radiation Therapy

Isolated cases of the following conditions have been reported following noncutaneous irradiation, mostly for internal neoplasms: Stevens-Johnson syndrome,[63] pemphigoid,[64] dermatophytosis,[65] eccrine poromas,[66] and keratotic miliaria.[67] Pandya and co-workers[68] reviewed the literature and described a case of erythema multiforme appearing 2 weeks after radiotherapy for lung cancer. The first three cases were reported by Arnold.[69] Del Giudice and Gerstley[70] reported a patient with a sunburn of the arms who developed a radiation-recall reaction in the radiation port area of his gluteal region, which was not exposed to ultraviolet radiation. Similar recall reactions are sometimes seen when antineoplastic antibiotics (e.g., dactinomycin) are administered after completion of radiation therapy.

Genetic Effects

In contrast to somatic effects of ionizing radiation that occur in exposed individuals themselves, genetic or inheritable effects are manifested in subsequent generations. Since relevant human data are not available, all estimates of radiation-induced genetic changes are based on results obtained with other species. At the dose range involved in medical applications of ionizing radiation, heritable effects are considered to be stochastic, and no safe threshold dose is assumed. When reproductive cells are irradiated, changes may be produced in the genes or in the chromosomes of these cells and subsequently transmitted to the descendants of the irradiated individual. These genetic changes may include: (1) gene mutations; that is, alterations in the function of individual genes, (2) gross morphologic chromosome aberrations resulting from breakage and reorganization of the chromosomes, and (3) changes in the number of chromosomes.[4,5,42] Some of these effects may result in offspring suffering abnormalities that may range from mildly detrimental to severely disabling, or they may be lethal disorders.

Gonadal Dose Measurements

Measurements of gonad doses for different types of dermatologic radiation therapy were published by several investigators (see Goldschmidt and Sherwin[8]). For most indications in dermatologic radiotherapy, genetically significant doses are well within the recommended limits of the BEIR report,

TABLE 4.1. Annual whole-body dose rates in the United States (1970).[a]

Source	mrem/year
Environmental	
Natural	102
Global fallout	4
Nuclear power	0.003
Subtotal	106
Medical	
Diagnostic	72
Radiopharmaceuticals	1
Subtotal	73
Occupational	0.8
Miscellaneous	2
Subtotal	2.8
Total	182

[a] From ref. 5.

provided that appropriate radiation protection measures are used. The measured doses are significantly lower than the maximum permissible dose to critical organs of 300 mrem per week for radiation workers. It is understood, of course, that radiotherapy should not be given for any benign condition during pregnancy. For the general population, current radiation protection guides take 5 rem as the 30-year limit, which corresponds to 170 mrem per year. These maximum doses apply to accidental or avoidable exposures without medical benefit to the exposed subject; there is currently no stated limitation on population exposure from medical practice.

Radiation Protection and Shielding

Radiation protection measures are used to reduce to a minimum avoidable hazards of radiation. For comparison, annual whole-body dose rates and recommendations on limits of exposure to ionizing radiation are listed in Tables 4.1 and 4.2.

Routine Protection Measures

Special protection of all radiosensitive organs is imperative; this applies especially to the eyes, thyroid region, and gonads. Scattered radiation can be minimized by the use of metal cones, which confine the beam to the area to be treated. It can be reduced further by lead shielding of 0.5- to 1-mm thickness on the treatment table, and by placing lead shielding over the patient's body. The shielding ability of lead rubber, lead vinyl, and other materials is expressed in terms of "lead equivalent." This term denotes the thickness of lead affording the same attenuation. A 1-mm thick lead shield will reduce dermatologic radiation qualities by 99%. For gonad protection, a lead vinyl sheet is placed over the lower half of the body from the umbilicus to the knees. The thyroid area is protected by a separate lead shield (Fig. 4.1). An alternative approach is the use of a long lead vinyl sheet extending from the neck to the knees (Fig. 4.2). Eye shields are applied whenever significant direct or indirect radiation may reach the facial area. (Lead sheets, eye shields, and gonadal shields are

TABLE 4.2. Recommendations on limits for exposure to ionizing radiation from NCRP.[a]

A. Occupational exposures (annual)		
1. Effective dose equivalent limit (stochastic effects)	50 mSv	(5 rem)
2. Dose equivalent limits for tissues and organs (nonstochastic effects)		
a. Lens of eye	150 mSv	(15 rem)
b. All others (e.g., red bone marrow, breast, lung, gonads, skin, and extremities)	500 mSv	(50 rem)
3. Guidance: cumulative exposure	10 mSv $\times$ age	(1 rem $\times$ age in years)
B. Public exposures (annual)		
1. Effective dose equivalent limit, continuous or frequent exposure	1 mSv	(0.1 rem)
2. Effective dose equivalent limit, infrequent exposure	5 mSv	(0.5 rem)
3. Remedial action recommended when:		
a. Effective dose equivalent	>5 mSv	(>0.5 rem)
b. Exposure to radon and its decay products	>0.007 Jhm^{-3}	(>2 WLM)
4. Dose equivalent limits for lens of eye, skin and extremities	50 mSv	(5 rem)
C. Negligible individual risk level (annual)		
1. Effective dose equivalent per source or practice	0.01 mSv	(0.001 rem)

[a] From ref. 71.

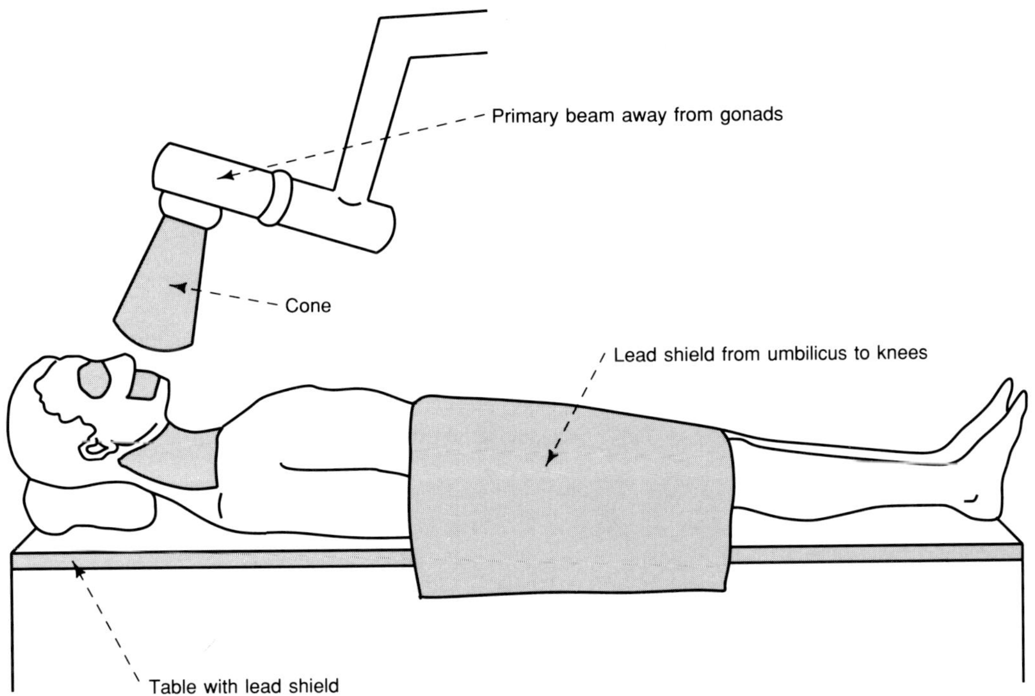

FIGURE 4.1. Radiation protection measures. Separate lead vinyl sheets in thyroid and gonad regions. (From Goldschmidt H, Sherwin WK. Reactions to ionizing radiation. *J Amer Acad Dermatol*. 1980;3:551–579.)

available form Nuclear Associates, Inc., Westbury, N.Y.). Scattered radiation to the gonadal areas can be reduced further by directing the beam away from the gonads. In order to reduce radiation exposure during treatment of facial lesions, the head is placed on a pillow and immobilized with sandbags while the patient lies supine on the treatment table. Scattered radiation can also be reduced by selecting a quality of radiation properly suited to the actual depth of the pathologic process, especially by application of the half-value depth (D½) concept. Unnecessarily penetrating radiation will increase scattered radiation.

Specific Shielding Procedures

Cones and overlay shielding are used as protection against the direct therapeutic beam of the radiation. This is especially important during radiotherapy of skin cancers, when large doses are delivered to the skin. The recent review by Gladstein[72] describes various radiation protection measures and illustrates specific shielding techniques in detailed step-by-step fashion. In general, the field

of radiation is limited by a cone and lead shields with a margin of safety of 0.5 to 1.0 cm around the visible and palpable borders of the lesions. The x-ray cones are usually tipped with lead glass to permit better visualization of the lesion. Because tumors are rarely perfectly round, cut-out lead shields are used in addition to the available cylindrical lead glass cones. The diameter of the cone should always exceed the largest diameter of the cut-out area in the shield. A lead cutout should be applied even if a cone with the exact size of the desired field is available. The added lead shield will prevent irradiation of normal tissue in case the patient moves during treatment. Most dermatologists use overlay shielding with lead sheeting of 0.9-mm thickness, which absorbs 99% of a radiation with an HVL of 0.9 mm Al. This material can easily be cut to the desired size and contour with scissors, and molded to fit the surfaces of unusual lesions. Thinner 0.5-mm lead foil will absorb more than 95% of the radiation and is frequently used for lesions with irregular contours. Specific shielding techniques for skin cancer in various anatomic locations are described in Chapter 7.

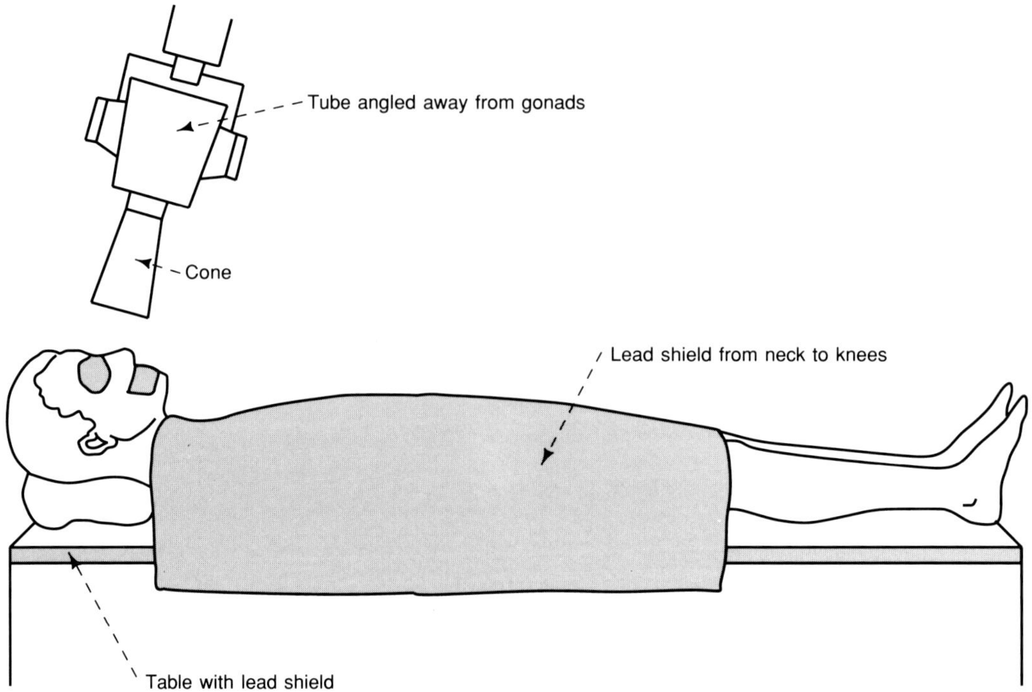

FIGURE 4.2. Radiation protection measures. Lead vinyl sheet from neck to knee. (From Gladstein,[72] by permission.)

Other Safety Measures

Radiation safety also includes the necessity for frequent calibrations of the x-ray machine. This is best carried out by a radiophysicist.

The current attitude of United States government agencies concerning the use of ionizing radiation for benign diseases in all medical specialties is reflected in the recommendations of a committee of the National Research Council—National Academy of Sciences (NRC-NAS) that were endorsed by the Food and Drug Administration in 1980 (Table 10.1, p. 140).[73]

Many of the commonly used therapeutic modalities in dermatology are associated with degrees of risk, especially when used without discrimination. For more than three decades, most dermatologists using ionizing radiation therapy have followed guidelines similar to the recommendations proposed in the NAS report. The foregoing detailed discussion of the methodology, and results of various scientific studies on low-dose radiation effects, confirm again that injudicious use of ionizing radiation can be associated with serious hazards. It also indicates that the inherent risks of properly applied dermatologic radiation therapy are small when appropriate radiation protection measures are used.[74]

References

1. Upton AC, Albert RE, Burns FJ, et al. *Radiation Carcinogenesis.* New York, NY: Elsevier; 1986.
2. Merriam GR Jr., Focht EF. Radiation dose to the lens in treatment of tumors of the eye and adjacent structures. *Am J Roentgenol.* 1958;71:357–360.
3. Kopf AW, Grisewood EN, Bart RS, Petratos M, Wingate C. X irradiation of ocular tissues measured by thermoluminescence dosimetry. *J Invest Dermatol.* 1967;49:512–516.
4. UNSCEAR (1977), United Nations Scientific Committee on the Effects of Atomic Radiation. *1977 Report to the General Assembly, Sources and Effects of Ionizing Radiation, UN E77.IX.1.* United Nations, New York, 1972.
5. National Academy of Sciences-National Research Council. The effects on populations of exposure to low levels of ionizing radiation. *Report of the Advisory Committee on the Biological Effects of Ionizing Radiation (BEIR).* Washington, DC: US Government Printing Office, 1972.
6. Low-level radiation risk climbs in new estimates. *Med World News.* Jan 22, 1990; 31:24–25.

7. Furst CJ, Lundell M, Holm LE, et al. Cancer incidence after radiotherapy for skin hemangioma: a retrospective cohort study in Sweden. *J Natl Cancer Inst.* 1988;80:1387–1392.

8. Goldschmidt H, Sherwin WK. Reactions to ionizing radiation. *J Am Acad Dermatol.* 1980;3:551–579.

9. NCRP (1985). National Council on Radiation Protection and Measurements: *Induction of thyroid cancer by ionizing radiation.* NCRP Report No. 80, Bethesda, MD; 1985.

10. Schottenfeld D, Gershman ST. Epidemiology of thyroid cancer. *CA.* 1978;28:66–86.

11. Mortensen JD, Bennett WA, Woolner LB. Incidence of carcinoma in thyroid glands removed at 1000 consecutive routine necropsies. *Surg Forum.* 1954;5:659–663.

12. Sampson RJ, Woolner LB, Bahn RC, et al. Occult thyroid carcinoma in Olmsted County, Minnesota: prevalence at autopsy compared with that in Hiroshima and Nagasaki, Japan. *Cancer* 1974;34:2072–2076.

13. Crile G Jr, Hazard JB. Relationship of the age of the patient to the natural history and prognosis of carcinoma of the thyroid. *Ann Surg.* 1953;138:33–38.

14. Crile G Jr. Changing end results in patients with papillary carcinoma of the thyroid. *Surg Gynecol Obstet.* 1971;132:460–468.

15. Pochin EE. Why be quantitative about radiation risk estimates? NCRP Lecture 2, Washington, DC; 1978.

16. Hempelmann LH, Pifer JW, Burke GJ, Terry R, Ames WR. Neoplasms in persons treated with x-rays in infancy for thymic enlargement. A report on the third follow-up survey. *J Natl Cancer Inst.* 1967;38:317–341.

17. Hempelmann LH. Risk of thyroid neoplasms after irradiation in children. *Science* 1968;160:159–163.

18. Jablon S, Belsky JL, Tachikawa K, et al. Cancer in Japanese exposed as children to atomic bombs. *Lancet.* 1971;1:927–932.

19. Conard RA, Dobyns BM, Sutow WW. Thyroid neoplasia as a late effect of exposure to radioactive iodine in fallout. *JAMA.* 1970;214:316–324.

20. Crile G, Esselstyn LB, Hawk WA. Needle biopsy in the diagnosis of thyroid nodules appearing after radiation. *N Engl J Med.* 1979;301:997–999. Editorial.

21. Modan B, Baidatz D, Mart H, Steinitz R, Levin SG. Radiation induced head and neck tumours. *Lancet.* 1974;1:277–281.

22. Albert R, Omran A, Brauer E, et al. Follow-up study of patients treated by x-ray epilation for tinea capitis. Part II. *Arch Environ Health.* 1968;17:919–934.

23. Albert RE, Omran AR. Follow-up study of patients treated by x-ray epilation for tinea capitis. *Arch Environ Health.* 1968;17:899–918.

24. Shore RE, Albert RE, Pasternack BS. Follow-up study of patients treated by x-ray epilation for tinea capitis. Resurvey of posttreatment illness and mortality experience. *Arch Environ Health.* 1976;31:17–24.

25. NCRP (1980). National Council on Radiation Protection and Measurement: *Influence of dose and its distribution in time on dose-reponse relationships for low-LET radiations.* NCRP Report No. 64, Washington, DC; 1980.

26. Silverman C, Hoffman DA. Thyroid tumor risk from radiation during childhood. *Prev Med.* 1975;4:100–105.

27. Petratos MA, Grisewood EN, Wingate C. Measurement of scattered radiation to body areas during radiotherapy of basal cell epitheliomas. *Derm Int.* 1969;8:10–13.

28. Goldschmidt H, Lassen M, Gorson RO. Dermatologic radiotherapy and thyroid cancer. Dose measurements and risk quantification. *Arch Dermatol.* 1983;119:383–390.

29. Idsoe O, Guthe T, Willcox RP, DeWeck AL. Nature and extent of penicillin side-reactions, with particular reference to fatalities from anaphylactic shock. *Bull WHO.* 1968;38:159–188.

30. Wilson R. Analyzing the daily risks of life. *Technol Rev.* February, 1979;33:41–46.

31. Pochin EE. The acceptance of risk. *Br Med Bull.* 1975;31:184–189.

32. Pochin EE: Estimates of industrial and other risks. *J R Coll Phys Lond.* 1978;12:210–218.

33. Wanebo CK, Johnson KG, Sato K, et al. Breast cancer after exposure to the atomic bombings of Hiroshima and Nagasaki. *N Engl J Med.* 1968;279:667–671.

34. Maeeler FA Jr, Hempelmann LH, Dutton AM. Breast neoplasms in women treated with x-rays for acute postpartum mastitis. A pilot study. *J Natl Cancer Inst.* 1969;43:803–811.

35. Myrden JA, Hiltz JE. Breast cancer following multiple fluoroscopies during artificial pneumothorax treatment of pulmonary tuberculosis. *Can Med Assoc J.* 1969;100:1032–1034.

36. Mackenzie I. Breast cancer following multiple fluoroscopies. *Br J Cancer.* 1965;19:1–8.

37. Cook DC, Dent D, Hewitt D. Breast cancer following multiple chest fluoroscopy: the Ontario experience. *Can Med Assoc J.* 1974;111:406–409, 412.

38. Delarue NC, Gale G, Ronald A. Multiple fluoroscopy of the chest. Carcinogenicity for the female breast and implications for breast cancer screening programs. *Can Med Assoc J.* 1975;112:1405–1413.

39. Boice JD, Monson RR. X-ray exposure and breast cancer. *Am J Epidemiol.* 1976;104:349–350.

40. Wolfe JN. Mammography: a radiologist's view. *JAMA.* 1977;237:2223–2224.

41. Simon N. Breast cancer induced by radiation. *JAMA.* 1977;237:789–790.

42. ICRP (1977). International Commission on Radiological Protection. *Recommendations of the International Commission on radiological protection*. ICRP publication 26. Oxford: Pergamon Press Ltd; 1977.

43. Schwartz RA, Burgess GH, Milgrom H. Breast carcinoma and basal cell epithelioma after x-ray therapy for hirsutism. *Cancer.* 1979;44:5–9.

44. Goldschmidt H, Gorson RO, Lassen M. Dermatologic radiotherapy and breast cancer. *Arch Dermatol Res.* 1982;272:293–300.

45. McKenna RJ. Tumors of the major and minor salivary glands. *CA* 1984;34:27–39.

46. Preston-Martin S, Thomas DC, White SC, et al. Prior exposure to medical and dental x rays related to tumors of the parotid gland. *J Natl Cancer Inst.* 1988;80:943–949.

47. Benninger MS, Lavertu P, Linden MD, Sebek B. Multiple parotid gland primary neoplasms after radiation therapy. *Otolaryngol Head Neck Surg* 1988;98(3):250–253.

48. Belsky JL, Takeichi N, Yamamoto T, et al. Salivary gland neoplasms following atomic radiation. *Cancer.* 1975;35:555–559.

49. Schneider AB, Favus MJ, Stachura ME, et al. Salivary gland neoplasms as a late consequence of head and neck irradiation. *Ann Intern Med.* 1977; 87:160–164.

50. Seo IS, Warner TFS, Warren JS, et al. Cutaneous postirradiation sarcoma. *Cancer.* 1985;56:761–767.

51. Reyes CV. Radiation-induced soft tissue osteogenic sarcoma of the scalp. *Int J. Dermatol.* 1989;28:38–39.

52. Hatlinghus S, Rode L, Christensen I, Vaage S. Sarcoma following irradiation for breast cancer. Report of three unusual cases including one malignant mesenchymoma of bone. *Acta Radiol (Oncol).* 1986;25 (4–6):239–242.

53. Goette DK, Deffer TA. Postirradiation malignant fibrous histiocytoma. *Arch Dermatol.* 1985;121(4): 535–538.

54. Handfield-Jones SE, Kennedy CT, Bradfield JB. Angiosarcoma arising in an angiomatous naevus following irradiation in childhood. *Br J Dermatol.* 1988;118(1):109–112.

55. Sironi M, Marchini R, Taccagni GL, Cantaboni A. Juvenile cutaneous angiosarcoma following radiotherapy of a haemangioma. *Pathologica.* 1988;80 (1066):235–241.

56. Goette DK, Detlefs RL. Postirradiation angiosarcoma. *J Am Acad Dermatol.* 1985;12(5, Pt 2): 922–926.

57. Court Brown WM, Doll R. Mortality from cancer and other causes after radiotherapy for ankylosing spondylitis. *Br Med J.* 1965;5474:1327–1332.

58. Bross IDJ, Natarajan N. Leukemia from low-level radiation; identification of susceptible children. *N Engl J Med.* 1972;287:107–110.

59. Gibson R, Graham S, Lilienfield A, Schuman L, Dowd JE, Levin ML: Irradiation in the epidemiology of leukemia among adults. *J Natl Cancer Inst.* 1972;48:301–311.

60. Ron E, Modan B, Boice JD, et al. Tumors of the brain and nervous system after radiotherapy in childhood. *N Engl J Med.* 1988;319:1033–1039.

61. Burns FJ. Cancer risk associated with therapeutic irradiation of the skin. *Arch Dermatol.* 1989;125: 979–981.

62. Spallone A, Gagliardi FM, Vagnozzi R. Intracranial meningiomas related to external cranial irradiation. *Surg Neurol.* 1979;12(2):153–159.

63. Maiche A, Teerenhovi L. Stevens-Johnson syndrome in patients receiving radiation therapy. *Lancet.* 1985;2(8445):45.

64. Ernst TM, Marsch WC. Induktion eines lokalisierten Pemphigoids durch energiereiche Strahlen. *Dermatologica* 1982;164:73–81.

65. Maor MH. Dermatophytosis confined to irradiated skin. A case report. *Int J Radiat Oncol Biol Phys.* 1988;14(4):825–826.

66. Ullah K, Pichler E, Fritsch P. Multiple eccrine poromas arising in chronic radiation dermatitis. *Acta Dermatol Venereol (Stockh).* 1989;69(1):70–73.

67. Kossard S, Commens CA. Keratotic miliaria precipitated by radiotherapy. *Arch Dermatol.* 1988; 124(6):855–856.

68. Pandya AG, Kettler AH, Bruce S. Radiation-induced erythema multiforme. *Int J Dermatol.* 1989;28: 600–602.

69. Arnold H. Erythema multiforme following high voltage roentgen therapy. *Arch Dermatol Syphilol.* 1949; 60:143–149.

70. Del Giudice SM, Gerstley JK. Sunlight-induced radiation recall. *Int J Dermatol.* 1988;27:415–416.

71. NCRP (1987). National Council on Radiation Protection and Measurements: *Recommendations on limits for exposure to ionizing radiation.* NCRP Report No. 91, Bethesda, MD; 1987.

72. Gladstein AH. Radiation protection. In: Goldschmidt H, ed. *Physical Modalities in Dermatologic Therapy.* New York, NY: Springer Verlag; 1978:39–49.

73. Goldschmidt H: FDA recommendations on radiation of benign diseases. *Arch Dermatol.* 1978;114:1149.

74. Goldschmidt H. Dermatologic radiotherapy. The risk-benefit ratio. *Arch Dermatol.* 1986;122:1385–1388.

5

Treatment Planning: Selection of Physical Factors and Radiation Techniques

Herbert Goldschmidt

In radiotherapy, treatment planning refers to the process of selecting the tumor dose prescription, daily dose, fractionation schedule, and arrangement of the radiation beam to achieve the desired radiation dose distribution in a target volume. The radiation beam selected depends on the location and shape, in all three dimensions, of the target volume.

A review of older publications in the field of dermatologic radiotherapy shows a bewildering array of recommendations concerning the proper selection of physical factors. Recent advances in the technology of dermatologic radiotherapy units have made it possible to define more precisely which factors are most suitable for specific therapeutic purposes, resulting not only in greater therapeutic efficacy but also in a reduction of necessary variations. This simplification of modern therapeutic techniques has been a major factor in the elimination of potential technical or human errors, the main causes of unnecessary radiation sequelae. Standardization of therapeutic factors and the introduction of advanced x-ray units with sophisticated safety devices have largely eliminated these risks.

Since we recognize that there still is a great deal of individuality in the techniques of irradiation, we have attempted to include descriptions of various technical approaches, leaving to the individual reader the critical task of selecting the most appropriate method for the patient under consideration.

Basic physical considerations have been discussed in Chapter 1. Essential points will be repeated here briefly; special emphasis will be given to practical aspects of dermatologic radiotherapy and to specific recommendations concerning technical details. Some of these definitions have been discussed elsewhere in greater detail.[1-4]

Physical Factors

Milliamperage

The milliamperage of an x-ray machine determines its output. However, the quantity of radiation per unit time (dose rate) depends both on milliamperage (mA) and kilovoltage (kV). The penetrating power (quality) of an x-ray beam is not changed by altering the milliamperage alone if the kilovoltage remains constant. As the milliamperage of an x-ray tube is increased, the intensity of the x-ray beam changes almost in direct proportion. The increased milliamperage means that more electrons strike the target per minute, producing more x-ray photons per minute and therefore increasing the quantity of radiation per minute (i.e., its intensity). In modern dermatology, the amperage of an x-ray unit is usually not changed; most modern dermatologic units are calibrated at one standard amperage only (e.g., 5 mA or 25 mA). Older glass-windowed units often required two settings (e.g., 5 mA and 10 mA) to increase the relatively low output of these machines, thus adding another potential source of error.

Target-Skin Distance

Target-skin distance (TSD), depending on the source of ionizing radiation, also known as focus-skin distance (FSD) or source-skin distance (SSD), indicates the distance between the target of the x-ray tube or the radiation source and the treated skin area. For hard x rays, the intensity or dose rate of radiation at a given point is inversely proportional to its distance squared, as measured from the focal spot. In dermatology, the inverse square law applies only in principle. It cannot be used instead of actual measurements because soft x rays and grenz rays are partially absorbed in air. Theoretically, all x-ray machines (except grenz-ray units) could be used at any distance, limited only by low dose rates at long TSDs. Under practical conditions, however, the choice is usually reduced to only two distances. Modern rules of radiation protection require the use of cones in most circumstances and most manufacturers supply cones in sets of only two lengths. These metal cones confine the beam to the field to be treated and minimize direct and indirect exposure of other areas. Their sizes usually correspond to TSDs of 15 and 30 cm (or 20 and 40 cm). Consequently, calibration is necessary only for these two TSDs.

The selection of the TSD depends on the type of radiation used and the size of the field selected. To achieve homogeneous radiation over the entire area to be treated, it is important to select a TSD that is at least twice as large as the diameter of the field. When this is done, the difference in radiation intensity between the central beam and the periphery of the treated area is relatively small (e.g., the periphery receives 90% of the central dose). The peripheral dose could be only 50% when the TSD equals the field size; in this case, recurrences in the periphery of the portal may be expected. On the other hand, the periphery receives 95% of the central dose if the TSD corresponds to 3 times the diameter of the field[1]; this relation is preferred by many authors.[2,5] Because of the increased homogeneity of the x-ray beam, longer TSDs are also advantageous for carcinomas in curved or uneven anatomical regions (e.g., in the nasolabial fold). The larger TSD is always preferable unless the increased field size is associated with a marked reduction in dose rate (as in grenz-ray units or superficial x-ray machines with Pyrex windows). Because of their high dose rate per minute, this is not a major factor for machines with beryllium windows, and a TSD of 30 cm can be used in the treatment of all cutaneous cancers. This limitation to only one TSD also eliminates errors in the selection of calibration data because only one set of measurements is required and available.

Size of Field

Determination of the proper field size of the radiation beam is of critical importance in the treatment of cutaneous cancers. Ordinarily this presents no difficulty because most basal cell carcinomas have fairly well-demarcated clinical margins. If the lesion is poorly defined, the physician may either estimate its extent or, preferably, do multiple biopsies to determine its dimensions. Since many basal cell carcinomas extend laterally beyond what can be readily seen or felt, a margin of at least 5 mm of normal-appearing skin is always included in the area treated. Thus, if the maximum diameter of a well-defined lesion is 20 mm, the minimum diameter of the port used should be 30 mm. If the borders are indistinct (e.g., in morpheaform basal cell carcinomas),[6] a wider margin of up to 10 mm is used. An adequate margin of normal-appearing tissue is essential; nothing will be regretted more than the selection of a field size that is too small. When the chosen field size is too small it may cause a "geographical miss," the most common type of recurrence. In large clinical investigations[7] the percentage of marginal recurrences (indicative of inadequate field size) was much higher than the percentage of central recurrences (indicative of inadequate radiation penetration). It is much better to add an additional margin of 0.5 cm to the treated field; the additional cosmetic side effects will be minimal compared to the increased cure rate. The direction of the central beam depends on the treatment area and is usually perpendicular to the treated site.

As mentioned earlier, large field sizes are associated with increased backscatter, especially when more penetrating x rays are used. For identical exposures the intensity of radiation-induced skin reactions varies considerably with the field size (e.g., a field of 2 cm² can be exposed to a maximum fractionated dose of 15,000 cGy without serious sequelae, whereas an area of 4 cm² may tolerate a maximum of only 8000 cGy).[1]

Radiation Techniques

Tables 5.1 and 5.2 present a summary of x-ray therapy methods and x-ray generators that are currently used in dermatology and radiation oncology. A systematic classification is difficult because different physical and technical aspects were emphasized when new radiation methods were developed. Consequently, these modalities can be arranged according to depth of penetration (i.e.,

TABLE 5.1. Terminology of ionizing radiation.

Energy	Classification	Commonly used voltages	Type of generator
100 MeV			
	Megavoltage		
		20 MeV	Betatron
10 MeV	or	10 MeV	
			Linear accelerators
		4 MeV	
	Supervoltage		Isotope teletherapy machines (^{60}Co)
		2 Mev	
1 MeV		1 MeV	(γ rays)
(1000 kV)	Orthovoltage		
	or	250–600 kV	
	Deep x rays		
	Half-deep x rays	150–250 kV	
100 kV	Superficial x rays	50–100 kV	X-ray machines
	Soft x rays	20–50 kV	
10 kV	Grenz rays	10–20 kV	

deep x-ray therapy, intermediate x-ray therapy, and superficial x-ray therapy), or according to the type of x-ray generator used. In dermatology, the type of window is particularly important and x-ray units have been classified accordingly as glass-windowed (Pyrex) machines (high-voltage or low-voltage units), beryllium-window machines (soft x-ray units and modern grenz-ray machines), or Lindemann-window machines (older grenz-ray machines). Most x-ray machines function at TSDs varying from 15 to 40 cm. The major exception is the contact x-ray technique, which is also known as ultra-short-distance therapy (Chaoul and Philips units). In radiation oncology, modern therapy units have been subdivided into high-energy x-ray units, where x rays are produced with particle accelerators (e.g., Van de Graaff accelerator, linear accelerator, betatron), and teleisotope machines (telecurie therapy machines), where x rays are produced by isotopes (e.g., radium teletherapy, cesium 137, cobalt 60).

Tables 5.2 and 5.3 also emphasize the differences between radiotherapeutic and dermatologic concepts

TABLE 5.2. Radiation methods.

Type	Sources and synonyms	kV	TSD (cm)	Wavelength ($\overset{\circ}{A}$) (average)	HVL	D½ (mm tissue)
Megavoltage therapy	Betatron, particle accelerators	>1000	80	0.001	>10 mm Pb	200
Supervoltage therapy	γ ray Telecurie sources	400–800	50–80	0.03	5–10 mm Pb	80–110
Orthovoltage therapy	Deep x-ray therapy Conventional x-ray therapy	200–400	50–80	0.14	2–4 mm Cu	50–80
Intermediate x-ray therapy	Half-deep therapy	110–130	30	0.1	4 mm Al	30
Contact therapy	Ultrashort distance (Chaoul)	50–60	1.5–3.0	0.8	2–4 mm Al	4–30
Superficial x-ray therapy	Low voltage, standard x-ray therapy Pyrex window	60–100	15–30	0.5	0.7–2.0 mm Al	7–20
Soft x-ray therapy	Beryllium window	20–100	10–30	0.15	0.1–2.0 mm Al	1–20
Grenz-ray therapy	Ultrasoft therapy Supersoft therapy	5–20	10–15	2	0.03 mm Al	0.2–0.8

TABLE 5.3. Percentage depth doses for various radiation sources used in radiation oncology.[a]

Source	D90% (mm tissue)	D50% (mm tissue)	D10% (mm tissue)
Surface applicators (^{90}Sr)	0–3	1	2.5
Radium mold 10 cm²			
0.5 cm		10	40
1.0 cm		20	70
Electron beam 10 cm²			
5 MeV	14.5	21	25
10 MeV	28	42	51
20 MeV	61	83	100
X rays 10 cm²			
100 kV	2	9	40
125 kV	10	40	150
250 kV	25	70	180

[a] Adapted from Brady et al.[30]

TABLE 5.4. Different types of radiation used in dermatology offices in 1974.[a]

Type of equipment	No. of replies	Offices with x-ray equipment (%)[b]
Grenz-ray units (5–20 kV)	1361	604 (44.4)
Beryllium-window units (soft x-ray machines; 10–50–100 kV)	1095	141 (12.8)
Superficial low-voltage machines (Pyrex window; 60–120 kV)	1589	984 (61.9)
Contact therapy units	1025	14 (1.4)
Other x-ray machines	1008	71 (7.0)
Radium	1063	102 (9.6)
Other radionuclides	933	12 (1.3)

[a] From Goldschmidt,[11] with permission. © 1975, American Medical Association.

[b] The percentages add up to more than 100% because some offices are equipped with more than one type of x-ray machine.

and objectives. A chief aim of newer techniques in radiation oncology has been the development of generators that produce more penetrating ionizing radiation in order to treat tumors at greater depth. At the same time, efforts have been made to reduce cutaneous side effects that often prevented the delivery of therapeutically effective doses to deeper tissues. Major achievements in this area are exemplified by new megavoltage treatment units that combine great penetration with a "skin-sparing" effect, thereby reducing both the acute and chronic radiation reactions that had been a serious problem in the treatment of internal carcinomas with previous techniques. It is obvious that the great penetration of modern x-ray generators used by radiation oncologists makes them less suitable for most dermatologic purposes. In contrast, dermatologists have been instrumental in developing x-ray units with less penetrating qualities, particularly when it became clear that only absorbed doses have any therapeutic effect and after it had been established that softer x rays have the same therapeutic effects as harder x rays. Limited penetration was considered essential to achieve absorption in the skin itself instead of in deeper tissues. The first improvement in dermatologic x-ray therapy was the introduction of so-called superficial (low voltage) x-ray machines with Pyrex (glass) windows. These machines are still in use and are suitable for most dermatologic purposes. The designation "low voltage superficial x-ray units" derives from the fact that their effect on the skin was more superficial and that they employ a lower voltage than did previously used deep (orthovoltage) x-ray generators. Very low voltages with even more superficial radiation could be used when grenz-ray machines became available.

The construction of an x-ray tube with a window of lithium borate glass by Lindemann permitted the therapeutic use of very long wavelengths. The advantages of grenz-ray machines in dermatologic therapy were described by Bucky and other authors,[8,9] starting in 1925. The grenz-ray technique was revived when beryllium windows became available; all modern grenz-ray machines are now supplied with beryllium windows.

If one uses the half-value depth as a criterion for the selection of x-ray machines for dermatologic purposes, a glance at Table 5.2 shows that there was still a large difference between the tissue depths that could be treated properly with superficial x rays or with grenz rays (i.e., between 1 and 7 mm, where most skin diseases are located). An attempt to bridge this gap was the introduction of the contact x-ray technique by Chaoul and Wachsmann[10] who used extremely short TSDs to simulate the fall-off ratio of radium corpuscular radiation. Its main limitation was the limited field size. The technologic gap between superficial x-ray units and older grenz-ray machines was finally closed with the introduction of modern beryllium-window tubes (10–100 kV), which made it possible for the first time to build x-ray machines for the intermediate range of penetration, which are suitable for all dermatologic purposes.

TABLE 5.5. Dermatologic x-ray machines: advantages and disadvantages.

X-ray machine	Advantages	Disadvantages
Grenz-ray units (ultrasoft)	Relative safety	Useful only for very superficial dermatoses
Soft x-ray units (beryllium window)	Useful for all dermatologic purposes	May need shielded treatment room
Superficial (conventional) x-ray units	Useful for most dermatologic purposes	Often too penetrating; shielded treatment room may be required
Contact therapy units	Useful in cancer therapy	Field size very limited due to short TSD

X-Ray Machines and Radiation Sources

Good therapeutic results can be achieved with various types of radiotherapy units. Table 5.4 lists x-ray equipment used by dermatologists. The statistical data were derived from a 1974 nationwide survey that was answered by 2000 dermatologists.[11] No new data have been published since 1974; it is clear, however, that the current numbers and percentages are much lower. Table 5.5 summarizes advantages and disadvantages of various dermatologic x-ray machines. Figures 5.1 to 5.4 illustrate some commercially available x-ray machines (Table 5.6).

Superficial X-Ray Units

In the United States and Canada, the most commonly used x ray machine is the superficial x ray unit with a Pyrex window. Unfiltered, low-voltage x-ray therapy is eminently useful in the treatment of moderately deep cancers.[12] The half-value depth ($D\frac{1}{2}$) starts at 6 to 7 mm and the lowest half-value layer (HVL) is 0.6 mm Aluminum (Al). Filtered, superficial x-ray therapy (with 1–2 mm added Al filter) yields radiation that is often too penetrating for cutaneous cancers (HVL 2–3 mm Al; $D\frac{1}{2}$ 12–20 mm).

Soft X-Ray Units

Modern beryllium-windowed soft x-ray machines are most suitable for dermatologic therapy because

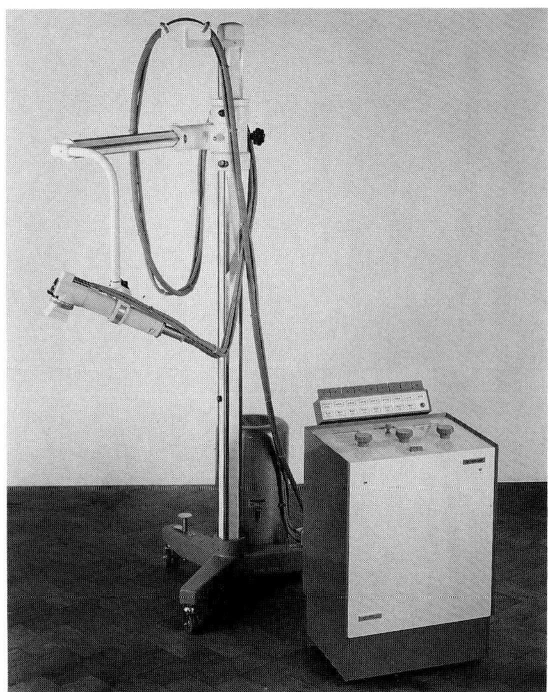

FIGURE 5.1. Philips RT 100 soft x-ray unit. Courtesy of Philips Medical Systems, Shelton, CT.

their softer radiation qualities allow an even greater adaptation of the penetration of x rays to the depth of the treated tissue. In recent years, this technique has played an increasingly important role in dermatoradiotherapy.[13–15] Table 5.7 shows calibration data of a 50-kV beryllium-windowed x-ray unit, arranged by increasing depth of penetration.

Grenz-Ray Machines

Ultrasoft x rays (grenz rays) are used widely for benign dermatoses but are less useful for cancer of the skin; they can be used only for the treatment of epidermal lesions extending no more than 1 to 2 mm in depth because the intensity of x rays produced at low voltage (10–20 kV) decreases rapidly within the tissue.[16] Multiple superficial basal cell epitheliomas are often suitable for grenz-ray therapy. The proper dosage should be selected with great care (see Chapter 12). Very large, single doses (>1500 R) and excessive total doses may result in superficial atrophy even when grenz rays are used.

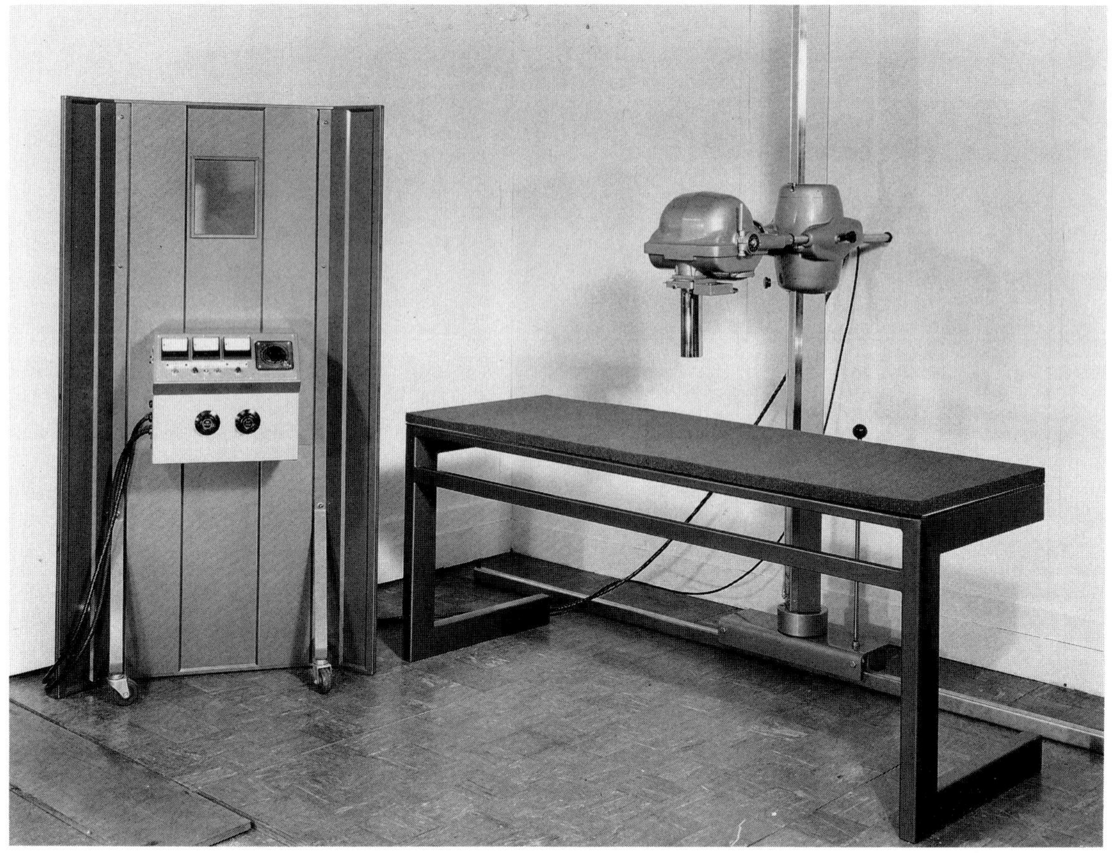

FIGURE 5.2. Bucky dermatologic combination therapy unit. Courtesy of Bucky X-ray International Ltd., New York, NY.

Contact X-Ray Machines (Chaoul)

Contact x-ray machines used to offer distinct advantages in the treatment of smaller cancers of the eyelids and other areas.[17] Because of the short TSD (2–4 cm), the size of the field was often too small for larger tumors. In these cases, overlapping grid techniques were recommended. Contact x-ray machines have now been superseded by modern soft x-ray units with beryllium windows, which offer the same therapeutic advantages, even for large field sizes, and offer greater safety to the patient and operator.

Orthovoltage (Deep Therapy) Units

Orthovoltage x-ray machines operate at potentials of 150 to 500 kV, usually in the range of 200 to 300 kV with a tube current of 10 or 20 mA. With the use of added filters, such as the Thoraeus filter (a combination filter consisting of thin sheets of tin, copper, and aluminum), deep x-ray units yield a HVL of 1 to 4 mm Cu at a TSD of 50 cm. Because of their deep penetration ($D_{\frac{1}{2}}$ 50–70 mm), they are rarely needed in dermatologic therapy but they are valuable in the treatment of rare cancers involving bones or lymph nodes or for cancer with unusual complications.[18–21]

Radium and Other Radionuclides

The application of radioactive sources to the surface of the skin (or of sources used at a short distance from the body area to be treated) is now called brachytherapy (Gr. brachys = short); this

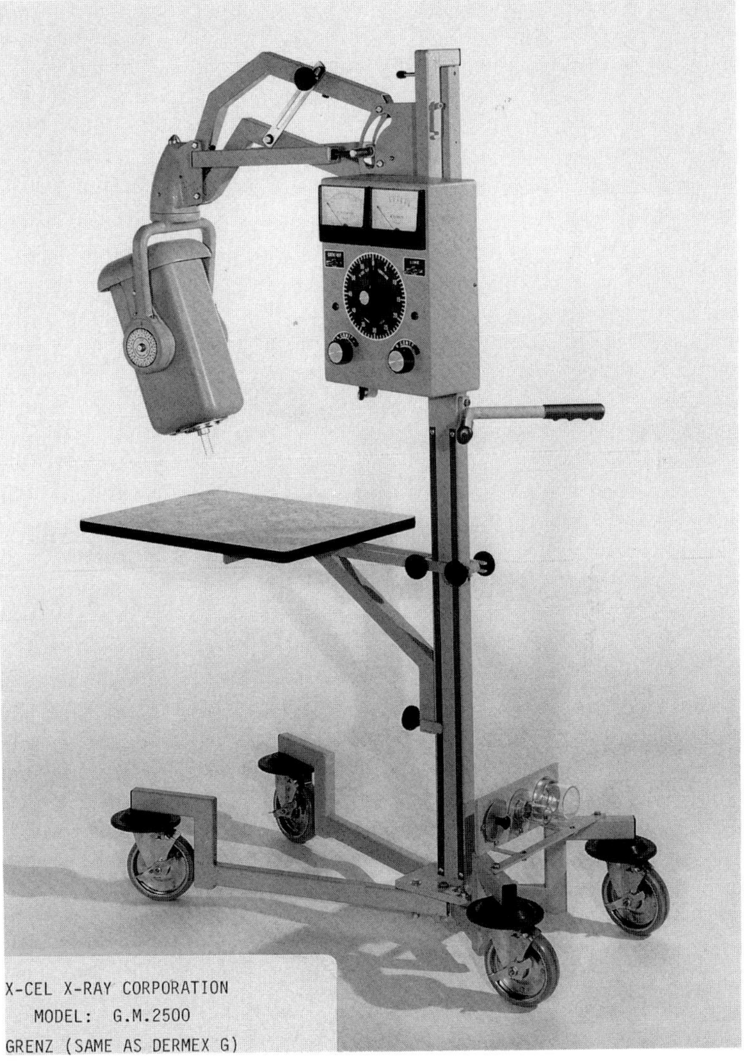

FIGURE 5.3. X-Cel GM 2500 grenz-ray unit.

contrasts with teletherapy techniques where the source is at a greater distance from the object of irradiation. In the past, excellent results have been achieved in the treatment of cutaneous malignancies with various forms of radium 226 and with other radionuclides used in interstitial radiation methods.[12,22] Temporary (removable) implants with radium or cobalt 60 needles, iridium 192 ribbons, and permanent implants with gold 198 or radon seeds are now used only rarely for uncomplicated skin cancers because of the hazards of exposure to medical personnel, operative trauma, expense to the patient, and uncertainty of geometric uniformity of dosage.[23]

Moss and colleagues[21] compared the effectiveness of roentgen therapy with both radium and radon used as molds or interstitially. They concluded that roentgen therapy provides the greatest flexibility in adjusting quality, size of field, and fractionation. They also stressed that roentgen therapy is the most convenient mode for most radiation oncologists and that it entails considerably fewer radiation hazards to the patient and operator.

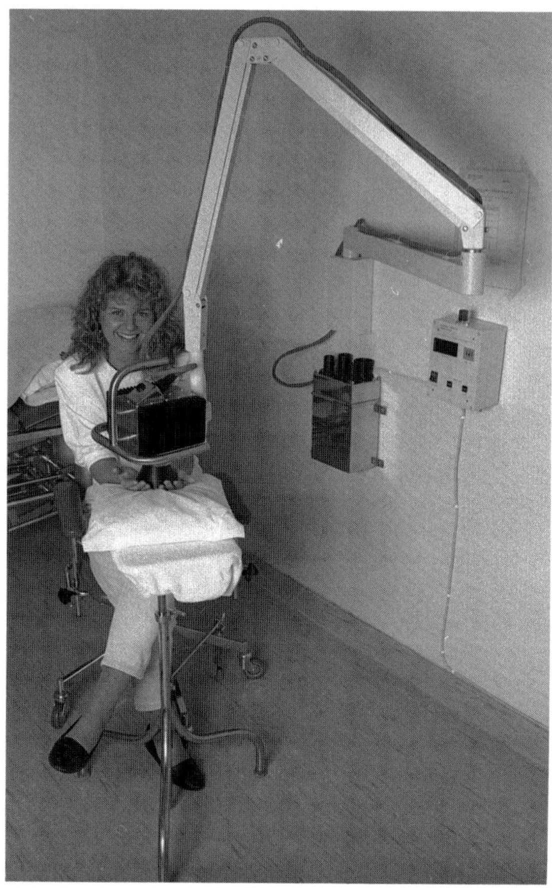

FIGURE 5.4. Progressus Medica grenz-ray unit. Courtesy of Progressus Medica.

Supervoltage Units

The development of supervoltage and isotope therapy units has drastically altered hospital radiation therapy. However, their main advantage, deep penetration (cobalt 60 has a D½ of 100 mm and caesium 137 has a D½ of 70 mm of tissue), makes these machines unsuitable for most dermatologic purposes.

Linear Accelerators (Megavoltage Units)

Since its first introduction in 1953, the design of high-energy medical linear accelerators has been improved so much that they are now the dominant radiation therapy units in the world; in 1987 more than 50% of all operational megavoltage treatment units were linear accelerators.[24] In the x-ray mode, accelerated electrons strike a target, producing bremsstrahlung of x rays with a tissue D½ of 150 to 200 mm. Obviously, these x rays are rarely indicated in dermatology. In contrast, electrons produced by linear accelerators in the electron beam mode are theoretically ideal for the treatment of skin disorders. Because of their sharp dose falloff, the penetration of electrons can be limited to pathologic tissue much more accurately than even soft x rays. Treatment of cancers of the skin with low-energy electron beams is therefore a rational form of treatment. However, since there is a significant skin-sparing effect at energies below 18 MeV, bolus (usually 1 cm thick) has to be added to

TABLE 5.6. Beryllium-windowed x-ray units.

Manufacturer	Model	mA	kV	HVL (mm Al)	D½ (mm tissue)
Philips Medical Systems 710 Bridgeport Avenue P.O. Box 484 Shelton, Conn 06484	RT 100	8–10	10–100	0.025–2.5	0.2–20
Bucky X-ray International 30 East 81st Street New York, NY 10028	Dermatologic combination therapy machine	5–10	5–100	0.02–3.0	0.2–35
X-Cel X-Ray Corporation 4220 Waller Drive Crystal Lake, IL 60012	GM2500 Grenz-ray unit	5–10	12–15	0.02–0.04	0.2–0.5
Progressus Medica AB Fornuddsvagen 109 135 52 Tyreso Sweden	Grenz-ray unit	10	10	0.02	0.2

TABLE 5.7. Calibration data of a 50-kV beryllium-window unit.

$D\frac{1}{2}$ (mm tissue)	HVL (mm Al)	kV	Filter (mm Al)	mA	TSD (cm)	Dose rate (R/min)
0.2	0.02	10	–	25	30	100
3.0	0.15	29	0.3	25	30	100
7.5	0.40	43	0.6	25	30	100
13.0	0.75	50	1.0	25	30	100
18.0	1.40	50	2.0	25	30	45

increase the skin dose.[24] Although local electron beam therapy has many theoretical advantages, it is not used widely because it is more expensive, complex, and difficult to apply than x rays.[25] Electron-beam therapy is commonly used for certain large cutaneous cancers that cannot be treated surgically without great difficulty, especially for large carcinomas of the scalp where routine megavoltage therapy may cause side effects on the brain, for cancers of the lip, chest wall, neck, breast, and lymph nodes.

The use of electrons in the treatment of local skin disorders is discussed in more detail in Chapter 11. Total body electron-beam therapy for widespread cutaneous T-cell lymphomas and other disorders is also described in this chapter.

Quality of Radiation

The heterogeneous beam produced by dermatologic x-ray units consists of x rays of varying wavelengths. The proportion of shorter wavelengths (hard x rays) versus longer wavelengths (soft x rays) determines the penetrating effect (quality) of radiation.

The penetration of x rays is largely determined by two factors: voltage and filtration. The combined effect of these factors is usually expressed as "half-value layer" (HVL). This term has recently been replaced by the newer designation, half-value thickness (HVT), but most textbooks of dermatology and radiation oncology continue to use HVL as a standard definition of radiation quality.[3,21,24]

Half-Value Layer (Half-Value Thickness)

The HVL is defined as the thickness of a given filter material (in dermatology, usually aluminum) that reduces the intensity of a narrow beam of photons to 50% of the original exposure (Fig. 5.5). A beam of hard quality requires a greater thickness of aluminum for 50% attenuation than does a beam of soft quality. Therefore, the more penetrating beam has a greater HVL. In dermatologic therapy the HVL usually varies from 0.01 (grenz-ray range) to 2.0 mm Al; more penetrating x-ray qualities are rarely indicated in skin disorders. The HVL of radiation is influenced by several factors. For practical purposes, however, only two of these are important: kilovoltage and additional filtration.

Kilovoltage

Most dermatologic x-ray machines are operated within a range of 10 to 100 kV. When the kilovoltage applied to the x-ray tube is increased, the intensity (quantity) of the radiation is increased. In addition, the speed and kinetic energy of the electrons are increased and the resulting x rays contain photons of higher energy. Consequently, an x-ray beam produced by higher kilovoltage has a shorter wavelength and greater penetrating power. Depending on which window material is used in the x-ray tube, longer wavelengths can be absorbed by the inherent filtration of the window itself. For this reason, older glass-window (Pyrex) units are rarely used below 50 kV because their inherent filtration is approximately 0.5 mm Al. Modern beryllium-window tubes have an inherent filtration of only 0.1 mm Al, and allow utilization of a wider range of x rays of different penetration (10–100 kV).

Filtration

A filter is a sheet of metal (usually aluminum, in dermatologic therapy, and in radiation oncology often copper) that is placed in the x-ray beam to change its quality. Cellulose acetate or polyethylene filters are occasionally used in grenz-ray therapy. The beam is attenuated by absorption and

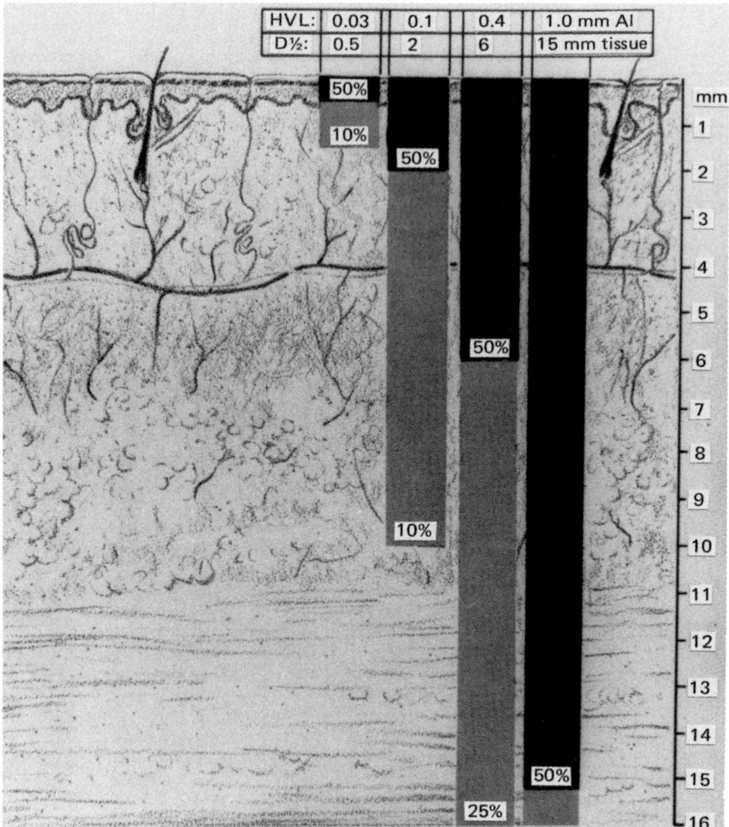

FIGURE 5.5. Percentage depth doses with D½ and HVL of various x-ray qualities. (From ref. 36, with permission.)

scattering so that its intensity is diminished by the filter. With a given kV and mA, the thicker the filter and the higher its atomic number the greater the reduction in beam intensity. Thus, 1 mm of copper reduces beam intensity more than 1 mm of aluminum does because copper has a higher atomic number, and 1.0 mm of aluminum reduces intensity more than does only 0.1 mm of aluminum. Since the x-ray beam is heterogeneous in wavelength and the lower energy photons are more readily removed from the beam by the filter than are the higher energy photons, there is a relative increase in the percentage of high-energy photons in the emerging beam and its average penetration power is increased. The resulting actual reduction in output is usually compensated by an increase in kilovoltage.

Selection of a filter thickness suitable for the desired depth of penetration is an important step in treatment planning. The choice is limited by the fact that most manufacturers provide only four to five different thicknesses of aluminum filters (e.g., 0.1, 0.25, 0.5, and 1 mm). In the interest of standardization, this limitation is desirable to avoid confusion and error. Only a limited number of different combinations of filter and kV are needed in daily practice.

Selection of Physical Factors

Since many physical factors can now be standardized, the basic decisions before treatment deal only with the quantity of radiation (dose) and its quality (HVL). The x-ray penetration should correlate with the depth of the pathologic process. When very soft radiation qualities are used, there may be too great a difference between the doses received by the upper and lower levels of the lesion. Conversely, when the selected x rays are too penetrating, the normal tissue below the lesion may receive an excessive dose. A compromise is usually necessary so that the depth dose below the actual lesion falls off as rapidly as possible. Data on actual penetration of a given x-ray beam can be obtained from isodose curves or depth dose tables, which give the dose on the central axis of the beam as a percentage of the surface dose (Figs. 1.12 and 1.14).

Half-Value Depth

The selection of the appropriate combination of kilovoltage, filter, and HVL is the most important decision in treatment planning. The introduction of the half-value depth (D½) as a guideline in the selection of radiation qualities has simplified this process immensely.[26] Its main advantage is that its routine application makes roentgen therapy safer and more effective; in addition, it eliminates confusing arithmetic computations. Instead of using several sets of depth dose charts for different combinations of radiation factors, the modern dermatologic radiotherapist takes advantage of calibrations based on the D½. The D½ (or HVD) is the tissue depth (expressed in mm) at which the absorbed dose is 50% of the surface dose (Fig. 5.5). Proposed and elaborated by Jennings[27] and Wachsmann,[1] this biologic concept has achieved greater significance for the dermatologist than has the physical term HVL. Another logical term, half-dose depth (HDD, or D½), was proposed by Kopf and associates.[28] The practical importance of the D½ concept was emphasized by Schirren[26] for treatment of skin cancers and by Goldschmidt[29] for benign dermatoses.

Since the attenuation of the incident radiation with depth is approximately exponential, it is impossible to deliver an adequate dose to the base of the lesion and still achieve the ideal condition in which no radiation reaches the underlying structures. Hence, one must compromise between adequate dosage and the possibility of damage to deeper structures. According to Jennings and Schirren, the most satisfactory compromise is to deliver 50% of the surface dose to the lesion's base.

The main significance of the D½ concept is that most of the radiation is absorbed in the pathologic process and is therefore of greater therapeutic benefit. In addition, it is assumed that the selection of softer radiation qualities with reduced absorp-

tion of ionizing radiation in the underlying healthy dermis will be associated with fewer late radiation sequelae, such as vascular changes (telangiectasia, atrophy, sclerosis) and changes in pigment (hyper- and hypopigmentation), than following administration of more penetrating x rays. Of course, radiation can also be therapeutically effective when qualities are used that are either too superficial or more penetrating than the tissue depth would warrant. Traditionally, skin cancers have often been treated with very penetrating radiations. Yet, only a small percentage of the surface dose is absorbed in the tumor itself and a disproportionately high percentage penetrates to deeper uninvolved tissues, thus increasing the possibility of undesirable radiation sequelae. On the other hand, ultrasoft x rays have been found effective in some inflammatory cutaneous disorders of much greater tissue depth than the maximum D½ of grenz rays (usually not more than 0.5 mm of tissue). This therapeutic response may be explained by the release of unknown factors from the epidermis and uppermost dermis, which may reduce the inflammatory reaction in tissue depths not reached by ultrasoft x rays. It should also be noted that routinely used individual doses for grenz-ray therapy are 2 to 3 times higher than are individual doses recommended for superficial x rays; this also accounts for a relatively deeper effect.

In either case, the selection of radiation qualities corresponding to tissue depth seems to be a more reasonable choice. Figure 5.6 illustrates this concept for skin cancers and premalignant tumors. Figure 5.7 demonstrates the same for benign dermatoses. An example of a typical calibration based on the D½ concept is given in Table 5.6. (Since the D½ is influenced by field size, TSD, and HVL, different sets of calibrations should be available.) Table 5.7 presents calibration data of a beryllium-window machine with five radiation qualities that have proved adequate for the treatment of most cutaneous carcinomas. Kilovoltage and filtration have been arranged to produce the same dose rate (100 roentgen (R)/min) for the first four calibration steps. This feature will reduce potential errors, particularly in beryllium-window machines with fixed kilovolt-filter combinations. In our experience, these five standard combinations of kilovoltage and filtration have been satisfactory for 95% of routine dermatologic radiation treatments.

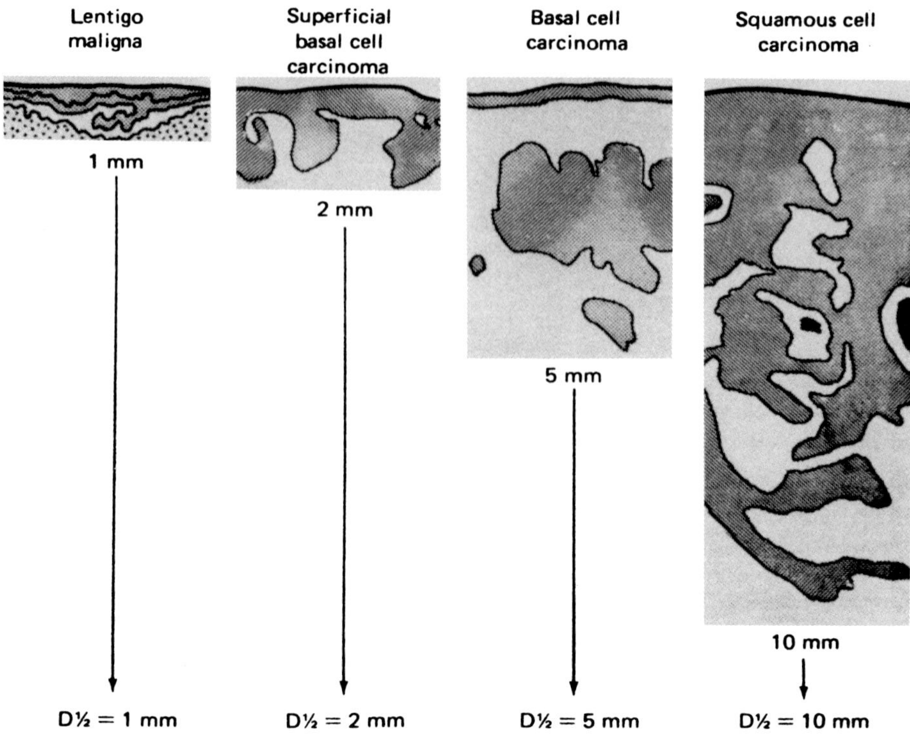

FIGURE 5.6. Selection of D½ for skin cancers and premalignant tumors. (From refs. 14 and 36 with permission.)

Instead of calculating the dose that will reach the depth of the treated lesion, the physician consulting this set of data will easily locate the depth at which 50% of the surface dose is absorbed and select the other physical factors accordingly. Calibrations based on D½ can easily be provided by a radiophysicist; detailed depth dose data have been published by several authors.[27,30] Accurate measurements of the actual depths of various skin diseases have been published by Zoon and Werz,[31] and can serve as the basis for selection of adequate D½s (Table 5.8). Atkinson[32] has correlated depths of skin cancers and dose homogeneities.

In addition to providing for an optimal tissue depth, the adoption of the D½ concept offers practical advantages in the calculation of required surface doses for lesions of varying depth. When the D½ is chosen properly, the base of the lesion receives exactly 50% of the surface dose; the necessary individual and total surface doses can then be computed easily for each required tissue depth by doubling the depth dose (e.g., if the base of a skin cancer is to receive 2500 cGy, a surface dose of 5000 cGy will be required). The known HVL of any radiation can easily be converted to the corresponding D½ value from available charts and

TABLE 5.8. Anatomical depth measurements.[a]

	Depth (in mm)
Normal skin	
Epidermis	0.03–0.25
Stratum corneum	0.015–0.5
Corium	3.0–4.0
Hair papilla	2.5–3.5
Eccrine sweat glands	2.0–3.0
Benign dermatoses	
Dermatitis, eczema	0.8–2.1
Psoriasis vulgaris	0.7–3.2
Lichen simplex chronicus	1.1–4.4
Lichen planus	0.4–2.1
Folliculitis, acne vulgaris	3.0–5.0
Cutaneous tumors	3.0–10 (rarely deeper)

[a] Adapted from Zoon and Werz,[31] with permission.

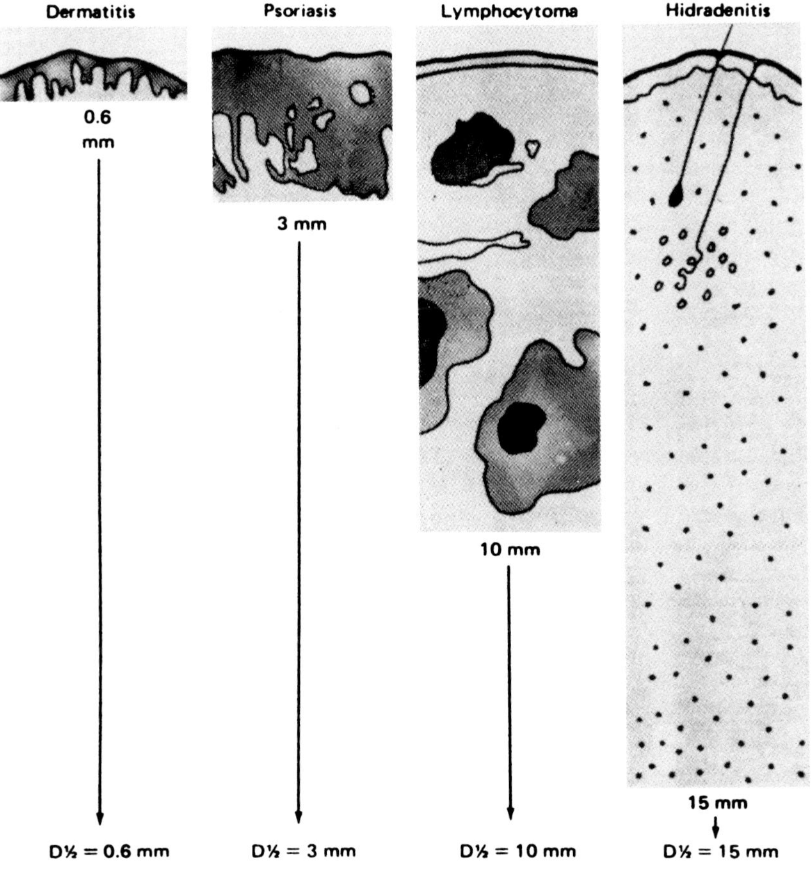

FIGURE 5.7. Selection of D½ for benign dermatoses. (From refs. 14 and 36 with permission.)

curves (see Fig. 1.15 in Chapter 1).[34-36] Recent measurements by Harley and colleagues[33] permit accurate determination of D½ values.

Definitions of Radiation Doses

Exposure

The quantity of radiation delivered to an area can be expressed by several different terms. The "exposure" (formerly called air dose) refers to the amount of ionization produced in a small volume of air under certain specified conditions. Historically, the unit of exposure has been the roentgen (R). The roentgen was originally defined as the exposure required to produce one electrostatic unit of charge (esu) per cubic centimeter of air at standard temperature and pressure (0°C, 760 mmHg). However, the International Commission on Radiation Units and Measurements (ICRU) recommended in 1975 that a new set of radiation units be adopted in order to bring research work and applications in the radiologic and health sciences into conformity with the units being used in other scientific fields. These new units are termed Systeme International (SI) units. In SI units the exposure dose of one roentgen is expressed in terms of coulombs (C) per kilogram of air: $1\ R = 2.58 \times 10^{-4}$ C/kg of air at standard temperature.

Absorbed Dose

The concept of "absorbed dose" is of greater biological relevance than that of exposure. The biological effect of any radiation depends on the actual quantity of radiation absorbed, chiefly through the process of ionization. Most medical textbooks use the term "rad" as the standard term for the absorbed, or tissue, dose.[5,34–36] One rad is equivalent to the absorption of 100 ergs of energy per gram of absorbing material. In dermatologic therapy the difference between one roentgen and one rad is usually insignificant, although in deep x-ray therapy the values for roentgen and rad may be at great variance. It should be pointed out that it is difficult to measure directly the dose absorbed in tissue. However, for x rays, the absorbed dose at any point is proportional to the exposure at that point. The absorbed dose in tissue can be estimated from the measurable exposure by taking into account the difference between the x-ray absorbing co-efficients of air and the absorbing tissue in question. Older dose recommendations by various authors have been given in air doses (R); their data can be translated into surface doses by multiplying the air dose (now known as "exposure") by the "backscatter" factor. In dermatologic therapy, this factor ranges from approximately 3% for small lesions and soft radiation to 20% for penetrating radiation, especially for sizes larger than 20 cm². [5,34] Because of the backscatter, the "surface dose" is higher than the "air dose"; the final "skin dose" (expressed in rad) is then reduced by multiplication with the roentgen to rad conversion factor (which varies from 0.87 to 0.9 for water or skin). For small lesions the resulting dose in rad is usually 5% to 10% lower than the air dose. For very large lesions it could be slightly higher than the air dose.[34] Since the ICRU has recommended adoption of the SI system by 1985, most medical journals are now using this new system of units.

The new unit for absorbed dose is the joule (J) per kilogram, or one gray (Gy). One gray is equivalent to 100 rad; one centigray (cGy) is equivalent to one rad. The use of centigray in daily clinical practice serves as a practical means of implementing the introduction of the gray into radiation therapy during a transition period. No numerical changes thus need be introduced into dose prescriptions or into the records of doses accumulated by patients during a treatment regimen.

In the recommended style for SI usage, names of units are not capitalized: meter, becquerel, sievert. Symbols for units are capitalized if they are based on a person's name: A, Gy, Bq, Sv. They are not capitalized otherwise: m, kg.

References

1. Wachsmann F. Physikalische Grundlagen der Röntgentherapie und Dosimetrie. In: Meyer-Mattes G, ed. *Die Strahlentherapie*. Stuttgart: Georg Thieme Verlag; 1949.
2. Storck H, Ott F, Schwarz K. Haut. In: Zuppinger A, Krokowski E, eds. *Handbuch der Medizinischen Radiologie*. Heidelberg: Springer-Verlag; 1972:17–160.
3. Helm F. *Cancer Dermatology*. Philadelphia, Penn: Lea & Febiger; 1979.
4. Goldschmidt H, Sherwin WK. Reactions to ionizing radiation. *J Am Acad Dermatol*. 1980;3:551–579.
5. Storck H. Radiotherapy of cutaneous cancers and some other malignancies. *J Dermatol Surg Oncol*. 1978;4:573–584.
6. Bart RS, Kopf AW, Gladstein AH. Treatment of morphea-type basal cell carcinoma with radiation therapy. *Arch Dermatol*. 1977;113:783–786.
7. Bart RS, Kopf AW, Petratos MA. X-ray therapy of skin cancer: evaluation of a "standardized" method for treating basal cell epitheliomas. In: *Proceedings of the Sixth National Cancer Conference*. Philadelphia, Penn: JB Lippincott; 1968.
8. Bucky A, Combes FC. *Grenz Ray Therapy*. New York, NY: Springer Publishing Co, 1954.
9. Hollander MD. *Ultrasoft X-Rays*. Baltimore: Williams & Wilkins; 1968.
10. Chaoul H, Wachsmann F. *Die Nahbestrahlung*. 2nd ed. Stuttgart: Georg Thieme Verlag; 1953.
11. Goldschmidt H. Dermatologic radiation therapy: current use of ionizing radiation in the United States and Canada. *Arch Dermatol*. 1975;111:1511–1517.
12. Cipollaro AC, Crossland PM. *X-Rays and Radium in the Treatment of Diseases of the Skin*. 5th ed. Philadelphia, Penn: Lea & Febiger; 1967.
13. Schirren CG. Über die Bedeutung der Weichstrahlung für die dermatologische Röntgentherapie. *Arch Dermatol Syphilol*. 1955;199:578–609.
14. Goldschmidt H. Dermatologic radiotherapy: selection of radiation qualities and treatment techniques. *Int J Dermatol*. 1976;15:171–181.
15. Gladstein AH, Kopf AW, Bart RS. Radiotherapy of cutaneous malignancies. In: Goldschmidt H, ed. *Physical Modalities in Dermatologic Therapy*. New York, NY: Springer-Verlag; 1978.
16. Lewis HM. Grenz-ray therapy: regimens and results. In: Goldschmidt H, ed. *Physical Modalities in Dermatologic Therapy*. New York, NY: Springer-Verlag; 1978.

17. Domonkos AN. Treatment of eyelid carcinoma. *Arch Dermatol.* 1965;91:364.

18. Farina AT, Leider M, Newall J, et al. Modern radiotherapy for malignant epitheliomas. *Arch Dermatol.* 1977;113:650–654.

19. Farina AT. Radiotherapy for aggressive and destructive keratoacanthomas. *J Dermatol Surg Oncol.* 1977;3:177–180.

20. Farina AT. Radiotherapy for aggressive and destructive keratoacanthomas. *J Dermatol Surg Oncol.* 1977;3:177–180.

21. Moss T, Brand WM, Battifora H. *Radiation Oncology.* 5th ed. St. Louis, Mo: CV Mosby; 1979.

22. Lehmann CF, Pipkin VL. Radium in malignant cutaneous disease. *JAMA.* 1954;154:4–8.

23. von Essen CF. Skin and lip. In: Fletcher, ed. *Textbook of radiotherapy.* 3rd ed. Philadelphia, Penn: Lea & Febiger; 1980:271–285.

24. Perez CA, Brady LW: Introduction. In: Perez CA, Brady LW. eds. *Principles and Practice of Radiation Oncology.* Philadelphia, Penn: JB Lippincott; 1987; 1–45.

25. von Essen CF. Roentgen therapy of skin and lip carcinoma: factors influencing success and failure. *Am J Roentgenol.* 1960;83:556–570.

26. Schirren CG. Die Röntgentherapie gutartiger und bösartiger Geschwulste der Haut. In: *Jadassohn J, ed. Handbuch der Haut-und Geschlechtskrankheiten.* Suppl. Vol. V/2, Berlin: Springer-Verlag; 1959: 289–463.

27. Jennings WA. A survey of depth dose data for x rays from 6 to 75 kVp (half value layers from 0.01 to 1.0 cm Al. Br J Radiol. 1953;26:781.

28. Gladstein AH, Kopf AW, Bart RS. Radiotherapy of cutaneous malignancies. In: Goldschmidt H, ed. *Physical Modalities in Dermatologic Therapy.* New York, NY: Springer-Verlag; 1978.

29. Goldschmidt H. Röntgenbehandlung gutartiger Dermatosen. In: Jadassohn J, ed. *Handbuch der Haut-und Geschlechtskrankheiten.* Suppl. Vol. V/2, Berlin: Springer-Verlag; 1959:464–573.

30. Brady LW, Binnick SA, Fitzpatrick PJ. Skin cancer. In: Perez CA, Brady LW, eds. *Principles and Practice of Radiation Oncology.* Philadelphia, Penn: JB Lippincott; 1987, 377–394.

31. Zoon JJ, Werz VFC. The quality of x-ray in the treatment of skin diseases. *Arch Dermatol.* 1957;75: 733–739.

32. Atkinson HR. Skin carcinoma depth and dose homogeneity in dermatological x-ray therapy. *Aust J Dermatol.* 1962;6:208.

33. Harley HH, Kolber AB, Altmen SM, et al. Determination of half-dose depth in skin for soft x-ray. *J Am Acad Dermatol.* 1982;7:328–332.

34. Gorson RO, Lassen M. Physical aspects of dermatologic radiotherapy. In: Goldschmidt H, ed. *Physical Modalities in Dermatologic Therapy.* New York, NY: Springer-Verlag; 1978.

35. Johns AE, Cunningham HR. *The Physics of Radiology.* 3rd ed. Springfield, Ill: Charles C Thomas; 1969.

36. Goldschmidt, H. Treatment planning: selection of physical factors and radiation techniques. In: Goldschmidt H, ed. *Physical Modalities in Dermatologic Therapy.* New York, NY: Springer-Verlag; 1978.

6

Radiation Therapy of Cutaneous Carcinomas: Radiation Techniques and Dose Schedules

Herbert Goldschmidt

General Considerations

Carcinoma of the skin is the most accessible cancer; the diagnosis is readily made and the limits of the lesion are usually easy to define. No single treatment method is best for all cancers of the skin. The careless application of any method can produce a poor cosmetic effect or result in a recurrence. If the sole criterion of success is eradication of the lesion, surgery and radiotherapy yield similar results. However, the use of either of these methods to the point of exclusion of other methods is certain to yield less satisfying cosmetic and functional results than using each where it is best suited. Most cutaneous cancers are sufficiently sensitive to radiation to be eradicated by doses that are well tolerated by the surrounding normal tissue. Thus, radiation therapy, when skillfully applied, can result in the selective destruction of the tumor without permanent mutilation or dysfunction of normal tissue. The uncertainties and pitfalls encountered in the early years of x-ray therapy have been virtually eliminated by the development of modern equipment and techniques. If appropriate principles are followed and precautions are taken, x irradiation is a safe and effective method of therapy.

There is a general consensus that no single mode of therapy gives superior results in all clinical situations. Not too long ago, only surgery and radiotherapy were recommended for treatment of cutaneous cancers. Due to technical advances and increased training in specialized surgical techniques, the emphasis has now shifted toward the use of surgical methods both in training and clinical prac-

tice. This is true even for relatively complicated cutaneous cancers, which were once routinely treated with radiotherapy. Surgical techniques that require the use of skin grafts or the planning of flaps for primary closure are now used not only by plastic surgeons but also by specially trained dermatologic surgeons. Cryosurgery and Mohs stratigraphic surgery are also used more widely. These developments have been of great benefit to patients with cancers of the skin and have reduced the need for radiation therapy. Modern dermatologic radiation therapy still is an indispensable primary or alternative modality for the treatment of a small percentage of cutaneous cancers.[1,2] We describe techniques and results of modern dermatologic radiotherapy and emphasize indications and contraindications for cutaneous cancers in specific anatomic locations, especially on the nose, eyelid, ear, and lip. Our discussion is deliberately limited to radiotherapy of common cutaneous cancers of moderate size that can be effectively treated in any office equipped with a beryllium-window, superficial x-ray or contact-therapy unit. Larger and more complicated skin cancers should be referred to Mohs surgeons or radiation oncologists for treatment with higher kilovoltage, megavoltage, or electron-beam techniques or for implants with radioactive isotopes. These methods are described in detail in radiation oncology textbooks.[3-8]

Frequency of Usage

The former role of radiotherapy in the treatment of cutaneous cancers was emphasized in the last survey taken by the American Academy of Dermatology in 1974,[9] which showed that of more than 2000 dermatologists, 89% treated selected basal cell carcinomas with x rays or referred patients for x-ray therapy. Ninety percent of these dermatologist stated that radiation treatment was indicated in more than 20% of their cases. For squamous cell carcinomas, 80% recommended radiation treatment in special cases, and 9% suggested or used radiotherapy in more than 20% of their patients. The usefulness of radiotherapy in the management of cutaneous neoplasms is also emphasized in statistics gathered by large dermatologic centers where all modern therapeutic modalities (including cryosurgery and Mohs surgery) are available. Chernosky[10] reported his experiences with various modalities in the treatment of 3817 cutaneous cancers; more than 10% of these were treated in his office with x rays. At the New York Skin and Cancer Unit,[11-13] 19.7% of 1000 patients with cancer of the skin received radiation therapy. These figures were updated by Dubin and Kopf in 1983,[14] who reported recurrence rates for 2064 patients with 3531 basal cell carcinomas. Fifty percent of these patients were treated with curettage and electrodesiccation, 21% with x rays, and 14% with surgical excision. In Houston, Freeman and colleagues[44] treated 10% of 2288 skin tumors with x rays.

Indications for Radiotherapy

Theoretically, nearly all cutaneous cancers anywhere on the body can be treated successfully with x rays. However, experience over the past five decades has shown that cosmetic results of radiotherapy are less satisfactory in certain anatomic regions. The real superiority of irradiation over excision lies in its greater preservation of uninvolved tissue, but, when such preservation is not important, surgery is usually more expeditious. Regardless of the therapeutic modality used, adequate treatment requires that a margin of normal-appearing skin be included. In certain anatomical regions this may pose a problem for the surgeon but not for the radiotherapist, who can easily adjust the size of the field to the required area of treatment. Tumor margins may be made as generous as necessary without permanently removing normal tissue. In addition, the radiation port may be easily adjusted with lead shields for lesions with

irregular borders. Therefore, radiation is often the treatment of choice in areas where tissue cannot be readily sacrificed for cosmetic or functional reasons.

There is general agreement[2,15-19] that ionizing radiation is often preferable to other methods of treatment for cutaneous carcinomas of the eyelids, medial and lateral canthi of the eyes, nose, ears, and lips. Radiation therapy is also considered the treatment of choice by many dermatologists for carcinomas of the nasolabial fold and preauricular areas, which often show a tendency to deep invasion along embryonal fusion planes. Large cutaneous cancers of the cheek (or of other cutaneous areas where surgical excision may leave deformities) often respond to radiation therapy with minimal scarring. Conversely, the skin of the trunk and extremities has a greater tendency to develop unsightly radiation sequelae, particularly telangiectasias and changes in pigment, and radiation therapy is rarely advisable in these locations.[17,20,21] Paterson[22] listed anatomical sites in decreasing order of tolerance to x rays as follows: scalp, face and neck, trunk and proximal portions of limbs, ears and groin, extremities, hands and feet. In exceptional cases (e.g., large, multiple, superficial basal cell carcinomas of the trunk, inoperable tumors in any other cutaneous area, or in patients who refuse surgery), cautious radiotherapy may be useful even in these regions.

We find office radiotherapy particularly valuable for medium-sized tumors of 1 to 4 cm in diameter. Lesions smaller than 1 or 2 cm in diameter can often be treated equally well or better by surgery. Tumors larger than 4 to 8 cm in diameter are rarely seen in private practice and are best referred to radiation oncologists or to Mohs surgeons.

The age of the patient is also important when considering the use of x-ray therapy. To minimize the potentiating or additive hazards of solar irradiation in later years, sun-exposed areas in patients under 45 years of age should not be treated if equally effective alternative methods are available.[2,12] In elderly patients, irradiation may be a more favored option for several reasons. First, there is comparatively little danger of late radiation sequelae. X-ray therapy is also a less psychologically traumatic procedure for elderly patients, who often fear surgery of any type. The treatment is relatively painless and does not require hospitalization, thereby allowing the patient to continue his normal activities. Even patients who are relatively poor surgical risks because of their medical condition can generally tolerate radiation therapy. Finally, for complicated lesions in strategic anatomic locations, radiotherapy often affords the patient economic advantages over intricate surgical procedures.

Before radiation therapy of a lesion is begun, the diagnosis must be confirmed by biopsy. Histologic examination of the tissue serves to determine the type and radiosensitivity of the neoplasm. Tumors have been classified as radiosensitive (e.g., lymphomas), of intermediate sensitivity (e.g., most epithelial tumors) or radioresistant (e.g., tumors originating from the mesenchyma, soft tissues, and bone). In some instances, a full-depth biopsy may be used to measure the depth of a lesion. However, in cosmetically important areas, particularly the nose and cheeks, we prefer tangential biopsies, usually from the raised border of the lesion. These biopsies rarely leave scars, whereas punch biopsies, even with a small diameter, often leave permanent, visible, reddish, slightly depressed scars in an otherwise inconspicuous radiation site.[2]

Contraindications for Radiotherapy

In general we do not recommend office radiotherapy for cutaneous cancers that are located on regions other than the head and neck, are more than 4 cm in diameter, occur intraorally, extend from the upper lip into a nostril, or occur in osteomyelitis, chronic ulcers, and burn scars.[11,12,20,21] We also do not treat carcinomas secondary to chronic radiodermatitis or recurrent (residual) cancers following radiotherapy of skin cancers. In the past, second courses of radiation were occasionally recommended for selected recurrent carcinomas.[15] Since the cosmetic effects are often unsatisfactory and complications and recurrences are not uncommon,[23] modern forms of surgery, especially Mohs surgery, offer a superior therapeutic alternative approach.[24] Radiotherapy is only rarely indicated in the basal cell nevus syndrome[21] and contraindicated in xeroderma pigmentosum where ionizing radiation may even induce new neoplasms. Because of their poor response to radiation therapy, rare tumors, such as malignant sweat gland tumors, malignant atypical fibroxanthomas, adenoacanthomas, and clear cell acanthomas, should also not be considered for office radiation therapy. We advise against office radiation therapy of carcinomas involving bone or cartilage. Surgical methods or special techniques used by radiation oncologists offer a better chance of curing these tumors.[8,15,23,24] We would like to emphasize again that our discussion will be deliberately limited to x-ray therapy of medium-sized, uncomplicated basal cell carcinomas, squamous cell carcinomas, and keratoacanthomas that can be treated without complicated equipment.[2,12,13]

Selection of Radiation Quality

In some instances, there are substantial differences between radiation qualities recommended by dermatologists and radiation oncologists. Historically, relatively penetrating x rays were used by both specialties, mostly because of limitations in radiation equipment. The introduction of new x-ray units with beryllium-windowed Machlett tubes after 1945 has led to divergent views on the selection of optimal radiation qualities.

Radiation Qualities Recommended by Dermatologists

European dermatologists were among the first to investigate the new beryllium-windowed x-ray units created specifically for dermatologic radiation therapy. In central Europe and Scandinavia, most skin cancers were treated in university dermatology departments and by dermatologists in private practice; only a small percentage were treated by radiation therapists. In the 1950s, many papers were published by dermatologic radiotherapy centers with special emphasis on the advantages of softer x rays and the disadvantages of more penetrating x-ray qualities in the treatment of hundreds of skin cancers. Soon after, Jennings[25] in England, Wachsmann[26] in Germany, and Tuddenham[27] in the United States introduced the half-value depth (D½) concept (see Chapter 5) that was also applied to radiotherapy of cutaneous malignancies. Most dermatologists now recommend, as a rule of thumb, to select radiation qualities with a D½ corresponding to the depth of the tumor (Fig. 6.1). Most of the radiation will then be absorbed

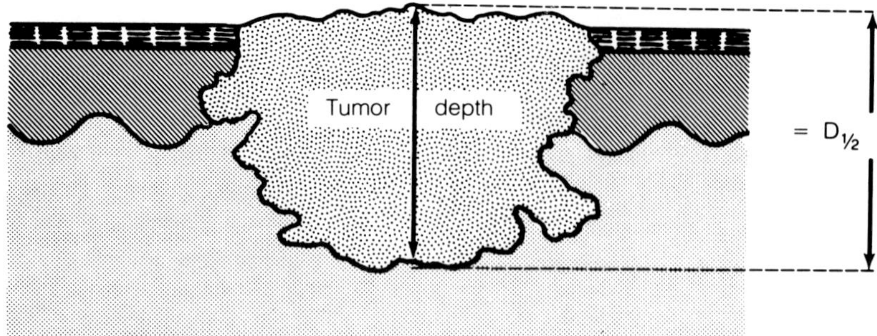

FIGURE 6.1. Proposed relationship between D½ and depth of tumor. (Reprinted by permission of the publisher from ref 2. Copyright 1983 by Elsevier Science Publishing Co., Inc.)

in the pathologic tissue (and will therefore be of greater therapeutic benefit), and the possibility of undesirable radiation effects to underlying uninvolved tissue will be markedly reduced. The depth of the tumor can be reasonably estimated by close inspection and palpation of the tumor. The biopsy specimen can then be used to measure the exact depth of the tumor. This method is not always reliable, however, because the depth of the tumor may be different in portions of the tumor that were not biopsied. Atkinson[28] correlated clinical findings and radiation quality by comparing depth of lesion and dose homogeneity in cutaneous carcinomas treated by x-ray therapy. He summarized the data on depth of lesions obtained by Strandqvist[29] (280 cases), Ebbehoj[30] (195 cases), and Polano[31] (170 cases) from biopsies of cutaneous cancers. He calculated that 50% of all basal cell carcinomas and selected squamous cell cancers infiltrate to a depth of only 2 mm or less, and 75% to 5 mm or less.

Newell[32] measured randomly submitted surgical excisions of basal cell epitheliomas and found that, of 67 tumors, 95.5% penetrated no deeper than 2.9 mm into the skin, and only 1.5% penetrated no deeper than 5 mm. Zacarian[33] also reported that 96% of 123 basal cell carcinomas did not extend below 3 mm, and only 0.8% exceeded a depth of 5 mm. This means that most "typical" and relatively superficially located basal cell carcinomas seen in private practice theoretically require a D½ of only about 5 mm (half-value layer [HVL], 0.2–0.4 mm Aluminum [Al]), and only 25% of all basal cell carcinomas are more deeply infiltrating, and these require a D½ of up to 10 mm of tissue (HVL, 0.8–1.0 mm of Al). More penetrating radiation qualities are rarely needed. In exceptional cases, referral to a radiation oncology department equipped for orthovoltage or electron-beam therapy may be considered.

Schirren[34,35] emphasized the advantages of relatively soft x-ray qualities for cutaneous malignancies; in his series of 1283 cutaneous cancers, 38% were treated with a D½ of only 3 to 4 mm (HVL, 0.15 mm Al), 31% with a D½ of 7 to 8 mm (HVL, 0.4 mm Al), 23% with a D½ of 10 mm (HVL, 0.7 mm Al), and only 8% with a deeper D½. Many other authors have recommended the D½ concept for the treatment of cutaneous cancers.[2,4,13,21,36-43] Even before beryllium-window, soft x-ray machines became available, many American dermatologists used superficial x-ray machines with thin Pyrex windows, applying radiation qualities that were not much more penetrating than the beryllium-window radiation qualities. For example, the "unfiltered superficial x-ray technique" utilized HVLs of 0.6 to 1 mm Al with good results.[44-49]

Superficial x-ray machines also were used with a "filtered technique" (100–140 kV, 1–2 mm Al added filtration) representing a HVL of 2 to 3 mm Al and a D½ of 12 to 20 mm of skin for deeper tumors. This radiation quality would now be considered too penetrating for ordinary and uncomplicated cutaneous cancers.

The only exception to the D½ rule applies to skin directly over bone or cartilage, which has a tendency to absorb more radiation in the soft-ray range. This is particularly important in areas with a relatively thin dermis (e.g., the pinna of the ear, bridge of the nose, and scalp). In these regions, the selection of softer radiation qualities is preferable. Even though soft x rays are strongly absorbed in bone, damage to bone is rarely seen after dermatologic radiation with soft x rays.

Radiation Qualities Recommended by Radiation Oncologists

Even though the D½ concept has been used successfully by dermatologic radiotherapists in thousands of skin cancers, most radiation oncologists in the United States have continued to use more penetrating radiation qualities. This is reflected in the recent radiation oncology literature. Moss and co-workers[8] and Brady and co-workers[3] recommend 0.25 to 0.5 mm Cu plus 1 mm Al filtration at 110 to 200 kV (D½ 24–42 mm tissue), Sharp and Birkley[50] recommend a HVL of 2.35 mm Al (D½ 20–24 mm tissue), and Fayos[51] recommends a HVL of 4.1 mm Al or 2.7 mm Cu (D½ 20–36 mm tissue). These empirical recommendations are based on the considerable clinical experience of these authors; in some instances, they are related to the lack of special dermatologic x-ray machines. The use of more penetrating x rays can also be explained by the fact that radiation oncologists treat larger and deeper tumors than those seen by dermatologists; in many desperate cases the radiation oncologist is the "last resort" for neglected skin cancers.[52,53] Moss and co-workers[8] suggest that all radiation qualities should be based on the assumption that cutaneous carcinomas are at least 1 cm thick. He reserves more penetrating radiations (e.g., Cobalt 60) for very thick tumors or for tumors close to bone or cartilage.

The preference for harder x rays also reflects the concept that homogeneous distribution of the radiation dose throughout the thickness of the tumor is needed for effective eradication of all cancer cells.[51] Since this principle was found useful in the treatment of internal neoplasms, it is also thought to be applicable to skin cancers. As mentioned earlier, Atkinson[28] calculated that 75% of cutaneous carcinomas infiltrate to a depth of only 5 mm. He used these data to emphasize that 75% of all basal cell carcinomas and 50% of unselected squamous cell carcinomas require a minimum HVL of only 0.35 mm Al when a 50% choice of homogeneity is selected (i.e., when the concept of D½ is applied), or a HVL of 0.8 to 1.4 mm Al when a 75% choice of homogeneity is preferred.

A more systematic approach has been attempted recently by von Essen,[54] who proposed a 70% to 80% depth dose for the selection of radiation qualities. This would mean that the base of the tumor would receive 70% to 80% (not 50%) of the maximum or surface dose and that the entire thickness of the tumor would be subject to more homogeneous radiation than with a 50% depth dose radiation. He published optimum factors for radiation therapy of superficial cutaneous tumors that were arranged in relation to estimated tumor depths and varied according to field size and target-skin distance (TSD). The recommended radiation qualities are listed in Table 6.1; corresponding D½ values were added according to the D½ tables published by Tuddenham.[27]

Recent publications by radiation oncologists indicate a trend away from penetrating radiation in favor of softer radiation qualities, especially for tumors of smaller size.[3,5,53] There is a good chance that the search for the optimal quality of radiation will ultimately be settled when electron-beam techniques have been refined further to permit wider use of their rapid fall-off ratio and minimal side effects to deeper tissues (see Chapter 11).

Radiation Dose

Time-Dose Relationship

Most authors recommend that the base of the tumor receive at least 2500 to 3000 cGy during fractionated therapy.[36] These doses can be administered in one single massive dose or in several fractions.

Massive Single Dose Therapy

In the early days of dermatologic radiation therapy, single massive doses (2000–2500 cGy) were applied to small tumors by many authors[53] (Miescher: 1500–1600 R,[55] Strandqvist: 2250 R[29]). Some modern radiation oncologists emphasize the convenience of this technique. Trott and associates[56] found single dose irradiation as effective as fractionated therapy for small tumors up to 1 cm diameter; 227 of 946 patients were treated with single doses ranging from 1200 to 2600 cGy. Hliniak and colleagues[57] irradiated 25 patients with single exposures of 2200 to 2600 cGy. Similar experiences were reported by Hale and Holmes.[58] Other authors have stressed that single massive doses often leave cosmetically unacceptable radiation sequelae[59] and are also associated with higher

TABLE 6.1. Optimum factors recommended by radiation oncologists for superficial cutaneous tumors.[a]

Tumor depth (mm)	Field area (cm²)	kV	TSD (cm)	HVL (mm Al)	Depth dose (%)	D½ (mm)
2	5	43	15	0.40	75	5.4
4	5	50	15	0.75	71	12
6	5	80	15	1.00	75	10
8	5	100	15	3.00	75	17
10	5	125	15	8.00	77	24
2	5–15	43	15	0.40	76	5.5
4	5–15	50	15	0.75	80	12
6	5–15	80	15	1.00	76	13
8	5–15	80–100	15	2.00	73	19
10	5–15	80–100	30	2.00	75	24
12	5–15	100	30	3.00	75	29
16	5–15	125	30	4.00	76	35
20	5–15	200	50	0.5 (mm Cu)	78	47
2	15–50	29	30	0.15	71	2.7
4	15–50	50	30	0.75	80	5.7
6	15–50	50	30	0.75	74	7
8	15–50	80	30	1.00	75	16
10	15–50	100	30	2.00	79	25
12	15–50	100	30	2.00	74	28
16	15–50	125	30	3.00	71	32
20	15–50	125	30	3.00	71	40
24	15–50	125	30	8.00	73	48
28	15–50	200	50	0.5 (mm Cu)	75	54

[a] Modified from von Essen,[54] with permission.

recurrence rates.[60] Fractionated dose schedules are now preferred by most radiation experts.

Fractionated Dose Therapy

Fractionation of radiation dosage is based on the assumptions that tissues recover at different rates from the effects of radiation and that tumor tissue recovers more slowly than normal tissue. When a given dose of radiation is divided into several increments and delivered over a period of several hours or days, the biological effect is usually less pronounced than that of the same radiation administered in a single dose. This lesser damage with daily fractionation appears to be related to cell recovery between increments and to the capabilities of recovering cells to adapt to radiation-induced alterations of the surrounding tissues (Fig. 6.2). The dependency of biological effectiveness on the degree of fractionation in classically referred to as the time-dose relationship.[60] Another factor used in describing time-dose relationships is "protraction," which refers to the length of time (in elapsed days) between the first and last dose.

Clinical Investigations

The first investigation of the correlation between radiation dose and time was undertaken in 1934 by Miescher,[55] one of the pioneers of dermatologic radiation therapy. He compared the effects of single high-dose therapy of skin cancers with various fractionated dose schedules. His study was followed in 1944 by Strandqvist,[29] who plotted the time-dose relationship of irradiated carcinomas on a log-log scale (Fig. 6.3). A line was drawn to separate the incidence of necrosis of skin from that of recurrences: doses above the line resulted in a complication of radiation, whereas those below the line were inadequate for control and resulted in recurrence of the tumor. (The usefulness of this curve can be demonstrated if the dose or time

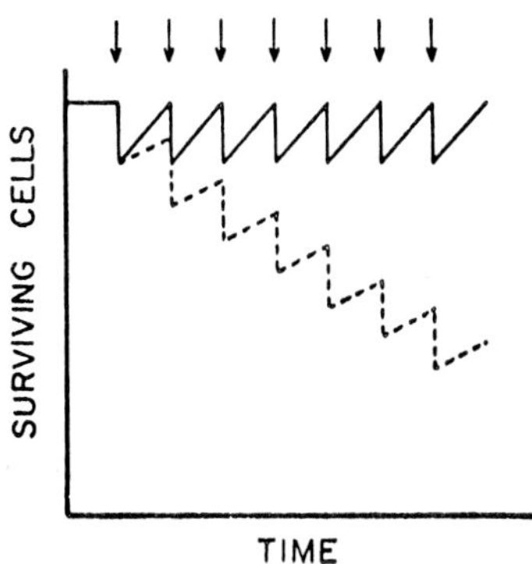

FIGURE 6.2. Differences in survival between tumor cells (broken line) and cells of surrounding normal tissue. (After von Essen[52]), with permission.)

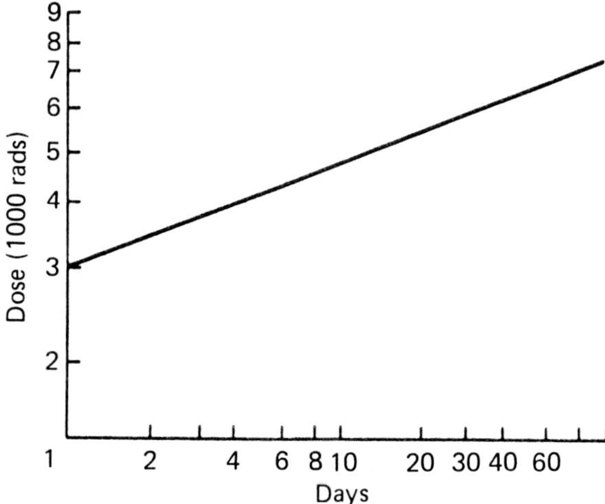

FIGURE 6.3. Strandqvist curve for carcinoma of the skin. (Reprinted by permission of the publisher from ref. 2. Copyright 1983 by Elsevier Science Publishing Co., Inc.)

factor of a treatment course is being changed. For example, if a tumor is usually treated with 3000 cGy in 4 days but for some reason a change in either the dose or the time is desired, the same effect might be obtained with 4000 rad in 11 days or 6000 cGy in 45 days.) The curves obtained are generally called the "Strandqvist plot": they have been used extensively in reports dealing with time-dose relationships of the skin and have also been applied to reactions of other tissues. Recent investigations have shown that Strandqvist's time-dose equations for cutaneous reactions produced by radiation therapy of cancer are of only limited value because they do not consider the influence of size of field, the extent of destruction of the skin by tumor, or the influence of treatment periodicity other than daily irradiation.[60-62]

Other Factors

Von Essen[52,60,63] emphasized the importance of the tumor volume of the irradiated tumor and prepared dose-effect curves by grouping together cancers of similar sizes. He concluded that larger tumors need higher doses than smaller tumors, and that more fractions are required for larger tumors because the use of an identical dose for a tumor of large volume results in more severe radiation sequelae than the same dose would cause in small tumors. This adverse effect can be reduced by using a higher number of smaller fractions over a longer period of time. Hliniak and colleagues[57] confirmed that larger tumors have a higher recurrence rate than small

tumors. Farina[64] summarized the relation between tumor size (volume) and dose by stating that the radiosensitivity of a tumor changes inversely with the size of the lesion and that the skin tolerance also changes inversely with the size of the field. A larger tumor needs a higher total dose, requires a longer delivery period of radiation, and needs a more penetrating radiation quality. Other factors are also important. One of these is the anatomical site of the tumor, which determines the total dose needed to eradicate the lesion.[8,61] The histology of the tumor also plays a significant role. Cancers of different cell types show different time-dose relationships. This is pertinent for different neoplasms treated by radiation oncologists.[60,62] On the other hand, the varying histology of common cutaneous neoplasms (basal cell carcinoma, squamous cell carcinoma, keratoacanthoma) does not play a major role in the radiosensitivity of these tumors, so most experts recommend similar doses for these neoplasms. Von Essen[52] also stressed that previously treated carcinomas (regardless of the modalities used) show a less satisfactory response to x rays than untreated primary tumors.

Treatment Dose and Total Dose

Much work has been done in an attempt to define optimum time-dose-volume relationships for carcinomas of the skin. There is no consensus as to the total dose needed to eradicate a cutaneous cancer and when to terminate radiotherapy. Different authors have recommended different dosages; the tendency at the present time is to use standardized schedules. Only a few authors use biologic responses as an end-point; for instance, by continuing radiotherapy regardless of the total dose until palpation shows that the tumor has disappeared completely.[35-37] An erosive and exudative reaction in the irradiated margin of normal skin in the periphery of the tumor has been regarded by other authors as an indication that a cancericidal dose has been reached.[35,65-67] This is based on the assumption that the cancericidal and epidermicidal dose are the same.[36] The New York Skin and Cancer Unit administers radiotherapy in a predetermined schedule and continues radiotherapy (with one or two more doses) only when the treated area shows no erythema after the recommended total dose has been administered.[12]

Dose Schedules and Results

In the treatment of most cutaneous tumors it has been established that better clinical results can be obtained by spreading the total treatment over a period of 2 to 6 weeks; possible schedules are once each day for 5 days per week, 3 times per week, or only once a week. The total exposure dose recommended by experts in dermatologic radiation for the treatment of cutaneous cancers ranges from 3400 to 6000 cGy. When larger individual doses are administered, the recommended total dose is usually smaller than in cases where smaller individual doses are used. This wide spectrum is surprising, even though some differences can be explained by variations in the quality of radiation, size of lesions, fractionation of dose, dose per treatment, total dose, intervals between treatment (number of treatments per week), and elapsed days between the first and last treatments. Table 6.2 outlines four commonly used dose schedules. The first three schedules represent x-ray techniques used by dermatologists. The fourth schedule is recommended by many radiation oncologists.

Dose Schedule A

In dose schedule A, doses of 500 cGy are administered 3 to 5 times per week over a period of 2 to 6 weeks up to a total dose of 4000 to 6000 cGy.

Doses and fractions are changed on an individual basis, depending on size and depth of the lesion. Smaller doses of 300 cGy are used for large tumors over a longer period of time. This is the most widely used dose schedule in the United States and in other countries. Treatment results have been reported by Cipollaro and Crossland,[46] Schirren,[34] Proppe,[36] Goldschmidt and Sherwin,[2] Braun-Falco and co-workers,[68] Wiskemann and co-workers, (95% 5-year cure rate),[40] Jansen,[47] Traenkle,[69] Nevrkla and Newton (129 cases, 94% cure rate),[48] Fischbach and colleagues,[70] Andrews and Domonkos,[71] Jacqueti (2117 cases, 95% cure rate),[42] Freeman and colleagues,[44] Jolly,[45] von Essen (565 cases),[72] Churchill-Davidson and Johnson (711 cases, 92.6% cure rate),[73] Moss and colleagues (821 basal cell carcinomas, 93% cure rate),[74] Andrews,[75] and Petrovich and co-workers (646 patients).[23] Our recommendations for office radiotherapy of cutaneous cancers in different anatomic regions in Chapter 7 are based on this schedule.

Dose Schedule B

Dose schedule B was developed at the New York Skin and Cancer Unit and is used by many dermatologists in the United States.[11-13] The standardized schedule advises five individual doses of 680 cGy (= 2 times "erythema dose") per treatment, with an interval of 2 to 3 days between treatments, up to a total dose of 3400 cGy (given over 9–11 days) for basal cell carcinomas. Eight treatments of 680 cGy (over 17–20 days) up to 5440 cGy are administered for squamous cell carcinomas. The cure rates (95%), cosmetic results, and regional differences obtained with this schedule have been described in detail by Kopf,[11] Bart and co-workers,[12] Gladstein and co-workers,[13] and Dubin and Kopf.[14]

Dose Schedule C

Dose schedule C was first used by Miescher[37] in Zurich and is now used by many dermatologists in Europe. Depending on the size of the tumor, three different treatment schedules are used. Cure rates of 94% were reported by Miescher and confirmed by Storck,[76] Schnyder,[21] and Panizzon.[77,78] A recent evaluation by Ballinari[79] of 433 basal cell carcinomas followed for 7.9 years revealed a cure rate of 94.9%, after basal cell carcinomas with histologic changes classified as sclerosing

TABLE 6.2. Dose schedules used at radiation therapy centers.

Schedule	Dose per fraction (cGy)	No. of fractions	Fractions per week	No. of weeks	Total dose (cGy)	TDF
A. <4 cm²	500	8	5	1½	4000	108
	500	10	5	2	5000	135
	400	12	5	2½	4800	115
>4 cm²	300	15	5	3	4500	92
	300	20	5	4	6000	123
	300	18	3	6	5400	102
	300	20	3	6½	6000	111
B. Basal cell carcinoma	680	5	2	2½	3400	94
Squamous cell carcinoma	680	8	2	4	5440	152
C. <2 cm	800	5	1	5	4000	109
2–8 cm	400	12	2	6	4800	96
>8 cm	200	26	2	13	5200	81
D.	300	15	5	3	4500	92
	300	18	5	3½	5400	111
	300	22	5	4½	6600	135
	200	30	5	6	6000	99
	200	34	5	6½	6800	112
	200	40	5	8	8000	132

basal cell carcinomas were eliminated from the statistical data.

Dose Schedule D

The data for dose schedule D illustrate two of the most common dose recommendations by radiation oncologists, usually administered with relatively penetrating radiation qualities. Two hundred to 300 cGy are administered 5 times a week in 20 or more sessions over a period of 3 to 6 weeks. For smaller carcinomas, 4500 to 5000 cGy are preferred; for larger tumors 6000 cGy are recommended.[6,74,51] Chahbazian and Brown[80] recommend a more protracted and fractionated course of therapy for larger lesions and for carcinomas in close proximity to bone, cartilage, and the eye. Recent publications show that many leading radiation oncologists find prolonged ultrafractionation over 7 to 8 weeks illogical and uneconomical for small uncomplicated cutaneous carcinomas.[3,6,15, 64,70,81,82]

Special Altered Dose Schedules

All commonly used dose schedules refer to daily treatments or treatment administered 1 or more times per week. Recently, clinical investigations have been undertaken with special altered dose schedules thought to be more effective than routine therapy. Among these are hypofractionation (a smaller number of large-dose fractions are given), hyperfractionation (a larger number of smaller than conventional dose fractions are given daily), accelerated multiple daily fractionation (normal fractions are given daily over a shorter total period), or split-course schedules (a rest period is inserted between treatments). Preliminary reports show promise for certain head and neck carcinomas but not for common cutaneous neoplasms.

Time-Dose-Fractionation Factor

Radiation experts have always searched for an optimal dose formula that will produce the maximal probability of tumor control with a minimal frequency of radiation sequelae. There is also a need for a means of comparing and summating tissue effects produced by different patterns of fractionation. It is now clearly established that comparisons are not meaningful when only the individual fractions and the total dose are reported. The number of fractions per week and the number of elapsed treatment days are equally important factors. As mentioned earlier, the histologic type of the tumor and the size and depth

TABLE 6.3. TDF factors of different dose schedules.[a]

Fractions per week	Dose per fraction (cGy)	No. of fractions	No. of weeks	Total dose (cGy)	TDF
5	500	6	1 1/7	3000	81
	500	8	1 3/7	4000	108
	500	9	1 4/7	4500	121
	500	10	2	5000	135
	400	10	2	4000	96
	400	11	2 1/7	4400	105
	400	12	2 3/7	4800	115
	400	14	2 4/7	5600	134
	300	15	3	4500	96
	300	16	3 1/7	4800	98
	300	18	3 3/7	5400	111
	300	20	4	6000	123
	250	20	4	5000	93
	250	24	4 4/7	6000	112
	250	26	5 1/7	6500	121
	250	28	5 3/7	7000	130
	200	25	5	5000	82
	200	30	6	6000	99
	200	35	7	7000	115
	200	40	8	8000	132
4	500	7	1 3/7	3500	92
	500	8	2	4000	105
	500	9	2 1/7	4500	118
	500	10	2 1/7	5000	131
	400	10	2 1/7	4000	93
	400	11	2 1/7	4400	102
	400	12	3	4800	112
	400	14	3 1/7	5600	130
	300	16	4	4800	96
	300	18	4 1/7	5400	107
	300	22	5 1/7	6600	131
	200	28	7	5600	90
	200	32	8	6400	102
	200	40	10	8000	128
3	700	4	1 1/7	2800	104
	700	5	1 2/7	3500	125
	700	6	2	4200	83
	600	6	2	3600	99
	600	7	2 1/7	4200	115
	600	8	2 2/7	4800	132
	500	7	2 1/7	3500	87
	500	8	2 2/7	4000	100
	500	10	3 1/7	5000	124
	400	10	3 1/7	4000	88
	400	12	4	4800	106
	400	14	4 2/7	5600	124
	300	16	5 1/7	4800	91
	300	18	6	5400	102
	300	22	7 1/7	6600	125
2	700	5	2 1/7	3500	98
	700	6	3	4200	118
	700	8	4	5600	157

TABLE 6.3. (*continued*)

Fractions per week	Dose per fraction (cGy)	No. of fractions	No. of weeks	Total dose (cGy)	TDF
2 (*cont.*)	600	6	3	3600	93
	600	7	3½	4200	109
	600	8	4	4800	124
	500	8	4	4000	94
	500	9	4½	4500	105
	500	11	5½	5500	129
	400	11	5	4400	91
	400	13	6½	5200	108
	400	15	7½	6000	125
	300	18	9	5400	96
	300	20	10	6000	107
	300	24	12	7200	128
1	800	4	4	3200	87
	800	5	5	4000	103
	800	6	6	4800	131
	700	5	5	3500	89
	700	6	6	4200	107
	700	7	7	4900	124
	600	6	6	3600	89
	600	8	8	4800	112
	600	10	10	6000	140

[a] Excerpted from Orton and Ellis,[84] with permission.

(volume) of the lesion also influence treatment results. Ellis[83] suggested in 1969 that it would be advantageous for comparing different techniques to use one number representing the dose of radiation that reached normal tissue tolerance. Because of the difficulty in using radiobiologic data derived from irradiated cell cultures, Ellis used human data based on skin tolerance and curability of squamous cell carcinomas. First he attempted to correlate the number of fractions with the dose and total time of a treatment series. He introduced the concept of the nominal single dose (NSD), which might be considered as the single dose equivalent of a total dose-protraction-fractionation scheme. These data permit the comparison of various treatment schemes and the changing of a given scheme to a different one of equivalent biological effectiveness. The NSD is given by the formula NSD = Dose $\times$ F$^{-0.24}$ $\times$ T$^{-0.1}$, where Dose is the total dose in cGy, F is the number of fractions delivered, and T is the number of treatment days. The unit of the NSD is the "ret," which stands for rad equivalent therapy. Typical treatment schedules deliver doses between 1700 and 1950 ret. Since the NSD formula did not take into account the number of treat

ment days per week, Orton and Ellis[84] later published another formula based on the factors of time, dose, and fractionation. Using their formula, the time-dose-fractionation factor (TDF) is given by the equation TDF = n $\times$ d$^{1.538}$ $\times$ X$^{-0.169}$ $\times$ 10^{-3}, where n is the number of fractions, d is the dose per fraction, and X is the function of the number of treatment days per week. When the fractional doses (varying from 200–1000 cGy), number of fractions (varying from 4–40), and number of treatments per week (varying from 1–5 times per week) are known, the TDF factor can be read directly from published tables (Table 6.3).[84]

Review of Recent Literature

The TDF concept is applied by radiation oncologists as a guide to treatment planning for normal tissue tolerance. For instance, the TDF values for the mandible and temporal bone are generally lower than those for the soft palate, tongue, and buccal mucosa.[6] The TDF formula can also be used to determine optimal dose schedules. Table 6.3 presents excerpts of Orton and Ellis' tables, with special emphasis on dose schedules with TDF values between 90 and 130. According to Ellis, the optimal factor for irradiation of carcinomas lies between 90 and 110. When the factor is smaller than 90, the malignancy may be undertreated; when it is larger than 110, the malignancy may be overtreated.[85] With overtreatment, there is a risk of a poor cosmetic result; with undertreatment there is the risk of recurrence. Even though there is no conclusive evidence that this theoretical formula can be applied to cutaneous cancers as it is to some internal malignancies, Storck[85] was the first to apply this formula to dermatologic therapy. For comparison, Table 6.2 also lists the TDF values for radiation schedules used at leading university centers. Only a limited number of comparative studies are available to determine the clinical usefulness of the TDF concept. Landthaler and Braun-Falco[109] compared long-term results of 290 irradiated cancers and confirmed that the TDF can be applied to skin cancer; 148 carcinomas treated with a TDF of 106 showed the same cure rates as 144 cancers treated with a TDF of 123.

Some radiation oncologists recommend higher TDF values. Wang,[6] at the Massachusetts General Hospital, summarized his clinical results in the treatment of cutaneous carcinomas and emphasized the importance of tumor size. He concluded that small squamous cell carcinomas respond well to radiation with a TDF of 110 to 120 (administered in 32 daily fractions over 6.5 weeks), whereas larger tumors require a TDF factor between 120 and 140. His suggestions are based on clinical experience; comparative data were not available. Hliniak and colleagues[57] compared radiation reactions and clinical results in the treatment of 497 skin cancer patients with four different dose schedules, based on their standard schedule of delivering 5100 cGy in 17 fractions of 300 cGy in 23 days. They concluded that the application of the NSD concept is useful to predict tumor control. Results with 7000 cGy in 47 daily fractions were equivalent to 4200 cGy in 11 days and to 5000 cGy in 23 days, all corresponding to NSD values of almost 1750 ret. Among other factors influencing cure rates were tumor size (large tumors recurred more often than small tumors when identical treatment factors were used), histologic type of carcinoma (the response of squamous cell carcinomas was less satisfactory than that of basal cell carcinomas), and overall treatment time (the recurrence rate of

squamous cell carcinoma was more favorable for treatment administered over 70 days than over 45 days). Good therapeutic responses were also recorded for 67 patients with carcinomas smaller than 30 cm^2, treated with only eight fractions of 525 cGy in 9 to 13 days.

At this time, the clinical usefulness of the TDF concept for dermatologic cancer therapy is not established with certainty. Careful long-term comparative studies with cancers of similar histologic type, volume, and location are needed to evaluate the influence of variations in each of the basic TDF components. However, since the original reports on time-dose effects were based on data derived from investigations of human skin tolerance and the therapeutic response of human squamous cell carcinomas, it is not improbable that skin cancers (squamous cell carcinomas and basal cell carcinomas) are suitable for radiation schedules based on TDF factors. Until more research data and reliable clinical comparisons are available, we do not suggest that older, clinically tested treatment techniques should be abandoned in favor of TDF schedules.

The selected TDF factors in Table 6.3 should be useful to clinicians theoretically interested in the biologic equivalency of various dose schedules. The table also facilitates altering established radiation schedules to accommodate patients with limited time (either total treatment time or feasible number of fractions per week), or when a change in dose per fraction is necessary. Orton and Ellis have also published special dose schedules for patients who have to interrupt treatments because of an intercurrent illness or for other reasons.[84]

Time-Dose-Fractionation Concept and Bioequivalent Dose Schedules

If we accept the validity of the TDF concept, we must decide whether protracted treatment with low doses (e.g., 200 cGy) over several weeks has advantages over shorter dose schedules with higher individual doses (e.g., 400–500 cGy). So far, there is no convincing evidence that one of the cited dose recommendations yields more cures or better cosmetic results than any of the others.[85] Only a limited number of clinical data are available to answer these questions. An often cited early landmark study on side effects of high individual doses was published by Trankle.[86] He saw 4 times as many necroses in skin cancers treated with four to five doses of 1000 cGy at weekly intervals than in tumors treated with 300 to 400 cGy 3 times a week for a total of 4000 to 5000 cGy. For some noncutaneous neoplasms there is early evidence (in need of further confirmation) that the following parameters might be important. Equivalency of two different time-dose regimens has been reported by Weissberg and associates[87] in 64 patients with advanced carcinoma of the head and neck. Patients were treated with five fractions of 200 cGy per week, increasing to 6000 to 7000 cGy in 6 to 7 weeks, or with 400 cGy daily, increasing to a total dose of 4400 cGy in 2 to 3 weeks. Acute skin and mucosal reactions occurred earlier in the patients receiving 400 cGy daily, but they were of the same intensity as those in patients receiving five fractions per week. Tumor control and other tissue reactions were similar in both groups. Higher fractions (730 cGy once a week) caused more severe sequelae than lower daily doses (250 cGy) in breast cancer.[88] Five fractions per week have yielded better curative results and fewer sequelae than three fractions or only one fraction per week in carcinomas of the larynx, uterus, and oropharynx.[89-92] Smaller daily doses (200 cGy) gave better results than higher daily doses (400 cGy) in bronchial carcinoma and in head and neck carcinomas.[87,93]

These observations seem to favor radiation therapy with multiple small daily fractions (e.g., 200 cGy) over several weeks as a desirable alternative for special cases. Interestingly, similar experiences were also reported in the older dermatologic literature where daily doses of 200 cGy were suggested for best cosmetic results, especially to reduce to a minimum telangiectases and pigment changes.[36,55,85] The potential advantages of multiple small doses must be balanced against economic considerations; dose schedules requiring 20 to 30 office visits are not only more inconvenient to the patient but also much less cost effective in relation to the presumed slight increase in cosmetic benefits. As in all medical decisions, the choice of therapy should depend only on the patient's best interests. A 2- to 3-week course of therapy is probably just as effective for small tumors (<3 cm) as a prolonged course of treatment. However, for larger tumors, especially in areas of cosmetic importance, treatment of selected cases with daily small individual doses over several weeks may be a valuable therapeutic option.

Dosage for Different Types of Cutaneous Cancers

In contrast to internal neoplasms, there is no major difference in radiation schedules for treatment of basal cell carcinomas, squamous cell carcinomas, and keratoacanthomas.

Basal Cell Carcinoma

The recommended dose schedules for a basal cell carcinoma are applicable to all clinical and histologic variations with the exception of the sclerosing (morpheiform) basal cell carcinoma. Bart and associates[94] have demonstrated that these carcinomas are radioresponsive, especially when a large border is chosen. Panizzon[78] reported less favorable results and a recent review of therapeutic results in Zurich[79] revealed a recurrence rate of 21.7% in 23 partially sclerosing basal cell carcinomas and 31% of 13 sclerosing basal cell carcinomas during a follow-up period of 7.9 years. This high recurrence rate contrasted with a recurrence rate of only 5.1% for 297 nonsclerosing basal cell carcinomas. Superficial basal cell carcinomas do not need any adjustment in radiation dose. However, multiple tumors with a larger diameter have shown a higher recurrence rate than smaller tumors.[77,78]

Squamous Cell Carcinoma

The described dose schedules can also be used for squamous cell carcinomas without any change in dosage. To reduce the rare possibility of chondritis, Panizzon recommends higher fractionation for squamous cell carcinomas overlying cartilage.[78] Some authors prefer to add 500 to 1000 cGy to the total dose for squamous cell cancers.[12,13,45] Exophytic tumors can be shaved before radiotherapy is started. Metatypical carcinomas are regarded as squamous cell carcinomas for radiotherapeutical purposes. Carcinomas of sweat glands and sebaceous glands are not suitable for office radiotherapy. Most authors warn against the use of ionizing radiation in cases where cartilage and bone are already involved by the tumor, in patients with neoplasms of the mucous membrane (which can be treated in radiation oncology centers), and in tumors arising from damaged skin (e.g., burn scars or in scars of chronic discoid lupus erythematosus).[12,78]

Residual (Recurrent) Cutaneous Carcinomas

Recurrences of cutaneous carcinomas soon after excision or several years following surgical therapy can also be treated with the same radiation schedules. Radiation can be administered to selected patients several weeks after surgery when microscopic examination of the surgical specimen has shown that the cancer was incompletely excised or when the surgical margin around the tumor was inadequate; the techniques are the same as for primary tumors. The functional and cosmetic results of irradiation after excision are satisfactory and there is no increase in late sequelae because of prior surgery. In patients previously treated by curettage and electrodesiccation, ionizing radiation therapy can also be administered when the tumor has not been completely excised. In this case a full course of radiotherapy is indicated. We do not recommend routine treatment by curettage followed by lower doses of x-ray therapy as suggested by Ebbehoj[30] and other authors because we believe that a cutaneous cancer should be treated adequately either by surgical means or by radiotherapy but not by a combination of both modalities. In combining methods there is always the danger of going halfway with either, or of overtreatment.

Results of Radiation Therapy

Cure Rates for Primary Carcinomas

Most reports in the literature indicate cure rates of 90% to 100% for uncomplicated small (<3 cm^2) cutaneous carcinomas. These results are similar to those obtained with other therapeutic methods. Large invasive cancers or lesions previously treated without success are more likely to recur; for very large, deep tumors the recurrence rate may be as high as 30%.[57] Panizzon[78] and Churchill-Davidson and Johnson[73] also reported that tumors with a diameter larger than 5 cm recur more often than smaller tumors. Hliniak and colleagues[57] and Petrovich and colleagues[23] observed higher recurrence rates in squamous cell carcinomas than in basal cell carcinomas.

Specific statistical data for different anatomical sites will be presented in Chapter 7.

Review of Recent Literature

The 5-year cure rate published by the New York Skin and Cancer Unit for 500 histologically proved basal cell carcinomas was 93%.[12] In contrast, the cumulative recurrence rate for 468 basal cell carcinomas treated by surgical excision was 6.8%, with the highest recurrence rates in the periocular areas, scalp, nose, and perinasal areas.[94] Dubin and Kopf[14] updated these results in 1983 when they reported recurrence rates for 2064 patients with 3531 basal cell carcinomas. Twenty-one percent were treated by radiotherapy, with a recurrence rate of 9.3% (18% for curettage and electrodesiccation, and 9% for excision). The overall recurrence rate was 15.2%. Recent publications by radiation oncologists quote similar results. Brady and co-workers[3] reported 4-year cure rates of 95.9% for 444 basal cell carcinomas and 92.3% cure rates for 156 squamous cell carcinomas. Other authors report higher recurrence rates for squamous cell cancer.[23,57] The most comprehensive investigation of long-term recurrence rates for primary basal cell carcinomas was carried out by Rowe and co-workers,[95] who systematically reviewed the literature over the past 40 years. They employed 5-year life table analyses (which adjust recurrence rates for the number of patients lost to follow-up each year) and compared therapeutic results of all modalities. Unfortunately, many larger scale favorable therapeutic reports from European dermatologic radiotherapy centers were not included in their evaluation. Five-year recurrence rates were as follows: surgical excision, 10.1% (264 of 2606 patients); curettage and electrodesiccation, 7.7% (274 or 3573 patients); radiation therapy, 8.7% (410 of 4695 patients); cryotherapy, (insufficient data) 7.5% (20 of 269 patients); Mohs micrographic surgery, 1.0% (73 of 7670 patients). The weighted 5-year average recurrence rate for all non-Mohs modalities was 8.7% (968 of 11,143 patients). Even though important radiotherapeutic results were missed, the large number of reported cases makes it likely that the average 5-year recurrence rate of 8.7% for patients treated with x rays is realistic and represents prevailing cure rates. Many of the reports not included in the review quote similar overall recurrence rates. A fair evaluation of treatment results of different modalities is difficult to accomplish when one considers that a certain degree of patient selection, usually in favor of the subspecialty of the author, is unavoidable. In reference to the radiotherapeutic data, one must also recognize that modern dermatologic radiotherapists limit their treatment to special, more difficult cases (e.g., eyelids, nose, ears, lips), where alternative methods are either not indicated or associated with special problems.

Cure Rates of Recurrent (Residual) Carcinomas

Menn and colleagues[96] have emphasized the high incidence of recurrences following treatment of recurrent skin cancers. The overall re-recurrence rate was 47%; the re-recurrence rate after radiotherapy of recurrent cutaneous cancers was 27%. The re-recurrence rates after excision, and especially after curettage and electrodesiccation, were higher still (40% and 59%, respectively). Mohs surgery, with a cure rate of more than 90% for recurrent basal cell carcinomas, was the most effective therapeutic modality. Rowe and co-workers[24] examined recurrence rates of recurrent (previously treated) basal cell carcinoma by reviewing numerous papers on 3748 patients treated since 1945 with various modalities. The overall 10-year re-recurrence rate was 8.2%. The specific 10-year weighted average re-recurrence rates were as follows: Mohs surgery, 5.6% (1634 of 3009 patients); radiation therapy, 9.8% (10 of 102 patients); surgical excision, 17.4% (91 of 522 patients); curettage and electrodesiccation, 40.0% (46 of 150 patients). They concluded that Mohs surgery is the best treatment for recurrent basal cell carcinoma and pointed out that radiation therapy is a viable alternative, especially for smaller carcinomas. The authors also stress that longer follow-up times are needed for all modalities to evaluate treatment success. Less than one-third of all recurrences appeared in the first year following treatment, only 50% appeared within the first 2 years, and only 66% within the first 3 years. Eighteen percent of recurrences appeared between the fifth and tenth year following treatment. They concluded that life-time follow-up is necessary to detect both recurrences and new primary tumors.

Cosmetic Results

Although it is relatively easy to determine cure rates for various radiation methods, it is much more difficult to judge cosmetic late effects of such treatments. More attention has been paid to this important aspect of radiotherapy in recent publications. Bart and associates[12] have emphasized that cosmetic results tend to worsen with time after radiation therapy and advise against radiotherapy in patients under 40 years of age. Excellent or good cosmetic results were observed in 74% of 500 lesions within the first year after treatment, in 68% in the third to fifth years after treatment, and in 49% in the ninth to 12th years. Churchill-Davidson and Johnson[73] evaluated 664 irradiated patients and found 15.8% excellent and 76.5% good cosmetic results. They stated that excellent results cannot be expected in very penetrating lesions and in lesions larger than 5 cm². Brady and co-workers[3] followed 130 patients with basal cell carcinomas and reported fair or poor cosmetic results after 5 years in only eight cases. Schneiter and Krebs[110] followed 117 basal cell carcinomas and judged cosmetic results after 9.1 years as good or very good in 57.2%, as average in 24.8%, and as bad in 11.1%. Results were better when only facial cancers were evaluated: 66% showed good or very good results, 21.6% average results, and only 4.1% poor results. The best results were seen in the nasal region (especially the tip of the nose) and in the orbicular area. Average results were noted on the forehead (hypopigmentation) and cheeks (telangiectases); unsatisfactory results occurred in some patients on the neck region, trunk, and extremities (telangiectases, atrophy).

Radiation Sequelae

Radiation effects and side effects are discussed in Chapters 3 and 4. The following descriptions represent a brief review of these findings with special emphasis on early and late cutaneous effects following radiation therapy of skin cancers.

Early Radiation Effects

Acute Radiodermatitis

The epithelial reactions during and immediately following radiation treatment have been classified into 4 groups[52]: first degree or erythema, second degree or dry desquamative epidermitis, third degree or moist desquamative (erosive, exudative) epidermitis, and fourth degree or necrosis (ulceration). Necroses can now be avoided by selection of appropriate radiation techniques and fractionation of tumor doses. The duration and severity of the acute radiation reactions vary considerably with different radiation schedules. When a typical 2-week daily treatment schedule with 500 cGy fractions is administered, erythema appears in the treated area during the first week of treatment, gradually developing into a dry scaling or erosive, crusted reaction by the end of the second week. The exudative reaction continues, reaching a peak 1 to 2 weeks after the last treatment. The wound is gradually re-epithelialized, and healing is usually complete 3 to 4 weeks after the last treatment (5–6 weeks after the first dose). Under unusual circumstances (large or deep cancers in special anatomical locations) longer healing times may be observed. Parker[97] summarized the factors affecting radiation reactions as follows: the severity of the reaction increases in proportion to an increase in radiation quality (due to increased absorption), the irradiated area (due to backscatter), and the total dose, and a decrease in the overall period of therapy (when the same total dose is applied).

The appearance of an erythematous, dry, or erosive epitheliolytic reaction is an unavoidable radiation effect. In some cases, plain water compresses or bland salves are soothing, or antibiotic ointments may be used to prevent secondary bacterial infection. An additional benefit of such treatment is cleansing and lubrication of the affected area, which makes it easier to observe the continuing radiation reaction. During this stage it is extremely important to avoid exposure to the sun, excessive heat, cold, friction, or infection. The mucous membranes of the mouth and nose tend to develop an erosive reaction at an even earlier stage. When treating the nose, the mucous membrane of the nose often reacts rather vigorously and small hemorrhagic crusts can be noted during the second and third week of treatment, even though the treated skin area (e.g., the ala of the nose) will not develop a vigorous exudative reaction until 2 weeks later.

Comedones

In some patients comedones are noted several weeks after irradiation of cutaneous cancers on the nose, cheeks, and ears, predominantly in the peripheral portions of the exposed field.[98] The so-called "comedo reaction" may persist for several months and usually disappears spontaneously. Preparations of retinoic acid accelerate this healing process.[99,100]

Pseudorecidives

In rare cases, keratosis-like nodular lesions appear in the treated area, usually in the periphery, several weeks after the initial cancer has disappeared. Even though they do not resemble the original tumor, a recurrence is often suspected. Rapid spontaneous disappearance is the rule.[101-104] However, if the new growth does not show any tendency to improve after several weeks, it must be differentiated from a recurrence of the original tumor by histologic examination. The microscopic examination of pseudorecidives shows marked epidermal acanthosis and sometimes pseudoepitheliomatous proliferation.

Delayed Tumor Regression

In rare instances, there is no immediate visible effect on the tumor and the possibility of a radioresistant carcinoma is considered. A biopsy may still show evidence of the original tumor. In these cases, it is often advisable to follow the recommendations by Gladstein and colleagues[13] to observe the area monthly for not more than 6 months after completion of therapy, provided the tumor is slowly shrinking or at least not clinically enlarging. Sufficient radiation may have been absorbed to render it incapable of growth and to induce slow resolution after several weeks or months. Should the tumor still show no noticeable improvement after 6 months, it should be considered radioresistant and other therapeutic modalities, preferably Mohs surgery, should be initiated.[13]

Late Radiation Effects

Chronic Radiodermatitis

Different degrees of chronic radiodermatitis can be anticipated in all irradiated areas, especially atrophy, dyschromia (hypo- and hyperpigmentation), and telangiectasias. Traenkle[105] suggested the term "late cutaneous radiation damage" because of the usual absence of histologic changes suggestive of a dermatitis in the damaged skin area. In sun-exposed areas these changes are more common because of the additional damaging effects of ultraviolet radiation on the atrophic radiation scar. Most telangiectases can be treated easily by electrodesiccation. Hypopigmented lesions and areas of irregular increased pigmentation can be camouflaged effectively with cosmetic preparations, especially because the original contour of the treated anatomical area is not damaged in most lesions.

Alopecia

X-ray therapy for basal cell carcinomas always produces permanent alopecia. Patients must be warned about this effect when the eyebrows, eyelashes, bearded areas, and scalp are exposed. Resulting cosmetic deficiencies can often be minimized with make-up, hair pieces, and long hair styles. Hair transplantation can be used for the scalp and eyebrows.

Delayed Ulceration – Combination Damage

An erosive or ulcerative reaction is usually seen at the end of a course of radiation therapy before the treated area starts to re-epithelialize. In rare instances erythema, scaling, shallow erosions or crusted ulcerations, and necroses (delayed postradiation ulcer, late radiation necrosis) may develop in the treated area several months or years after complete healing.[101,105,106] In the European literature, these reactions are called "combination damage"[35] because they are often triggered by excessive exposure to sunshine, cold, mechanical injury, or infections. Most cases are self-limited and heal slowly after several months. Permanent necrosis is a rare event that may require surgical intervention. In the past, these late radiation sequelae were observed following radiotherapy with massive dose increments or after single massive doses; they are extremely uncommon with modern radiation techniques.

Radiogenic Carcinomas

In contrast to the well-established potential carcinogenic effect of excessive irradiation in repeated small doses over longer periods of time (as given in the past for certain benign skin diseases), the development of new secondary neoplasms (especially squamous cell carcinomas) in irradiated areas is extremely rare following treatment of cutaneous cancers where much higher cancericidal doses are administered over a short period of time.[12,13,66,105] This appears surprising and paradoxical but is not unexpected. Investigations of experimental radiation carcinogenesis in animals have demonstrated that the dose-response relationship rises to a peak and then declines at higher doses. This may reflect the reduced numbers of cells at risk for carcinogenesis, caused by the cell-killing effects of radiation.[107] Ehring and Honda[108] reported that only one of 2005 patients irradiated for basal cell carcinoma developed a second tumor 40 years after the initial therapy. In contrast, 106 (5%) of these patients were treated for basal cell carcinoma originating in areas of chronic radiodermatitis caused by previous radiation therapy of benign skin conditions (lupus vulgaris, folliculitis barbae).

References

1. Braun-Falco O, Lukacs S, Goldschmidt H. *Dermatologic Radiotherapy.* New York, NY: Springer-Verlag; 1976.
2. Goldschmidt H, Sherwin WK. Office radiotherapy of cutaneous carcinomas. *J Dermatol Surg Oncol.* 1983:9:31–76.
3. Brady LW, Binnick SA, Fitzpatrick PJ, Skin cancer. In: Perez CA, Brady LW, eds. *Principles and Practice of Radiation Oncology.* Philadelphia, Penn: JB Lippincott; 1987:372–394.
4. Fletcher S. *Textbook of Radiotherapy.* Philadelphia, Penn: Lea & Febiger; 1980.
5. Murphy WT. Ionizing radiation. 1. X-ray therapy. In: Helm F, ed. *Cancer Dermatology.* Philadelphia, Penn: Lea & Febiger; 1979:365–409.
6. Wang CC. *Radiation Therapy for Head and Neck Neoplasms.* Boston, Mass: John Wright, PSG Inc; 1983.
7. Del Regato JA, Spjut HJ. *Ackerman and Del Regato's Cancer: Diagnosis, Treatment, and Prognosis.* 5th ed. St. Louis, Mo: CV Mosby; 1977.
8. Moss T, Brand WM, Battifora H. *Radiation Oncology.* 5th ed. St. Louis, Mo: CV Mosby; 1979.
9. Goldschmidt H. Dermatologic radiation therapy: current use of ionizing radiation in the United States and Canada. *Arch Dermatol.* 1975;111:1511–1517.

10. Chernosky ME. Squamous cell and basal cell carcinomas: preliminary study of 3,817 primary skin cancers. *South Med J.* 1978;71:802–806.

11. Kopf AW. Therapy of basal cell carcinoma. In: Fitzpatrick TB, Eisen AZ, Wolff K, Freedberg IM, Austen KF, eds. *Dermatology in General Medicine.* New York, NY: McGraw-Hill; 1971.

12. Bart RS, Kopf AW, Petratos MA. X-ray therapy of skin cancer: evaluation of a "standardized" method for treating basal cell epitheliomas. In: *Proceedings of the Sixth National Cancer Conference.* Philadelphia, Penn: JB Lippincott; 1968.

13. Gladstein AH, Kopf AW, Bart RS. Radiotherapy of cutaneous malignancies. In: Goldschmidt H, ed. *Physical Modalities in Dermatologic Therapy.* New York, NY: Springer-Verlag; 1978.

14. Dubin N, Kopf A. Multivariate risk scores of cutaneous basal cell carcinomas. *Arch Dermatol.* 1983;119:373–377.

15. Murphy W. X-ray therapy. In: Helm F, ed. *Cancer Dermatology.* Philadelphia, Penn: Lea & Febiger; 1979:322–324.

16. Wiskemann A, Pippert HD, Lotz GR. Röntgentherapie der Basaliome, Spinozellularenkarzinome und Keratoakanthome. In: Braun-Falco O, Marghescu S, eds. *Fortschritte der Praktischen Dermatologie und Venerologie.* Berlin: Springer-Verlag; 1976.

17. Storck H. Radiotherapy of cutaneous cancers and some other malignancies. *J Dermatol Surg Oncol.* 1978;4:573–584.

18. Schirren CG. Die Röntgentherapie gutartiger and bösartiger Geschwulste der Haut. In: Jadassohn J, ed. *Handbuch der Haut- und Geschlechskrankheiten.* Suppl Vol. V/2. Berlin: Springer-Verlag; 1959:289–463.

19. Gladstein AH, Kopf AW, Bart RS. Radiotherapy of cutaneous malignancies. In: Goldschmidt H, ed. *Physical Modalities in Dermatologic Therapy.* New York, NY: Springer-Verlag; 1978.

20. Miescher G, Pluss J, Weder B. Die Röntgenteleangiektasie als Spätsymptom. *Strahlentherapie.* 1954; 94:223–233.

21. Schnyder VW. Vor- und Nachteile der Röntgenweichstrahltherapie der Basaliome. *Therap Umschau.* 1976;33:524–528.

22. Paterson R. *Treatment of Malignant Disease by Radium and X-Rays.* Baltimore, Md: William & Wilkins; 1948.

23. Petrovich Z, Kmisk H, Langholz B, et al. Treatment results and patterns of failure in 646 patients with carcinomas of the eyelids, pinna and nose. *Am J Surg.* 1987;154:447–450.

24. Rowe DE, Carroll RJ, Day CL. Mohs surgery is the treatment of choice for recurrent (previously treated) basal cell carcinoma. *J Dermatol Surg Oncol.* 1989;15:424–431.

25. Jennings WA. A survey of depth dose data for x rays from 6 to 75 kVp. *Br J Radiol.* 1953;26:781–794.

26. Wachsmann F. Physikalische Grundlagen der Röntgentherapie und Dosimetrie. In: Meyer-Matthes G, ed. *Die Strahlentherapie.* Stuttgart: Georg Thieme Verlag; 1949.

27. Tuddenham WJ. Half-value depth and fall-off ratio as functions of portal area and target-skin-distance. *Radiology.* 1957;69:79–87.

28. Atkinson HR. Skin carcinoma depth and dose homogeneity in dermatological x-ray therapy. *Aust J Dermatol.* 1962;6:208–212.

29. Strandqvist M. Studien über die kumulative Wirkung der Röntgenstrahlen bei Fraktionierung. *Acta Radiol.* 1944;(suppl 55).

30. Ebbehoj E. Bucky rays and other ultrasoft rays. *Acta Dermatovenereol.* 1952;32:117–128.

31. Polano MK. Investigations on optimal dosage in the treatment of skin carcinoma. *J Belg Radiol.* 1958;41:1–37.

32. Newell GB. Depth of basal cell epitheliomas. Personal communication to S.A. Zacarian, cited in: Cryosurgery of skin cancer: fundamentals of technique and application. *Cutis.* 1975;16:449–460.

33. Zacarian SA. Cryosurgery of skin cancer: fundamentals of technique and application. *Cutis.* 1975; 16:449–460.

34. Schirren CG. Uber die Bedeutung der Weichstrahlung fur die dermatologische Röntgentherapie. *Arch Dermatol Syphilol.* 1955;199:578–609.

35. Schirren CG. Die Röntgentherapie gutartiger und bösartiger Geschwulste der Haut. In: Jadassohn J, ed. *Handbuch der Haut- und Geschlechtskrankheiten.* Suppl Vol. V/2. Berlin: Springer-Verlag; 1959:289–463.

36. Proppe A. Spezielle röntgenbehandlung. In: Gottron HA, Schonfeld W, eds. *Dermatologie und Venerologie.* II/1. Stuttgart: Georg Thieme Verlag; 1958:26–132.

37. Miescher G. Zur Entwicklung der dermatologischen Röntgentherapie. *Akt Probl Dermatol.* 1959; 1:426–453.

38. Helm F. The treatment of skin cancer: indications for selection among the various therapeutic methods. *Dermatol Digest.* 1968;1:70–75.

39. Hansen PB, Jensen MS. Late results following radiotherapy of skin cancer. *Acta Radiol.* 1968;7:307–319.

40. Wiskemann A, Lippert HD, Lotz GR. Röntgentherapie der Basaliome, spinozellulären karzinome und Keratoakanthome. In: Braun-Falco O, Marghescu S, eds. *Fortschritte der Praktischen Der-*

matologie und Venerologie. Berlin: Springer-Verlag; 1976.

41. Rubisz-Brzezinska J, Musialowica D, Zebrocka T. Treatment of basal cell epitheliomas. *Dermatol Digest.* 1976;9:10–15.

42. Jacqueti G. Treatment of skin epitheliomas. *Dermatol Ib Lat Am.* 1969;4:59–78.

43. Prieto JG, Del Pozo GJ. Tratmento de los epiteliomas cutaneos con radioterapia. *Med Cut.* 1966;1:51–60.

44. Freeman RG, Knox JM, Heaton CL. The treatment of skin cancer. *Cancer.* 1964;17:535–542.

45. Jolly HW, Jr. Superficial x-ray therapy in dermatology. *Int J Dermatol.* 1978;17:691–697.

46. Cipollaro AD, Crossland PM. *X-rays and Radium in the Treatment of Diseases of the Skin.* 5th ed. Philadelphia, Penn: Lea & Febiger; 1967.

47. Jansen GT. Treatment of basal cell epitheliomas and actinic keratoses. *JAMA.* 1976;245:1152–1154.

48. Nevrkla E, Newton KA. A survey of the treatment of 200 cases of basal cell carcinoma (1959–1966 inclusive). *Br J Dermatol.* 1974;91:429–433.

49. Andrews GF, Domonkos AN. Roentgen irradiation in the treatment of epithelioma. *JAMA.* 1954;154:21–22.

50. Sharp GS, Birkley FC. The treatment of carcinoma of the skin. *Presented at the 32nd Annual Meeting of the American Radium Society,* New York, May 1950.

51. Fayos JV. Radiotherapy in the treatment of carcinomas of the skin. *Dermatol Digest.* 1969;2:46–50.

52. Farina AT, Leider M, Newall J, et al. Modern radiotherapy for malignant epitheliomas. *Arch Dermatol.* 1977;113:650–654.

53. Farina AT, Leider M. Treatment of complicated cutaneous malignant neoplasms by modern radiotherapy. Principles, practice, and results. *J Dermatol Surg Oncol.* 1978;4:759–763.

54. von Essen, CF. Skin and lip. In: Fletcher S, ed. *Textbook of Radiotherapy.* 3rd ed. Philadelphia, Penn: Lea & Febiger; 1980:271–285.

55. Miescher G. Erfolge der Karzinombehandlung an der dermatologischen Klinik Zürich. Einzeitige Höchstdosis und frankationierte behandlung. *Strahlentherapie.* 1934;49:65–81.

56. Trott KR, Maciejewski B, Preuss-Bayer G, et al. Dose response curve and split-dose recovery in human skin cancer. *Radiother Oncol.* 1987;2:123–129.

57. Hliniak A, Maciejewski B, Trott KR. The influence of the number of fractions, overall treatment time and field size on the local control of cancer of the skin. *Br J Radiol.* 1983;56:596–598.

58. Hale CH, Holmes GW. Carcinoma of the skin: influence of dosage on the success of treatment. *Radiology.* 1947;48:563–569.

59. Miescher G. Tierexperimentelle Untersuchungen über den Einfluss der Fraktionierung auf den Späteffekt. *Acta Radiol.* 1935;16:25–38.

60. von Essen CF. Radiation tolerance of the skin. *Acta Radiol Ther Phys Biol.* 1969;8:311–329.

61. Cohen L. The statistical prognosis in radiation therapy: a study of optimal dosage in relation to physical and biological parameters for epidermoid cancer. *Am J Roentgenol.* 1960;84:741–749.

62. Cohen L. Radiation response and recovery. In: Schwartz EE, ed. *The Biological Basis of Radiation Therapy.* Phildelphia, Penn: JB Lippincott; 1966.

63. von Essen CF. A practical time-dose formula for x-ray therapy of skin cancer. *Br J Radiol.* 1969;42:474–480.

64. Farina AT. Current concepts in the use of radiotherapy for malignant epitheliomas of the skin. In: Robins P, Bennett RG, eds. *Current Concepts in the Management of Skin Cancer.* New York, NY: Clinicom; 1979.

65. Proppe A. Spezielle Röntgenbehandlung. In: Gottron HA, Schönfeld W, eds. *Dermatologie und Venerologie.* Stuttgart: Georg Thieme Verlag; 1958.

66. Suter L. Radiotherapy of neoplasms of the facial skin. *Laryngol Rhinol Otol (Stuttg).* 1986;65(10):533–537.

67. Storck H, Att F, Schwartz K. Haut. In: *Handbuch der Medizinischen Radiologie.* Heidelberg: Springer-Verlag; 1972:17–160.

68. Braun-Falco O, Lukacs S, Goldschmidt H. *Dermatologic Radiotherapy.* New York, NY: Springer-Verlag; 1976.

69. Traenkle HL. Management of skin cancer: basal cell epithelioma. *NY State J Med.* 1968;68:863–865.

70. Fischbach AJ, Sause WT, Plenk HP. Radiation therapy for skin cancer. *West J Med.* 1980;133:379–382.

71. Domonkos AN. Radiation therapy. In: Domonkos, Andrews. *Diseases of the Skin.* Philadelphia, Penn: WB Saunders; 1971.

72. von Essen CF. Roentgen therapy of skin and lip carcinoma: factors influencing success and failure. *Am J Roentgenol.* 1960;83:556–570.

73. Churchill-Davidson I, Johnson E. Rodent ulcers: an analysis of 711 lesions treated by radiotherapy. *Br Med J.* 1954;1:1465–1467.

74. Moss T, Brand WM, Battifora H. *Radiation Oncology.* 5th ed. St. Louis, Mo: CV Mosby; 1979.

75. Andrews GC. *Diseases of the Skin.* 3rd ed. Philadelphia, Penn: WR Saunders; 1946.

76. Storck H. Zur Strahlentherapie der Hautcarcinome, unter besonderer Berücksichtigung der fraktionierten Bestrahlung. *Z Hautkr*. 1977;53:67–74.

77. Panizzon R. Die Strahlentherapie des Basalioms. In: Eichmann E, Schnyder UW, eds. *Das Basaliom: Der häufigste Tumor der Haut*. Berlin-New York: Springer-Verlag; 1980:103–112.

78. Panizzon R. Modern radiotherapy of skin neoplasms. In: Kukita A, Seiji M, eds. *Proceedings of the XVI International Congress of Dermatology, Tokyo 1982*. Tokyo: University of Tokyo Press; 1983:482–489.

79. Ballinari M. *Die Röntgenweichstrahltherapie des Basalioms unter besonderer Berücksichtigung der Histologischen Wachstumsform*. Zürich: Medical Faculty of the University of Zürich; 1989. Inaugural dissertation.

80. Chahbazian CM, Brown GS. Radiation therapy for carcinoma of the skin of the face and/or neck. *JAMA* 1980;244:1135–1137.

81. Petrovich Z, Kuisk H, Tobochnik N. Carcinoma of the lip. *Arch Otolaryngol*. 1979;104:282–285 and 105:187–191.

82. Fitzpatrick PJ. Skin cancer of the head-treatment by radiotherapy. *J Otolaryngol*. 1984;13:261–266.

83. Ellis F. Dose, time and fractionation: a clinical hypothesis. *Clin Radiol*. 1969;20:1–7.

84. Orton CG, Ellis F. A simplification in the use of the NSD concept in practical radiotherapy. *Br J Radiol*. 1973;46:529–537.

85. Storck H. Radiotherapy of cutaneous cancers and some other malignancies. *J Dermatol Surg Oncol*. 1978;4:573–584.

86. Traenkle HL. Late radiation injury and cutaneous neoplasia. In: Helm F, ed. *Cancer Dermatology*. Philadelphia, Penn: Lea & Febiger; 1979:31–37.

87. Weissberg JB, Son YH, Percarpio B, et al. Randomized trial of conventional versus high fractional dose radiation therapy in the treatment of advanced head and neck cancer. *Int J Radiat Oncol Biol Phys*. 1982;8:179–185.

88. Turesson I, Notter G. The influence of fraction size in radiotherapy on the late normal tissue reaction. 1. Comparison of the effects of daily and once a week fractionation on human skin. *Int J Radiat Oncol Biol Phys*. 1984;10:593–598.

89. Kok G. The influence of the size of the fraction dose on normal and tumour tissue ^{60}Co. radiation treatment of carcinomas of the larynx and inoperable carcinoma of the breast. *Radiol Clin Biol*. 1971;40:100–115.

90. Wiernik G, Bleehen NM, Brindle J, et al. Sixth interim progress report on the British Institute of Radiology fractionation study of 3F/week versus 5F/week in radiotherapy of the laryngopharynx. *Br J Radiol*. 1978;51:241–250.

91. Singh K. Two regimens with the same TDF but differing morbidity used in the treatment of stage 111 carcinoma of the cervix. *Br J Radiol*. 1978;51:357–362.

92. Byhardt RW, Greenberg M, Cox JD. Local control of squamous carcinoma of oral cavity and oropharynx with 3 vs 5 treatment fractions per week. *Int J Radiat Oncol Biol Phys*. 1977;2:415–420.

93. Eichhorn HJ. Different fractionation schemas tested by histological examination of autopsy specimens from lung cancer patients. *Br J Radiol*. 1981;54:132–135.

94. Bart RS, Kopf AW, Gladstein AH. Treatment of morphea-type basal cell carcinomas with radiation therapy. *Arch Dermatol*. 1977;113:783–786.

95. Rowe DE, Carroll RV, Day LL. Long-term recurrence rates in previously untreated (primary) basal cell carcinoma: implications for patient follow-up. *J Dermatol Surg Oncol*. 1989;15:315–327.

96. Menn H, Robins P, Kopf AW, et al. The recurrent basal cell epithelioma. *Arch Dermatol*. 1971;102:628–631.

97. Parker RG. Selective use of radiation therapy for neoplasmas of the skin. *Clin Plast Surg*. 1980;7:337–348.

98. Stein K, Leyden JJ, Goldschmidt H. Localized acneiform eruption following cobalt irradiation. *Br J Dermatol*. 1972;87:274–279.

99. Larsen FS, Heyden Reich G, Christiansen JV. Comedo formation following cobalt irradiation. *Dermatologica*. 1979;158:287–289.

100. Graul EH. Über die "Comedonenreaktion" nach Chaoulscher Nahbestrahlung. *Strahlentherapie*. 1953;91:410–415.

101. Baer RL, Kopf AW. Complications of therapy of basal cell epitheliomas. In Baer RL, Kopt AW, eds. *Yearbook of Dermatology*, 1964–65. Chicago, Ill: Year Book Medical Publishers; 1965:7–26.

102. Nödl F. Das pseudorezidiv nach Röntgenbestrahlung. *Strahlentherapie* 1953;90:475–484.

103. Herold WC, Nelson LM. Pseudoepitheliomatous reactions (pseudorecidive) following therapy of epitheliomata. *Proceedings of the 11th International Congress of Dermatology*. Stockholm. 1957;2:426.

104. Poyzer KG, et al. Pseudorecidivism of irradiated basal cell carcinoma. *Aust J Dermatol*. 1975;15:77–78.

105. Traenkle HL. Late radiation injury and cutaneous neoplasia. In: Helm F, ed. *Cancer Dermatology*. Philadelphia, Penn: Lea & Febiger; 1979:31–37.

106. Traenkle HL. Management of skin cancer. *NY State J Med* 1968;68:863–865.
107. Burns FJ, Albert RE. Radiation carcinogenesis in rat skin. In: Upton AC, Albert RE, Burns FJ, Shore RE (eds): *Radiation Carcinogenesis*. New York, NY: Elsevier; 1986:199–214.
108. Ehring F, Honda M. Das Basalzell-Karzinoma auf röntgenbelasteter Haut. *Strahlentherapie.* 1967; 133:198–207.
109. Landthaler M, Braun-Falco O. Application of TDF-factor in soft-x-ray therapy. *Proceedings of the 17th World Congress of Dermatology.* Berlin: Springer-Verlag, 1988:928–930.
110. Schneiter M, Krebs A. Therapeutische, funktionelle und kosmetische Spätergebnisse von 103 Patienten mit mittels Weichstrahltherapie behandelten 117 Basaliomen. *Dermatologia* 1982;165: 342–351.

7

Radiation Therapy of Cutaneous Carcinomas: Indications in Specific Anatomic Regions

Herbert Goldschmidt

Carcinoma of the Nose

Carcinomas involving the nose and perinasal area are common; statistics from a large group of patients indicate that 20% to 25% of all facial cutaneous carcinomas occur in this anatomic region.[1] Several therapeutic modalities can be used effectively for these cancers. In our experience, the cosmetic and functional improvements following x-ray therapy of certain cancers of the nose are among the most gratifying results of dermatologic radiotherapy.

Most dermatologists have seen poor cosmetic results after simple excision with primary side-to-side closure because this method may bring about asymmetrical changes in the overall contour of the nose. Curettage and electrodesiccation may also yield unsatisfactory results because the nose has a stronger tendency to develop unsightly depressed scars with this method than other facial regions. Dermatologists aware of these therapeutic problems often refer patients with large cancers of the nose to plastic surgeons or to dermatologic surgeons for more extensive surgical procedures, including flaps, skin grafts, composite grafts, cryosurgery, or Mohs surgery. There is no doubt that these procedures can yield excellent results in skilled hands. However, in many elderly patients with medium-sized tumors, radiotherapy offers a valuable alternative that should be considered, and discussed with the patient, before extensive surgical procedures are contemplated. Radiotherapy is especially useful in patients with medical problems that might interfere with surgery, and in patients who refuse surgery. A recent analysis of 1620 basal cell carcinomas has shown that the relative risk for recurrent tumors is higher in the nasal region than in any other area.[2] In our experience, x-ray therapy is a valuable therapeutic alternative for carcinomas of the nose recurring after curettage or simple surgical excision. Recurrences after skin grafts or skin flaps are not suitable because the extent of the hidden tumor cannot be estimated properly.

Compared with many surgical techniques, radiotherapy is relatively easy to administer and is not associated with any major discomfort during or after treatment. The increasing emphasis on the cost-effectiveness ratio of various therapeutic modalities also favors dermatologic radiotherapy over complicated surgical procedures. Many dermatologic surgeons now recommend Mohs surgery even for relatively uncomplicated carcinomas, whether they are primary or recurrent tumors. Although there is ample evidence that Mohs surgery results in high cure rates, a leading dermatological cancer expert has argued that a maximal cure rate should not be the only factor to determine the choice of treatment.[3] Knox stated that the degree of tissue destruction, cost factor, aesthetic results, and time factor should also be considered; he specifically singled out the advantages of properly applied x-ray therapy for basal cell carcinomas in elderly patients. X-ray patients do not require hospitalization or anesthesia, nor do they require sophisticated reconstructive procedures. Cosmetic results are often excellent, primarily because radiotherapy does not change the contour of the treated area and preserves the normal surrounding tissue.[4-9] Surgery often requires the removal of fairly large lateral and deep margins that can preclude a

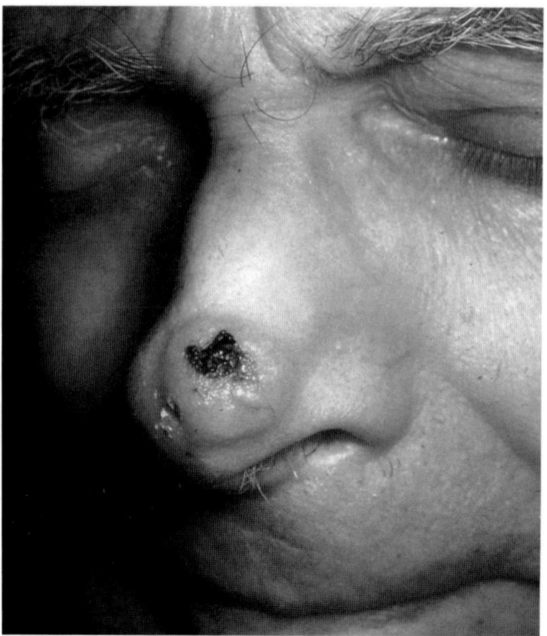

FIGURE 7.1. Markedly raised nodular basal cell carcinoma measuring 1.8 cm in diameter that had slowly enlarged over a period of years. (Reprinted by permission of the publisher from ref. 89. Copyright 1983 by Elsevier Science Publishing Co., Inc.)

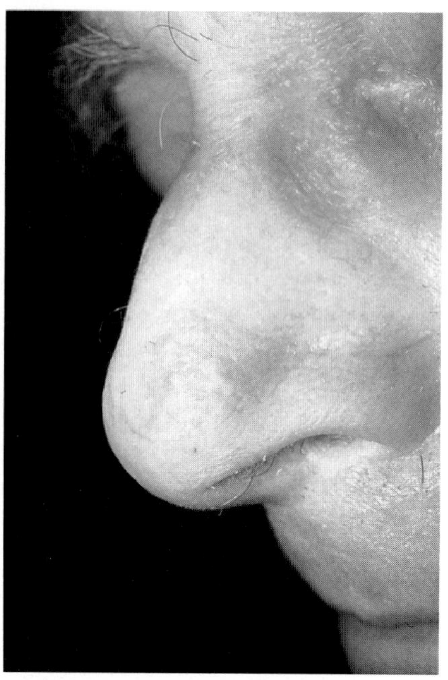

FIGURE 7.2. Resolution of the tumor with minimal cosmetic defect 2 years following radiation therapy. There is no change in contour. (Reprinted by permission of the publisher from ref. 89. Copyright 1983 by Elsevier Science Publishing Co., Inc.)

good cosmetic result.[10] In radiotherapy, the uninvolved margin can be as large as desired without significant cosmetic consequences; since carcinomas are more radiosensitive than normal tissue, only the tumor itself is eliminated and not the normal surrounding skin. Cosmetically disturbing radiation sequelae are uncommon on the nose, especially when proper radiation techniques are used. This was not the case several decades ago when carcinomas of the skin overlying nasal cartilages were treated with high doses of poorly fractionated and unnecessarily penetrating x rays. These obsolete radiation techniques sometimes resulted in painful chondritis or chondronecrosis and other undesirable sequelae. Modern radiotherapy with relatively soft x rays delivered in properly fractionated doses has reduced these problems to a minimum.[4-9]

Indications for Radiotherapy

Type of Carcinoma

Basal cell carcinomas are common on the nose and in the perinasal area and respond well to treatment.

Squamous cell carcinomas of the nose can also be treated effectively. Keratoacanthomas, especially rapidly growing giant keratoacanthomas, are also good indications for radiotherapy and a useful alternative in patients where Mohs surgery presents special problems because of the size of the tumor (see Chapter 8).

Age of Patient

Radiotherapy is recommended only for patients older than 45 years of age. Obviously, it is also an effective form of therapy for younger patients with unusual types of cancer or other unusual circumstances. However, because of the unavoidable additional solar damage to the irradiated area with the passage of time, surgical methods are preferred in younger patients.

Size of Tumor

Whereas previously untreated tumors smaller than 1 cm in diameter $(T_1 N_0 M_0)$[11] can be treated with x rays, we usually prefer surgical techniques or cryo-

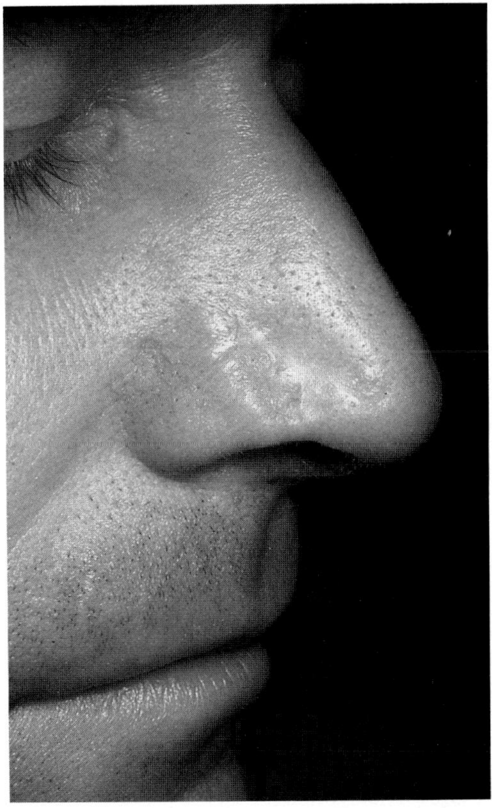

FIGURE 7.3. Nodular basal cell carcinoma measuring 2.6 × 1.7 cm with marked central depression following curettage and electrodesiccation.

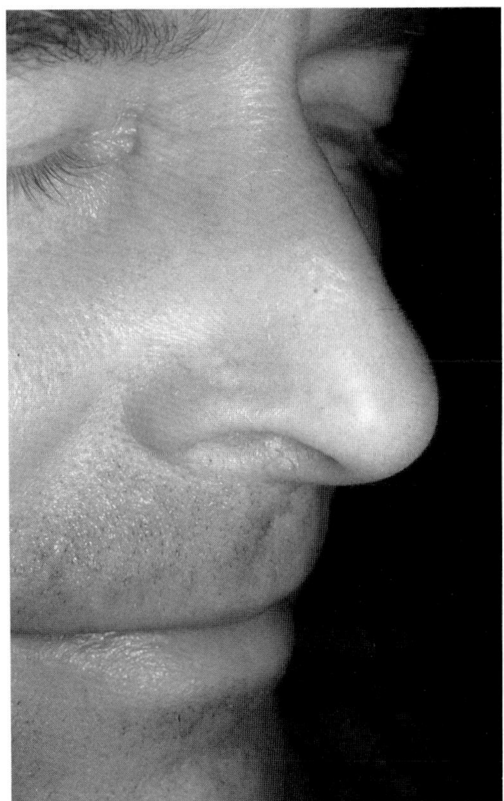

FIGURE 7.4. Excellent result 6 months following radiotherapy. Minimal hypopigmentation and telangiectasias are the only cosmetic defects.

surgery.[15] An exception to this preference are carcinomas on the tip of the nose. Because of the ease of treatment and good cosmetic results, even cancers smaller than 1 cm are suitable for radiotherapy in this location.

Radiotherapy should be considered for tumors ranging in size from 1 to 3 cm (the size seen in most patients) when simple resection techniques with primary closure are not feasible. Since the consistency of nasal carcinomas closely resembles that of cartilage, the borders of nasal cancers cannot always be determined with certainty. In these cases, multiple small biopsies are necessary to establish the true extent of the tumor. Radiotherapy of cancers with a diameter larger than 3 cm ($T_2N_0M_0$) may leave unsightly scars requiring plastic repair at a later date. For these patients primary surgical resection or Mohs surgery followed by reconstructive surgery is usually a better therapeutic choice.

Location of Tumor

Radiotherapy can be used for carcinomas located anywhere on the nose, and it is particularly suitable for cancers on the tip of the nose (Figs. 7.1 and 7.2), alae nasi (Figs. 7.3 to 7.9), and nasolabial folds (Figs. 7.10 and 7.11), where surgical techniques offer special problems. Radiation is also a useful alternative therapeutic modality for lesions on the sides, dorsum, and bridge of the nose in some patients in whom surgery would be problematic. In contrast to older techniques, radiochondritis is almost never encountered with modern radiation methods.[13]

Carcinomas involving the nasolabial fold deserve special consideration because many of these tumors invade deeply along embryonal fusion planes and require more penetrating radiation qualities. An ample margin of no less than 5 mm of

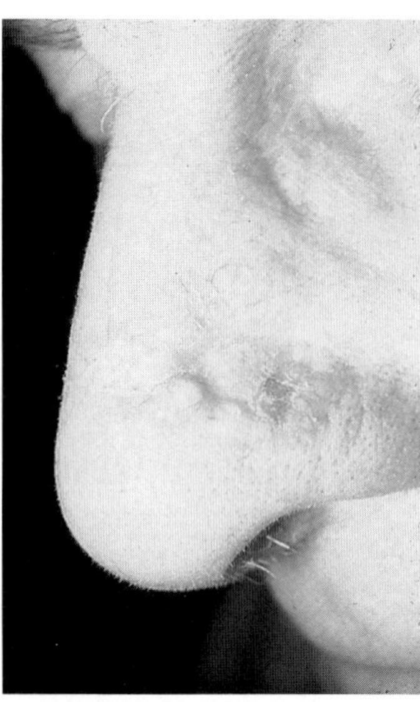

FIGURE 7.5. Large basal cell carcinoma measuring 3.0 × 2.4 cm that had recurred following plastic surgery several years previously. (Reprinted by permission of the publisher from ref. 89. Copyright 1983 by Elsevier Science Publishing Co., Inc.)

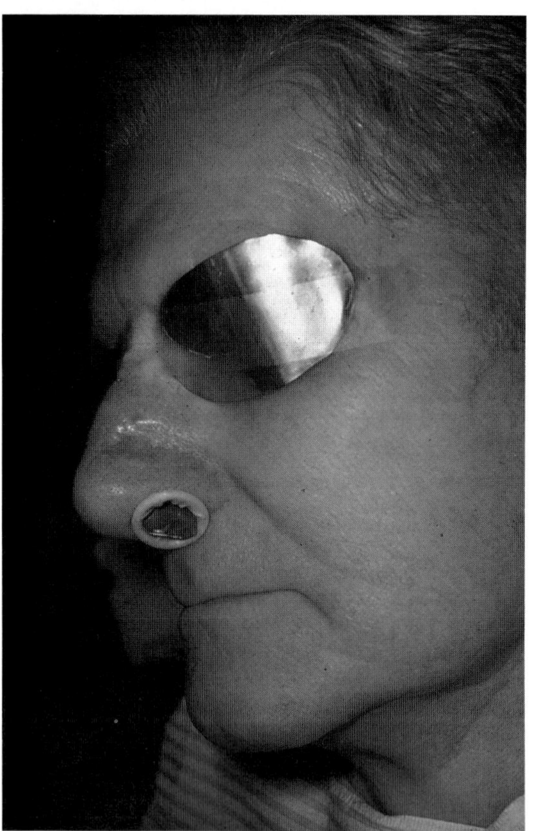

FIGURE 7.6. Same patient as Fig. 7.5. Lead shielding applied to both eyes and into left nostril; lead vinyl shield over neck region. (Reprinted by permission of the publisher from ref. 89. Copyright 1983 by Elsevier Science Publishing Co., Inc.)

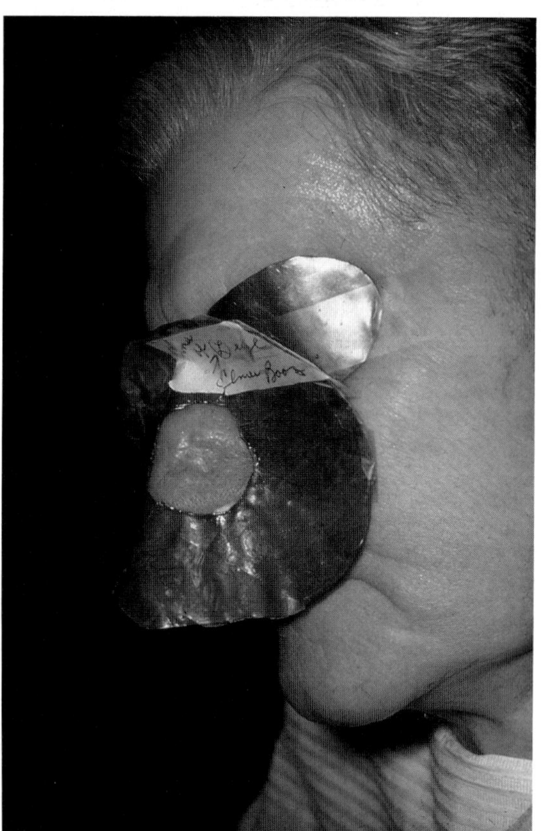

FIGURE 7.7. Overlay lead shield over normal skin in periphery of tumor. (Reprinted by permission of the publisher from ref. 89. Copyright 1983 by Elsevier Science Publishing Co., Inc.)

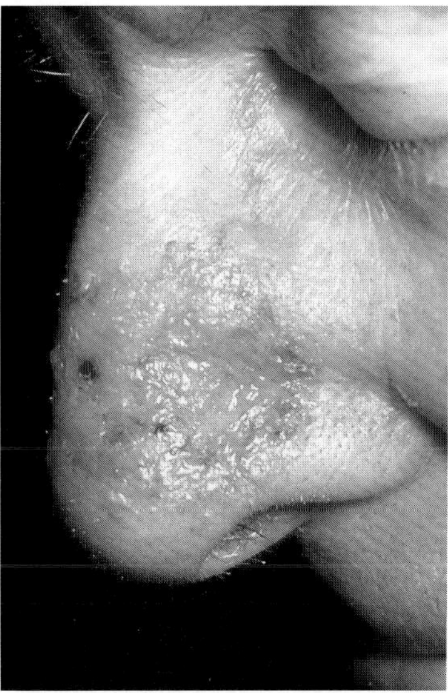

FIGURE 7.8. Exudative reaction 2 weeks after treatment with 14 400-cGy fractions of x irradiation (HVL 0.75 mm Al; D½ 12 mm). (Reprinted by permission of the publisher from ref. 89. Copyright 1983 by Elsevier Science Publishing Co., Inc.)

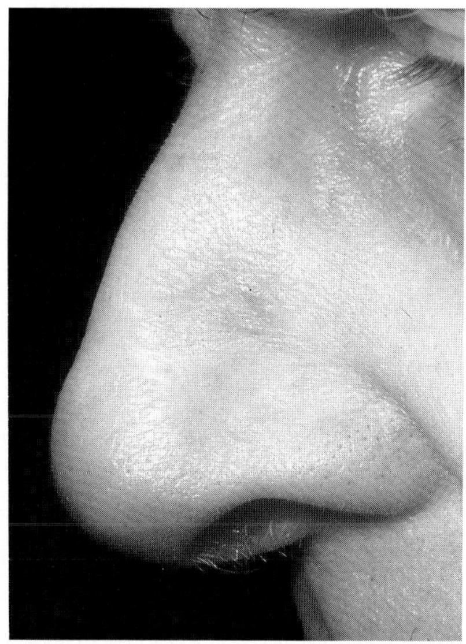

FIGURE 7.9. Very acceptable therapeutic and cosmetic results with retention of normal contour of nose 1½ years following treatment. (Reprinted by permission of the publisher from ref. 89. Copyright 1983 by Elsevier Science Publishing Co., Inc.)

apparently normal tissue should always be included in any irradiated site. Since carcinomas in this location often have poorly defined borders, a larger margin (up to 1 cm) should be used whenever feasible, even if apparently normal portions of the nose or upper lip must be included in the field of treatment.[14] Failures of radiotherapy in this anatomic region are mainly caused by improper techniques and fall mostly into two categories: insufficient field size (geographical miss) or incorrect appraisal of the depth to which the lesion extends. Nothing will be regretted more than the selection of an insufficient margin.[16-18] The only two recurrences in our own series of 70 carcinomas of the nose were caused by this error in judgment. In cancers recurring after x-ray therapy, Mohs stratigraphic surgery offers an excellent therapeutic alternative; previous radiotherapy does not interfere with the successful use of this surgical modality. Special considerations for cancers of the nose extending to the medial canthus are discussed under radiotherapy of the periocular area. Tumors involving the nasal vestibule, columella, and septum nasi need special techniques and are best referred to radiation oncologists.[19-22]

Recurrent Carcinomas

Radiotherapy yields highly satisfactory results in patients referred for radiotherapy with uncomplicated recurrences after inadequate surgical excision or incomplete curettage and electrodesiccation. Obviously, the scar from the previous operation will not disappear following radiotherapy. However, in some cases we have noted a definite cosmetic improvement of irregular surgical scars following radiotherapy. Large and complicated recurrent cancers are best treated by Mohs surgery with or without subsequent plastic repair. Radiotherapy is also not suitable for recurrences following reconstructive repair; Mohs surgery is the treatment of choice in these difficult cases where the border of the lesion is not clinically evident.

                    Herbert Goldschmidt

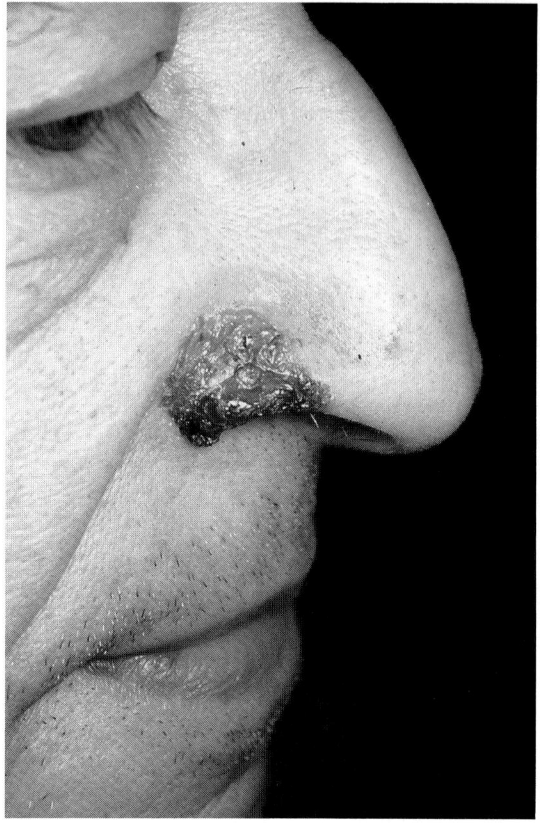

FIGURE 7.10. Large crusted nodular basal cell carcinoma of the nasolabial fold.

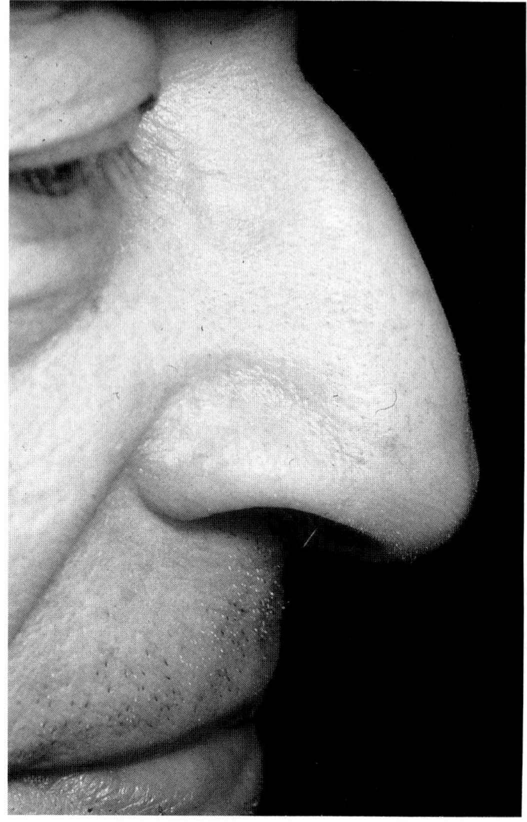

FIGURE 7.11. Good result with preservation of contour of ala nasi 3 months after treatment.

Contraindications

Tumors larger than 3 cm in diameter and carcinomas with deep involvement of cartilage or bone are not suitable for office radiotherapy. They should be referred to radiation oncology departments when surgical treatments are not feasible.[23,24] This also applies to tumors extending from the lip into the nasal orifice and to carcinomas involving the septum nasi, which often show early deep infiltration.[13,25] Cancers recurring after radiotherapy are also not suitable for radiotherapy.

Treatment Planning

Quality of Radiation

The radiation quality is adapted to the depth of the lesion (see Chapter 5). In most patients with early carcinomas of the nose, radiation qualities between 0.4 and 1 mm of Aluminum (Al) half-value layer (HVL) are satisfactory (half value depth [D½], 6–15 mm); more penetrating radiation is rarely needed.[6,18,24] Tumors in the nasolabial fold often extend deeper than clinically expected and a radiation quality of at least 1 mm Al HVL is usually preferred in this location. In smaller, relatively superficial carcinomas, the selection of a less penetrating radiation quality is not only possible but desirable because overly penetrating radiation is more likely to cause unsightly radiation sequelae. The poor cosmetic results of radiation therapy reported in the older literature were often due to poorly fractionated doses of penetrating x rays that damaged underlying cutaneous structures. Significant side effects on bony structures or cartilage can now be prevented by the proper choice of radiation quality.[16,24]

Dose

The most common treatment schedules are discussed in Chapter 6. In most of our patients with small carcinomas (1–3 cm in diameter), 400 to 500 cGy fractions are administered daily, 3 to 5 times per week, up to a total dose of 4000 to 5000 cGy. In exceptional tumors with diameters greater than 3 cm, we reduce individual doses to 300 to 400 cGy fractions given daily, 5 times per week, up to a total dose of 5000 to 6000 cGy. We administer the same dose for all types of cancers, although some treatment plans add 500 cGy to the total dose in the treatment of squamous cell carcinomas.[4,24,25] Other dose schedules are discussed in Chapter 6.

Protection and Shielding

Protection of the eyes with external lead or lead vinyl shields (0.5–1 mm of lead or equivalent) placed over the eyelids is mandatory (Fig. 7.6).[26] Lead shields or lead cups in the conjunctival sac are necessary when the tumor extends close to the inner canthus or when the inclusion of a border of normal skin may result in high scatter radiation to the lens. Whenever possible, the central beam of the radiation should be directed away from the eyes. Other measures for protection of anatomic areas (e.g., shielding of gonads and thyroid) are discussed in Chapter 4.

When the tip of the nose or the lateral surface of the lower half of the nose is treated (e.g., for lesions on the ala nasi), the septum and nasal passages are protected from the exit dose by insertion of a lead foil or a small tongue-shaped lead shield into the nostril; the shield is covered with a finger cot and lubricated with mineral oil (Fig. 7.6). More details on shielding procedures can be found in the excellent step-by-step descriptions provided by Gladstein and colleagues.[24,27]

Other Technical Factors

The selection of the proper target-skin distance (TSD) depends on the available x ray machine. Cones of lead glass facilitate treatment by defining the TSD and decreasing scattered radiation. In our practice, all treatments are administered with cones of 30 cm TSD and a cone diameter of either 1, 2, 3, or 4 cm. One end of the cone is attached to the x-ray tube and the other end is centered above a lead cutout molded over the nose (Fig. 7.7). A larger TSD (e.g., a 30-cm cone as opposed to a 15-cm cone) is especially useful when curved surfaces, such as the nose, are being treated because differences in radiation intensity between the center and the periphery of the field can thereby be reduced. Whenever possible, large lesions should be oriented so that their surfaces are flat and at right angles to the central beam. We always include a margin of at least 5 mm of normal skin around a lesion, or 1 cm when the border is indistinct. Small tumors require exposure of only one treatment field; for larger tumors, especially those involving both sides or the bridge of the nose, cross-fire techniques are indicated. Two separate oblique fields are treated on either side of the nose after applying a supplementary lead shield over one-half of the treated area. After the first half of the field has been treated, the supplementary shield is switched to the other side and the previously shielded half is irradiated.

Radiation Reactions

Acute Radiation Reaction

Most patients develop mild erythema of the treated site at the end of the first week of our treatment schedule. The erythematous reaction (acute radiodermatitis) intensifies during the second week of treatment and develops into an intensely erythematous, erosive, or exudative response 1 to 2 weeks after the last treatment (Fig. 7.8). A hemorrhagic crust often forms. The described acute radiation reaction subsides rapidly and re-epithelization is complete approximately 2 to 3 weeks after the last treatment, or approximately 4 to 5 weeks after the first treatment. Patients should be warned prior to therapy that this reaction is expected and is not a sign of any complication. In some patients the exit dose may cause a radiation reaction in the nasal mucous membranes. This usually occurs earlier than the reaction of the irradiated skin; it also subsides more quickly.

Chronic Radiation Sequelae

Following the resolution of the acute radiodermatitic reaction, the treated area usually shows an excellent cosmetic result without any evidence of radiation sequelae. After several years, especially following repeated excessive sun exposure, late radiation changes may develop in some patients. The most common sequelae are telangiectasias. Many patients are not even aware of their presence, but they can be treated by electrodesiccation if the patient finds them bothersome. Mild atrophy and hypopigmentation are also seen but are usually not of cosmetic significance because they can be easily covered with make-up. Hyperpigmentation is a rare side effect on the nose. Late radiation necrosis is almost never seen following the use of modern radiation techniques except in patients subject to severe sunburn, frostbite, mechanical injury, or infection. These changes usually subside after several weeks of treatment with bland salves. Permanent necrosis is extremely rare and surgical intervention is usually not needed. Patients should be advised always to protect themselves properly against the sun and to avoid sudden and excessive climatic changes.

An interesting and almost specific radiation effect following radiotherapy of the nose is the so-called comedo reaction, which becomes noticeable in the periphery of the treated area several weeks after irradiation.[28–30] Only the nose, the adjacent areas of the cheeks, and the ears show a strong tendency to develop comedones in radiation fields; other skin regions are affected only in exceptional cases. Treatment with retinoic acid preparations accelerates resolution of the comedo reaction. Even without therapy, spontaneous improvement after 6 to 12 months is the rule in most patients.

It should be stressed again that the avoidance of significant cosmetic side effects is the main reason many experienced dermatologists consider radiotherapy the therapy of choice for some neoplasms in the nasal region. The preservation of normal tissue and the absence of changes in the normal contour of the nose are significant arguments in favor of radiotherapy over surgical procedures, which often require complicated reconstructive techniques even for small tumors.[10,31]

Review of Recent Literature

Cure rates and other statistical data in relation to radiotherapy of cancers of the nose have been reported by several authors. Many of these publications include results of irradiation of large and complicated carcinomas of the nose. The incidence of side effects and recurrences is therefore higher than for the limited indications for radiotherapy suggested by us.

Wiskemann and colleagues[6] treated 97 cancers of the nose, mostly basal cell carcinomas, with soft x rays and reported a primary cure rate of 93%. Eighteen of these patients were irradiated for recurrent cancers following surgical methods; four of these recurred again after radiotherapy. Cosmetic results were very good in 72% of 82 patients and good in 21%; only 7% were unsatisfactory.

Rubisz-Brzezinska and co-workers,[32] achieved a cure rate of 98% in 54 patients treated with soft x rays (only one recurrence). Del Regato and Vuksanovich[1] observed three recurrences in 45 irradiated patients treated in a radiotherapy department, with a cure rate of 93%.

Jolly[4] recommended x-ray therapy for cancers in the nasolabial fold and the distal 40% of the nose, emphasizing that he had not seen necrosis of cartilage in any of the hundreds of cases he had treated with superficial x rays.

Bart and associates[33] reported a 5-year cure rate of 87.6% for 125 carcinomas of the nose and 88.8% for 69 cancers of the paranasal area treated with the standardized technique of the New York Skin and Cancer Unit.

Stoll and associates[34] achieved an 89.5% cure rate for superficial x-ray therapy in 276 previously untreated cases of basal cell carcinoma of the nose and a 94.5% cure rate in 62 patients with squamous cell carcinoma of the nose. Twenty-two percent of the cancers were located on the tip of the nose, 27% on the ala nasi, and 51% over the bridge of the nose. Most recurrences occurred during the first 3 years following treatment.

Mustafa[35] obtained a cure rate of 93% in 393 patients treated in a radiation therapy department. Eighty-five of these patients were irradiated for recurrent tumors. Six percent of the neoplasms occurred over the bridge of the nose,

33% over the dorsum, 37% on the alae nasi, 15% on the tip, 2% on the septum, and 4% on the nasal orifice. The author recommends x-ray therapy only for tumors whose diameters are smaller than 2.5 cm; recurrences were more frequent in larger tumors with or without involvement of cartilage. Storck[9] reported 96% good cosmetic results after radiation therapy of 316 basal cell carcinomas of the nose.

Fischbach and colleagues[36] treated 87 cancers of the nose in a radiation oncology department; seven recurred after a total dose of 4000 cGy. The authors emphasized that cartilage necrosis was not a significant problem. Preliminary results of electron-beam therapy with a betatron (7–15 MeV) were reported by Tapley and Fletcher.[37] Twenty-four patients with carcinoma of the nose were treated with good cosmetic results; three cancers recurred.

Petrovich and co-workers[25] treated 350 patients with carcinoma of the nose with 98% cure rates for tumors smaller than 2 cm in diameter. The recurrence rates were higher for larger lesions. The authors state that tumors overlying or even grossly involving the cartilage of the nose (and ear) can be irradiated successfully without significant complications such as cartilage necrosis.

Cure rates for primary excision of basal cell carcinomas of the nose and paranasal region are similar to the results obtained by radiotherapy. Bart and co-workers[38] reported a cure rate of 92.9% in 98 patients treated by scalpel excision at the New York Skin and Cancer Unit.

Carcinoma of the Eyelid

Collin[39] reported that one-sixth of all cutaneous cancers in a British plastic surgery service occurred in the orbital region. Seventy percent of these were basal cell carcinomas. The incidence of cutaneous cancer of the orbital region was 6.5/100,000 for males and 4.1/100,000 for females. The average age of those affected was between 60 and 69 years.

Differences in the location of basal cell carcinoma and squamous cell carcinoma were analyzed by Lederman,[40] who compared tumor locations in 630 patients with basal cell carcinomas and 59 patients with squamous cell carcinomas of the eyelids. He found that 11.7% of the basal cell carcinomas and 32.2% of the squamous cell carcinomas occurred on the upper lid, 61.3% of basal cell and 42.3% of squamous cell carcinomas on the lower lid, 24.3% of basal cell and 15.3% of squamous cell carcinomas on the inner canthus, and 2.7% of basal cell and 10.2% of squamous cell carcinomas on the outer canthus. Renfer[41] reviewed 182 cases in the literature and found that cancers involving the inner canthus represented 7% of all facial carcinomas and 36% of all periocular tumors. Green and colleagues,[42] of the New York Skin and Cancer Unit, listed the specific locations of 50 basal cell carcinomas of the periocular area and confirmed that the incidence was greatest on the lower lids, followed by the inner canthus and then by the upper lids and outer canthus.

The two accepted methods of treatment for carcinomas of the eyelids are surgery[38,39,43–45] (including cryosurgery[46–48] and chemosurgery[49] and radiation therapy. As for other cutaneous tumors of the face, the aim of any form of therapy should be to obtain the maximum cure rate with the least disfigurement or functional impairment. Unless the carcinoma has caused severe damage to the eyelid, the end result of treatment should be the restoration of a normally functioning eyelid; that is, minimal or no scarring, no shortening or deformity of the eyelid itself, and avoidance of either excessive or insufficient formation of tears. For many dermatologists the fear of radiation complications is the main reason for preferring surgery to radiotherapy in this anatomic site. Most of these fears are unwarranted when modern radiation techniques are used. Radiation sequelae resulting from older techniques were caused by penetrating x rays or lack of proper fractionation. Modern radiation techniques and protective measures have eliminated major side effects. In many cases the selection of the appropriate therapeutic modality will be based on the individual patient's age, general health, and cosmetic needs. Green and associates[42] and Gladstein[50] of the New York Skin and Cancer Unit list among advantages of radiotherapy of carcinomas of the eyelids the ease of therapy, lack of deformity, low incidence of complications, and high cure rates.

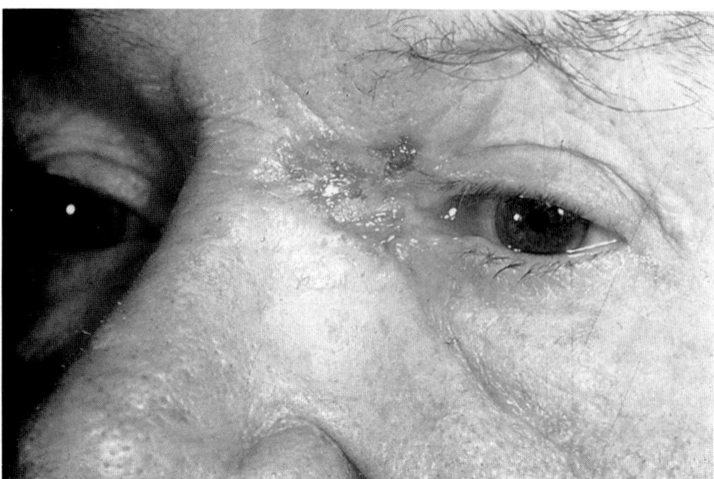

FIGURE 7.12. Large, irregularly shaped, ulcerative basal cell carcinoma, 3.0 × 2.7 cm, involving the nose, medial canthus, and upper and lower eyelids.

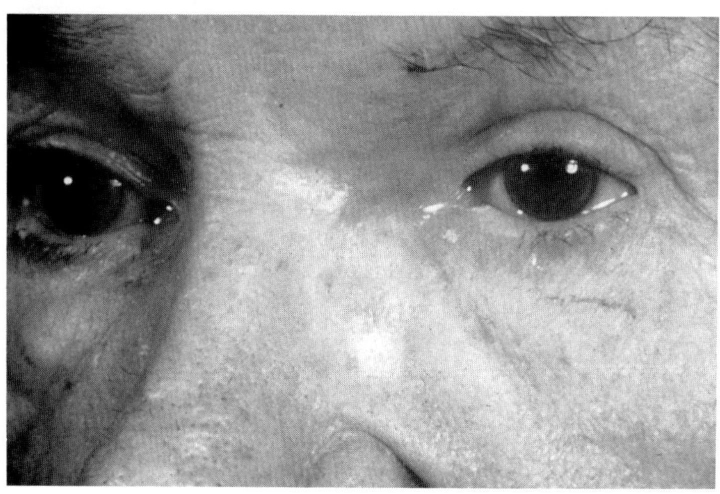

FIGURE 7.13. Good functional and cosmetic results 2 years after treatment with 6200 cGy administered in 400-cGy fractions.

Indications for Radiotherapy

Type of Carcinoma

Both basal cell and squamous cell carcinomas respond well to radiotherapy. Techniques for treatment are identical for these common types of eyelid cancer; keratoacanthomas can also be treated by similar radiation methods.

Age of Patient

As mentioned in Chapter 6, radiotherapy should be limited to patients older than 45 years of age. In younger patients the accumulation of solar damage to the irradiated area in the course of a lifetime may increase the incidence of late sequelae.

Size of Tumor

Small lesions (up to 5 mm in diameter) that involve the middle two-thirds of the eyelid can be excised with relatively good cosmetic and functional results. An exception to this rule are tumors of the inner canthus, where surgery may be difficult even for carcinomas smaller than 5 mm. In other locations on the eyelid small tumors are not considered primary indications for radiotherapy. It is usually easier and takes less time to treat these tumors by excision and closure, or cryosurgery.

Adequate excision of carcinomas larger than 5 mm often requires considerable margins in surface and depth. Therefore, good functional and aesthetic results after simple excision and closure

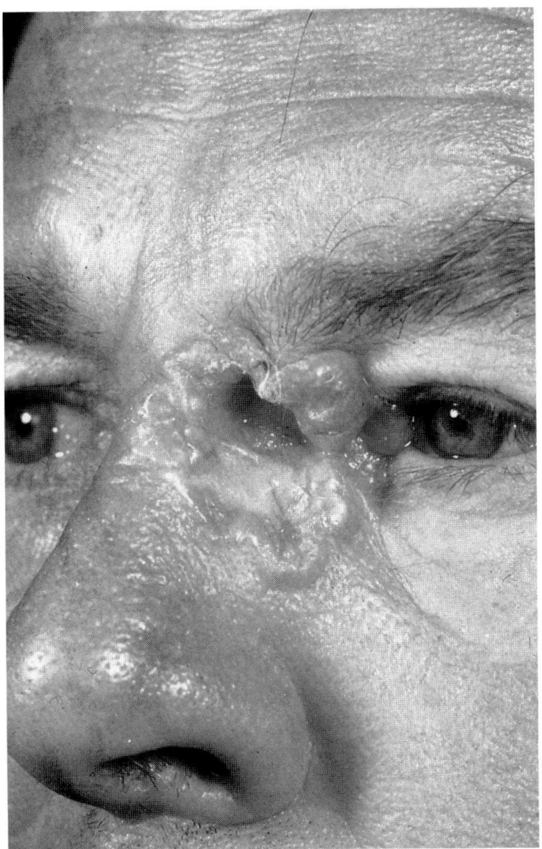

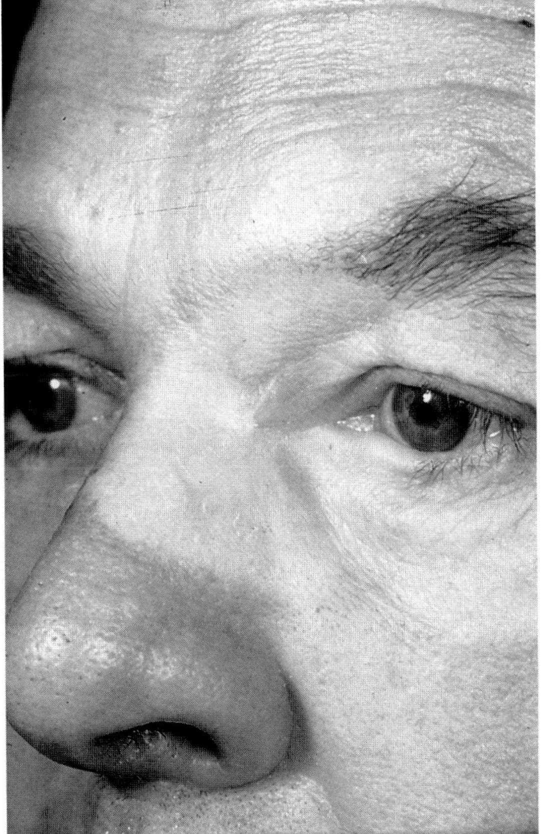

FIGURE 7.14. Very large basal cell carcinoma of the medial canthus and upper and lower eyelids with deep central ulceration. The patient was referred for radiation therapy by a plastic surgeon who felt surgery would be too disfiguring. (From ref. 90.)

FIGURE 7.15. Good functional result after treatment with 5700 cGy administered in 300-cGy fractions with a HVL of 1.4 mm Al (D½ 18 mm). Hypopigmentation is the only cosmetic side effect. (From ref. 90.)

are rare. Unusually high rates of incomplete excisions were reported by Henkind and Friedman.[51] Reconstructive surgery of the lower lid presents a major challenge to the oculoplastic surgeon. Even minor alterations in the architecture of the lower lid may result in ectropion, entropion, lagophthalmos, or epiphora.[44] In some patients, temporary tarsorrhaphy may be required to close the eyelids for several months. Radiation treatment offers a valuable therapeutic alternative for medium-sized tumors (0.5–1.5 cm) without deep tumor invasion or scarring ($T_1N_0M_0$). Properly administered modern radiotherapy yields highly satisfactory functional and cosmetic results without the need for later reconstructive surgery. Markedly raised exophytic carcinomas can be

"debulked" before radiotherapy either with a scalpel or with an electrocutting current.[52] This shortens treatment time and permits the use of softer radiation qualities.

Tumors larger than 1.5 cm in diameter, complicated tumors, or tumors with bone involvement are rarely suitable for office radiotherapy. Good functional and cosmetic results can be achieved even in large tumors by skilled oculoplastic and dermatologic surgeons by using skin flaps, grafts, or other reconstructive techniques after primary resection of the tumor.[38,39,43–45] For large and complicated tumors, the use of these more complicated, time-consuming, and expensive methods is well warranted because radiotherapy without subsequent plastic repair would not yield equivalent results.

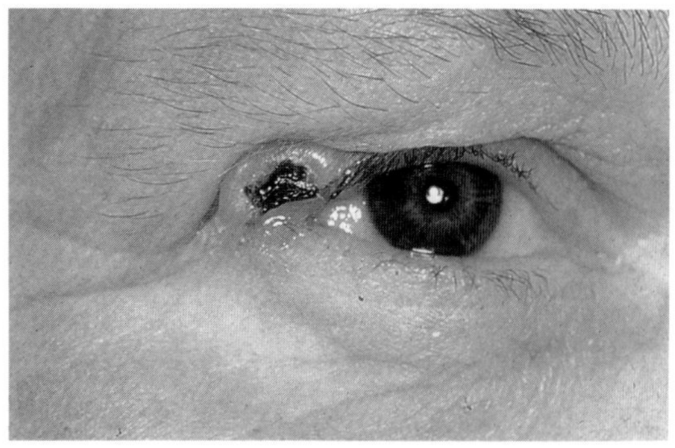

FIGURE 7.16. Large basal cell carcinoma involving the lateral margin of the upper eyelid and lateral canthus.

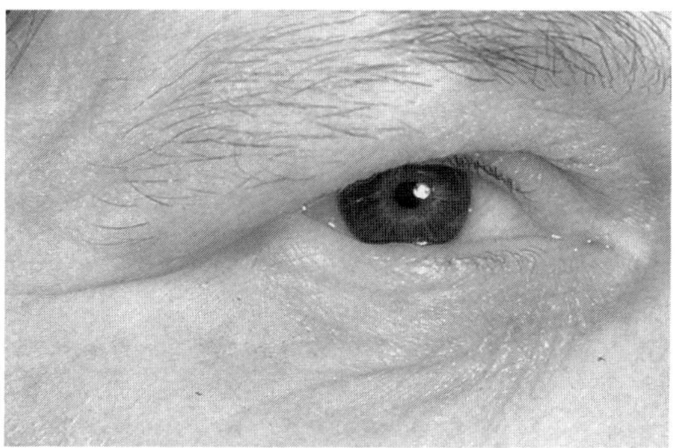

FIGURE 7.17. Excellent therapeutic and cosmetic results 2 years after radiation therapy.

Location of Tumor

There is no significant difference in techniques of treatment used in different anatomic locations of the periocular region. The principles discussed in Chapter 6 also apply to malignant tumors in this area. Special consideration is required in the area of the canthi, especially for lesions involving the inner canthus (Figs. 7.12 to 7.15), where carcinomas often extend more deeply than clinically suspected. Large field sizes and selection of a more penetrating x-ray beam are necessary in this area. This also applies to tumors of the lateral canthus (Figs. 7.16 to 7.19). Cancers of the lower lids need only routine techniques and respond well to treatment. For difficult tumors on the upper lids, especially in elderly patients, radiotherapy is preferred by some surgeons in order to eliminate the need for extensive reconstruction.[53]

Recurrent Carcinomas

Carcinomas recurring after simple surgical excision and closure can be treated successfully with x rays. Large field sizes and the selection of a sufficiently penetrating x-ray beam are important prerequisites for effective therapy.

Carcinomas recurring after any type of reconstructive surgery are not considered good indications for radiotherapy; Mohs surgery is the treatment of choice in these cases.

Recurrent cancers following previous irradiation are not an indication for radiotherapy. Robins and Bennett[53] report cure rates of 98.1% following Mohs surgery of primary periocular basal cell carcinomas and 93.6% for previously treated lesions. Tumors of the inner canthus recurring after previous radiotherapy had a higher risk of second recurrences after Mohs surgery than after other treatment modalities.

Contraindications

Radiotherapy is not indicated if the carcinoma invades deeply into cartilage and/or bone. Surgical methods or combined surgical and radiation oncology therapy are preferred in these cases.

Recurrences of any size after previous radiotherapy are not suitable for office radiotherapy.

Treatment Planning

Quality of Radiation

As explained in Chapter 6, the quality of the x-ray beam should be adapted to the measured or estimated depth of the lesion. Because of the anatomic structure of the eyelids, the dimensions of a tumor in the lower or upper lid can usually be visualized. The D½ and HVL of the radiation can then be selected according to the depth of the tumor. In our experience with medium-sized tumors, a HVL of 0.4 to 1.0 mm Al is satisfactory for most lesions. In contrast, lesions of the medial canthus (Figs. 7.12 to 7.15) are often deeply invasive; in these cases, the selection of a more penetrating x-ray beam is preferable. A HVL of at least 0.75 to 1.5 mm Al is usually necessary in this location.

Dose

Effective dose schedules are discussed in Chapter 6. The basic rules also apply to carcinomas of the

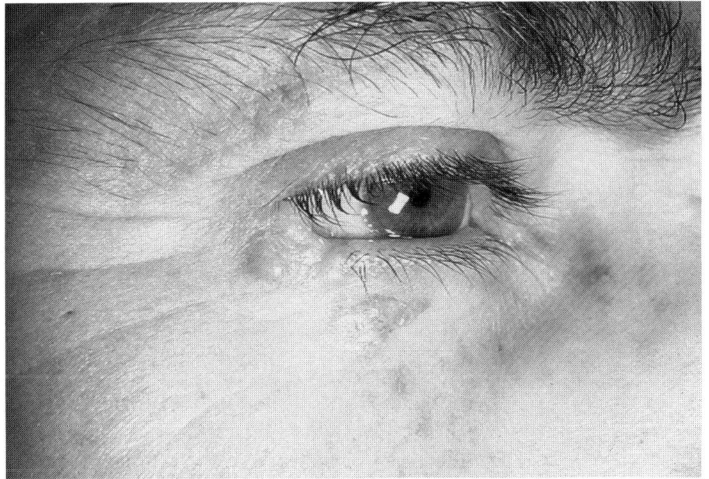

FIGURE 7.18. Large, multicentric basal cell carcinoma of the lower eyelid and lateral canthus. The patient refused surgery.

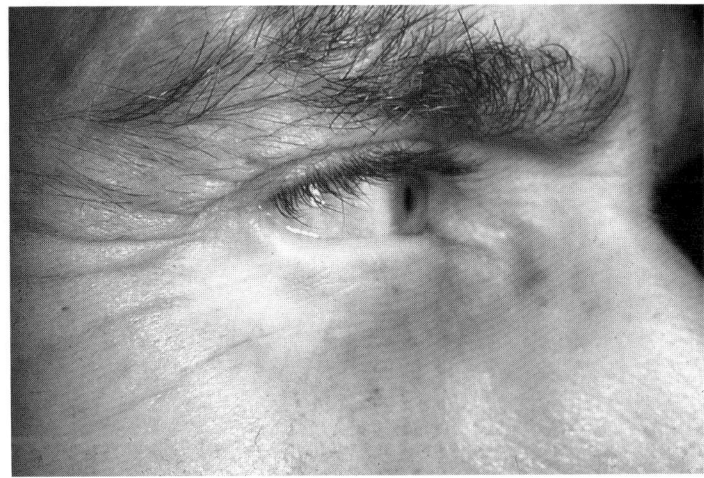

FIGURE 7.19. Good functional and cosmetic results 1 year after radiotherapy. Loss of eyelashes and some pigmentary changes are the only cosmetic side effects. (Reprinted by permission of the publisher from ref. 89. Copyright 1983 by Elsevier Science Publishing Co., Inc.)

eyelid. For small- to medium-sized tumors (up to 1.5 cm) we usually administer daily fractions of 500 cGy up to a total dose of 4000 to 5000 cGy. For exceptionally large tumors (for which we usually prefer plastic surgery or Mohs surgery), individual fractions should be reduced to 250 to 400 cGy. We use the same doses for basal cell carcinomas, squamous cell carcinomas, and keratoacanthomas. Other dose schedules are discussed in Chapter 6. Some authors recommend an additional dose of at least 500 cGy for squamous cell carcinomas.[24] Mendenhall and associates[21] recommend doses ranging from 4000 cGy in 10 fractions for lesions under 1 cm² to 6000 cGy administered over 7 weeks for larger lesions with cartilage or bone involvement.

Protection and Shielding

Meticulous shielding techniques are extremely important during radiotherapy of the eye region. The greatest (and completely avoidable) risk is the development of cataracts. A total dose of at least 350 to 400 cGy, administered in smaller fractions directly to the lens, is required to induce cataracts.[26] Modern shielding techniques have markedly reduced direct and scatter radiation to the lens. Kopf and co-workers[54] performed thermoluminescent dosimetry and calculated that, with their radiation technique for cutaneous cancers, only 27 roentgen (R) reach the lens during a full course of radiotherapy.

Shielding procedures for the eye are described and illustrated in detail by Gladstein and col-

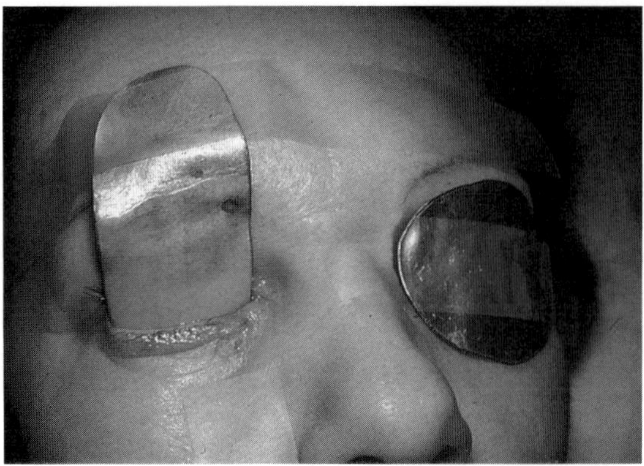

FIGURE 7.20. Lead eye shield shaped like a tongue blade and covered with a thin coating of paraffin is inserted into the lower conjunctival sac.

leagues.[24,50] Two types of eye shields are commonly used. Lead shields in the shape of a tongue blade are useful for lesions in the center of the upper or lower eyelid. For tumors involving the inner or outer canthi, the upper and lower eyelid must be exposed and brass, lead, or gold eye cups are preferred.

Tongue-Shaped Eye Shields

Tongue-shaped eye shields are used for carcinomas involving the central portion of the lower or upper lid. They were originally made of lead, 0.92 mm thick. The New York Skin and Cancer Unit has modified these eye shields to reduce the incidence of temporary benign conjunctival leukoplakia, which they observed as a result of radiation backscatter in a number of their cases. Backscatter from the eye shield to the palpebral conjunctiva could be reduced by 20% by using lead shields electroplated with 0.25 mm of copper and covered with 0.0075 mm of cadmium.[50,54,55] Before insertion of the eye shield into the palpebral cul-de-sac, a few drops of an ophthalmic anesthetic are instilled (e.g., Ophthaine, Squibb). The multilayered tongue-blade–shaped shield is carefully molded to fit comfortably into the upper or lower palpebral sac. Before use it is coated with heated paraffin and allowed to cool. The shield is then inserted and taped into position so that it is firmly secured (Fig. 7.20). Overlay shielding is then applied, which usually consists of a lead shield incorporating a cut-

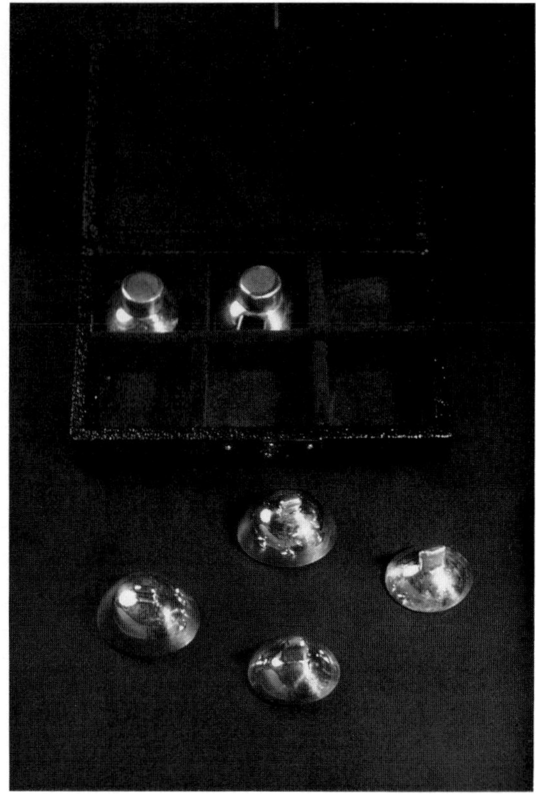

FIGURE 7.21. Set of eye shields of different sizes used to prevent cataract formation.

out area large enough to include a sufficient border of normal-appearing skin. After therapy the shields are removed gently and an ophthalmic antibiotic ointment is instilled. Since the eye is still anesthetized it is advisable to use an eye patch for 1 to 2 hours to prevent irritation by dust.

Cup-Shaped Eye Shields

Cup-shaped eye shields are used when the inner or outer canthal regions are irradiated. Tongue-shaped shields cannot be used in these locations because portions of both lids must be exposed during therapy. Formerly available commercial eye shields were made of silver-plated lead (Gougelman), brass, or gold[17] (Fig. 7.21). They are usually sold as sets with four pairs of shields fabricated of highly polished plated lead. Their lead thickness is approximately 2 mm, which permits less than 1% transmission (at 120 kV with 0.5 mm Al filtration)

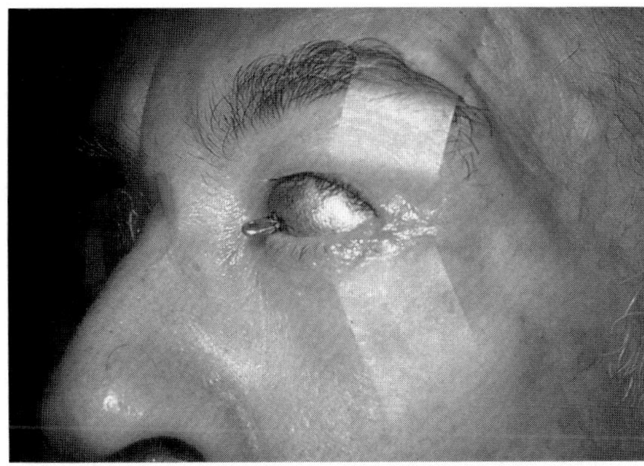
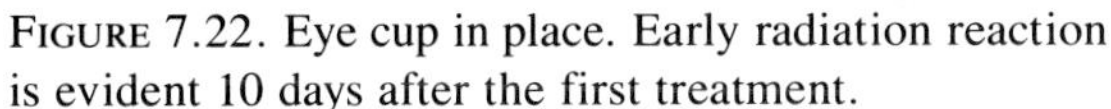

FIGURE 7.22. Eye cup in place. Early radiation reaction is evident 10 days after the first treatment.

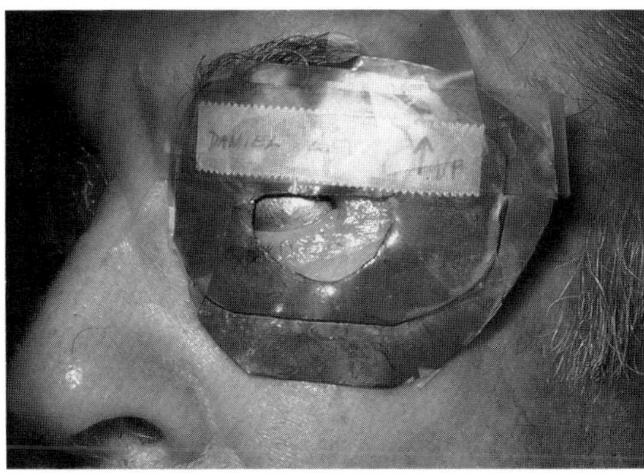

FIGURE 7.23. Overlay shielding is provided by a lead cutout with semilunar opening for the radiation portal.

(source: Victoreen Nuclear Associates, Carle Place, NY).

Gladstein[56] has recently designed a practical lead and bismuth eye shield with a handle at the end rather than in the center (Fig. 7.22). This cup is easier to insert and remove than older shield types, and the handle does not interfere with overlay shielding. After the local anesthetic has been instilled, the patient is instructed to look down and the cup is inserted under the upper lid; the lower eyelid is then pulled up over the shield. Before insertion we often apply a thin layer of paraffin or an ophthalmic antibiotic ointment to the inner and outer surfaces of the cup in order to reduce further the possibility of irritation to the cornea. The eye cup is taped into position to prevent accidental movement and is then overlaid with additional lead shielding (Fig. 7.23). Before treatment is started routine protection measures are used, especially lead shields over the noninvolved eye, as well as shielding of the thyroid and gonads (Fig. 7.24). The central beam is directed perpendicular to the area treated.

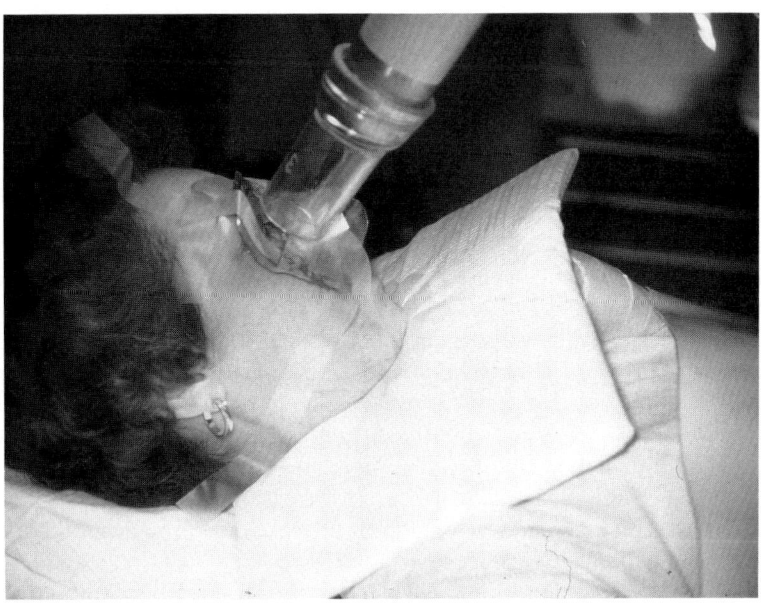

FIGURE 7.24. Additional lead shielding and thyroid protection in place prior to treatment.

Radiation Reactions

Acute Radiation Reaction

An acute radiation reaction invariably occurs after the suggested dose schedules. It is characterized by temporary erythema, erosion, and crusting. The nearby mucosal surface in the path of the x-ray beam often develops a temporary acute mucositis even before radiodermatitis of the treated skin area becomes apparent; however, it also subsides earlier. This reaction usually does not cause any major discomfort to the patient. Ophthalmic antibiotic ointments are soothing and help to reduce the possibility of secondary infections.

Chronic Radiation Sequelae

The cosmetic and functional results during the first year after treatment are usually highly satisfactory. Permanent alopecia of the eyelashes is a regular and expected effect of radiation treatments; in most patients this has no adverse functional consequences. Patients should be informed of this side effect before treatment is started. In some patients other sequelae may develop several years later, the most common of these being atrophy and telangiectasia. In a smaller percentage of patients, hypo- and hyperpigmentation and sclerotic changes may develop in later stages even though the functional results remain satisfactory.

Ectropion is a rare side effect in large tumors, where it is usually already present before therapy. It is extremely rare after appropriate radiotherapy of smaller lesions.

Epiphora (lacrimation) is rarely seen after treatment of carcinomas involving the inner canthus. In this location the tumor can affect the nasolacrimal punctum or the duct itself; obstruction of the nasolacrimal duct results in lacrimation over the border of the eyelid. Most experts agree that persistent tearing of the eyes occurs most often in patients with prior involvement and/or occlusion of the lacrimal duct, or after poorly fractionated radiotherapy with high total doses.[41] If the duct is involved only minimally by the tumor, it may reopen completely with the resolution of the tumor after the irradiation is completed. However, we feel that with pretreatment epiphora, office radiotherapy is usually not advisable. Slight temporary tearing following irritation by wind or cold may occur after treatment of carcinomas of the inner canthus in a small percentage of patients. This effect may also occur after surgery.[39] The occurrence of cataracts following radiation therapy can be completely prevented by the use of the suggested radiation protection methods.

Review of Recent Literature

Cure rates and complications of several large series of patients irradiated for cancers of eyelids have been reported by several authors. Many of these statistics summarize results of radiotherapy in large medical centers and include complicated, large, or neglected tumors.[57] Some of the statistics are also based on radiation techniques that are now considered outmoded. For these reasons the reported cure rates and frequencies of complications are obviously higher than for the uncomplicated, medium-sized tumors suitable for dermatologic office radiotherapy. Gladstein[50] describes x-ray therapy of basal cell carcinoma on periocular skin as "highly successful, easy to carry out, safe, and attended by cosmetic results that are good to excellent." He observed only two failures in 50 patients, obtained a cure rate of 96%, and consequently considers the results of x-ray treatment at least equal to other methods of treatment. The author attributes the good cosmetic results to the use of soft x-ray qualities and low total doses (3400–4080 cGy). He recommends the "standardized" New York technique with five to six individual doses of 680 cGy with a HVL of 0.9 mm Al. Minor side effects included five cases of temporary benign leukoplakia of the palpebral conjunctiva and three cases of epiphora (during cold weather[42]).

Lederman[40] reported cure rates obtained in a British radiotherapy department for basal cell carcinomas up to 4 cm in size. Ninety-five percent of 386 patients with carcinomas of the lower lid and 90.8% of 153 patients with carcinomas of the inner canthus did not show any recurrence after 4 years. No recurrences were seen after 15 years in 74 patients with basal cell carcinoma of the upper lid; only one recurrence was observed in 17 patients with cancer of the outer canthus. Three of 51 patients with squamous cell carcinomas died of complications of their carcinomas. Other complications were rare: 12% developed telangiectasias and/or changes in pigment, 7%

some deformity of lids, and 10% epiphora (mostly patients with a lid deformity).

Del Regato and Spjut[58] described treatment of 159 basal cell carcinomas of the orbit (representing 12% of all basal cell carcinomas of the skin of the face) in a radiation oncology department. Sixty five of these were located on the lower lid, 60 in the inner canthus, 17 in the outer canthus, and 17 on the upper eyelid. Treatment was administered in daily fractions of 150 to 250 cGy up to a total dose of 4000 to 5000 cGy over a period of 3 to 4 weeks. Only nine recurrences were observed after radiotherapy of 117 tumors of all sizes.

Wiskemann and associates[6] used soft x rays (D½, 6–11 mm) in 98 basal cell carcinomas of the periorbital region and achieved a cure rate of 96%. Temporary epiphora was noted in 5% of patients and slight ectropion in 2% of patients with larger tumors.

Fischbach and associates[36] treated 32 carcinomas of eyelids in a radiation oncology department and observed only one recurrence after a total dose of 4000 cGy. Contracture of an eyelid occurred in one recurrent carcinoma previously treated by surgery. Storck and colleagues[17] gave soft x-ray treatment to 271 patients, some with complicated tumors, and reported 25 recurrences. Most of these were located in the medial canthus. Occasional epiphora occurred in 5% to 10%; less than 5% developed an ectropion or entropion.

Fitzpatrick and co-workers[59] treated most of 565 tumors of eyelids (505 basal cell carcinomas, 36 squamous cell carcinomas) with only 3000 to 4000 cGy in 500 cGy daily fractions and a HVL of 0.7 mm Al. The series included large tumors encompassing both eyelids. All tumors were larger than 5 mm; the average tumor diameter was 12 mm. The recurrence rate was only 4.8%, and the cosmetic and functional results of 121 patients after 5 years were excellent in 93 patients (77%) and good in 21 patients (17%). Epiphora occurred in 21 patients; it existed prior to treatment in eight of these patients. This problem was successfully managed by dilating and syringing the lacrimal duct; only two patients required surgical repair. Severe telangiectasias were seen in seven of 565 patients (1%), and severe atrophy in 17 of 565 patients (3%). In 25% of their patients with small tumors, a single high-dose radiation exposure (2000–2250 cGy) seemed to be as effective in terms of cure, cosme-

sis, and functional result as more frequent fractionated doses.[59,60] Panizzon[14] reported 79% good cosmetic results in 251 patients with basal cell carcinomas of the eyelids. Petrovich and associates[25] irradiated 159 patients with eyelid cancers and found a much higher recurrence rate than in cancer of the nose. They attributed this to insufficient radiation margins related to fear of complications during administration of x rays.

Several authors reported results after contact therapy, some with less satisfactory cure rates.

Renfer[41] described the resolution of 25 carcinomas in and around the inner canthus region following radiotherapy with small individual fractions; his 5-year cure rate was only 85%. Most patients were irradiated with contact therapy units.

Saitmacher and Kropp[60] treated 109 carcinomas of eyelids with contact therapy and achieved a 5-year cure rate of 87.5%; the highest tendency for recurrence was observed in tumors of the medial canthus (23.8%). Functional and cosmetic results were considered good in more than 80% of all patients. Most recurrences occurred during the first 3 years; 91% were noticed during the first 5 years after therapy.

In contrast, Domonkos[61] reported results of various treatment modalities for 240 patients with carcinomas of eyelids, most of whom were treated by contact therapy. The cure rate was 97%.

The advantages of electron-beam therapy for tumors of eyelids were described by Tapley and Fletcher,[37] who treated 41 carcinomas of the eyelids and inner canthi with a 7-MeV betatron beam. Most patients received 6000 to 7000 cGy in 4 to 5 weeks. Only five out of 41 patients followed longer than 2 years (12%) developed recurrences, and most of these were in the inner canthus. Complications were infrequent and mild. The authors stressed the advantages of the sharp fall-off in dose beyond the selected depth and the relative protection of underlying structures. Side effects were more common with higher energy electron beams (11 MeV) and higher total doses. Radiation protection is more difficult for electron therapy than for x-ray therapy.

Collin[39] reported the following recurrence rates after surgery; 2.3% following primary surgery of 176 cases, 18.4% after surgery of irradiated cancers, 30% after surgery of previously operated cancers, and two deaths after surgery of previously

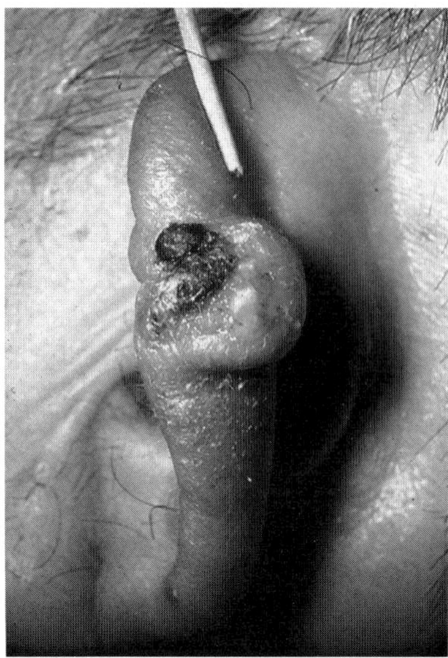

FIGURE 7.25. 1.8-cm nodular, ulcerated, and crusted squamous cell carcinoma of margin of ear.

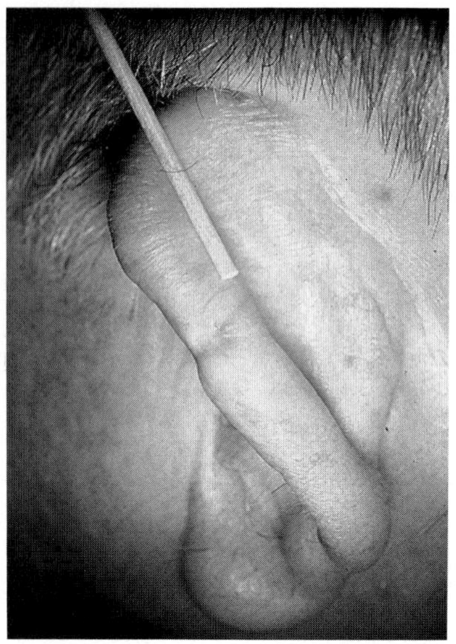

FIGURE 7.26. Good cosmetic result with slight "notching" 2 years after use of crossfire technique with 12 400-cGy fractions of x rays (HVL 0.75 mm Al; D½ 12 mm).

operated and irradiated cancers. He warned that basal cell carcinoma of the eyelid may develop into a potentially lethal condition; 3.5% of the patients in his series with recurrent large basal cell carcinomas in the medial canthus died of their disease.

Similar recurrence rates are observed following surgery; Bart and associates[38] reported an 87% cure rate following surgical excision of 23 basal cell carcinomas of the periocular region.

Carcinoma of the Ear

Carcinomas of the ear are not uncommon. Five percent to 10% of all cutaneous carcinomas occur in this area, and the incidence is higher in men than in women.[62] In contrast to older reports of poor therapeutic results or development of painful chondritis that have led many dermatologists to believe that it is unwise to irradiate cancers of the ear, most carcinomas of the ear do respond well to modern radiotherapy. Modern fractionated treatment techniques with soft x rays have replaced formerly used high-increment, penetrating radiation techniques and have reduced side effects to a minimum. Properly executed radiation therapy offers an excellent alternative to some forms of surgery where partial resec-

tion of the pinna followed by extensive reconstruction is the only therapeutic choice. In patients with other health problems, side effects from anesthetics and other complications can be avoided, and hospitalization is not required for radiotherapy. Radiation treatments also offer a useful alternative for patients who refuse surgery.

Indications for Radiotherapy

Type of Carcinoma

Basal cell carcinomas of the ear can be treated effectively by radiotherapy. Squamous cell carcinomas, although less frequent, are at least as radiosensitive as basal cell carcinomas. This applies both to well-differentiated and pseudoglandular tumors and to moderately to poorly differentiated squamous cell carcinomas. Some squamous cell carcinomas of the pinna have a definite tendency to metastasize to regional lymph nodes and some patients may die of secondary complications. Fitzpatrick[20] reported cervical node metastases in 12 patients (8%) with squamous cell carcinoma. Squamous cell carcinomas of the ear therefore should never be regarded as harmless tumors and the patient must be examined and followed closely.[62]

Size of Tumor

Small cancers (up to 1 cm) of the anterior or posterior surface of the pinna usually can be excised easily or treated with cryosurgery[63] or curettage and electrodesiccation. Primary excision and closure is more problematic in medium-sized tumors (1–3 cm), which are often seen in dermatologists' offices. In these cases simple surgical techniques often cause unsightly cosmetic defects; to prevent these, complicated grafting or flap techniques are required.[64,65] For this type of lesion $(T_1N_0M_0)$, radiotherapy offers a satisfactory therapeutic alternative; it is easy and usually affords good cosmetic results. Changes of the contour of the ear (often seen after surgical treatment) are rare, and unsightly chronic radiation sequelae are uncommon in this anatomic region. Even larger cancers (2–3 cm) with early invasion of cartilage respond well to radiation treatments[5]; however, when they are situated at the margin of the ear a slight "notching" defect can be seen after healing, which is limited to the actual area of the tumor and usually is much smaller than after simple surgical resection, where a considerable margin of healthy skin has to be sacrificed (Figs. 7.25 and 7.26). Various surgical methods are preferable in extensive lesions (larger than 3 cm) and in all tumors that are not moveable or where a satisfactory cosmetic result after irradiation is precluded by the destructive tendency of the tumor.[64,65] Radiotherapy seems of special importance, however, in medium-sized lesions (1–3 cm in diameter) where resection and/or reconstructive surgery would result in a noticeable cosmetic defect, or when patients object to more complicated surgical treatments. Cancers of any size with deep invasion of the cartilage are best treated with surgical methods even though some radiation oncologists report satisfactory therapeutic results without any complications in tumors overlying, or even grossly involving, cartilage.[25]

Location of Tumor

Cutaneous cancers in all locations of the ear can be irradiated effectively, including tumors of the concha, helix, antihelix, antitragus, lobule, rim, and posterior surface (Figs. 7.24 to 7.34). When the tumor involves both the ventral and dorsal surfaces of the ear, treatment with a "cross-fire technique" (50% of tumor dose given to both surfaces from front and back) is often advisable, particularly for "wraparound" lesions involving both surfaces of the helix or lobule (Figs. 7.25 and 7.26). Special considerations are necessary for cancers of the introitus of the ear and the retroauricular sulcus.

Introitus and Ear Canal

Radiotherapy of cancers in this location is not in the realm of dermatologic office radiotherapy. These tumors often extend more deeply than expected and should be referred to radiation oncology centers or otologic surgical experts.[5,58,66]

Retroauricular Sulcus

Like cancers of the nasolabial fold, tumors of the retroauricular sulcus may invade deeply and they have a high tendency to recur (Figs. 7.35 to 7.38). A plan to treat these tumors surgically must take this into consideration and the final results are not always pleasing cosmetically (the result is often "pinned down ears"). Radiotherapy offers a therapeutic alternative for patients in whom more complicated surgical techniques are not advisable. The dermatologic radiotherapist can often overcome these problems by selecting a more penetrating radiation quality (at least 0.75, and up to 1.5 cm Al HVL) and by including a large margin of apparently healthy skin (at least 8–10 mm).

Recurrent Carcinomas

Cutaneous cancers recurring after electrosurgery or simple excision and closure can be treated effectively by radiotherapy. Recurrences after reconstructive surgery are not suitable for office radiotherapy and are best treated by Mohs surgery; this applies especially to recurrent tumors in the retroauricular sulcus. Carcinomas recurring after radiotherapy should not be re-treated with x rays.

Contraindications

Radiotherapeutic methods are not indicated if there is involvement of deep cartilage or bone or if there is evidence of obvious structural deformities of the pinna. Carcinomas extending into the external ear canal also are not suitable for office radiotherapy. Patients with metastases should be referred to radiation oncology departments.

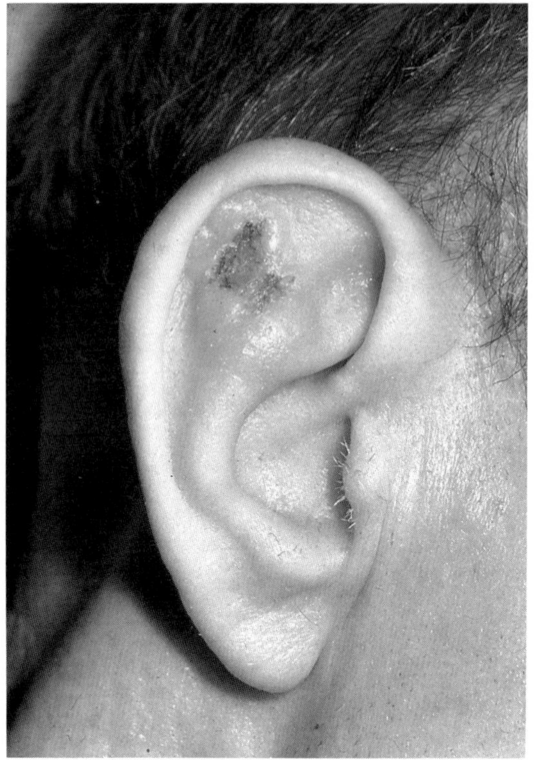

FIGURE 7.27. Squamous cell carcinoma of the ear measuring 2.5 × 1.5 cm that had recurred 3 times after curettage and electrodesiccation. Surgical excision would have required extensive reconstructive work.

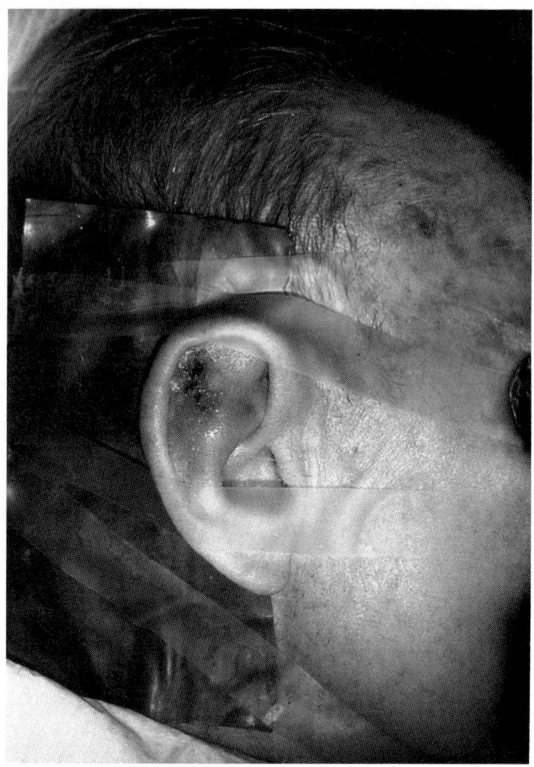

FIGURE 7.28. Lead shield applied between scalp and ear to prevent side effects (i.e., alopecia) related to exit dose.

Treatment Planning

Quality of Radiation

Principles of quality of radiation are discussed in Chapter 6. Small and superficially located cutaneous cancers can often be treated with a HVL of only 0.4 mm Al, which reduces the exit dose considerably and results in an even better cosmetic appearance of the treated area. More elevated tumors require at least a HVL of 0.75 to 1 mm Al. Markedly raised exophytic carcinomas can be debulked before radiotherapy with a scalpel or with an electrocutting current.[52] It has already been pointed out that tumors in the retroauricular region require radiation qualities of at least 0.75 to 1.5 mm Al.

Dose

Various effective dose schedules are discussed in Chapter 6. We use daily doses of 500 cGy, 5 times

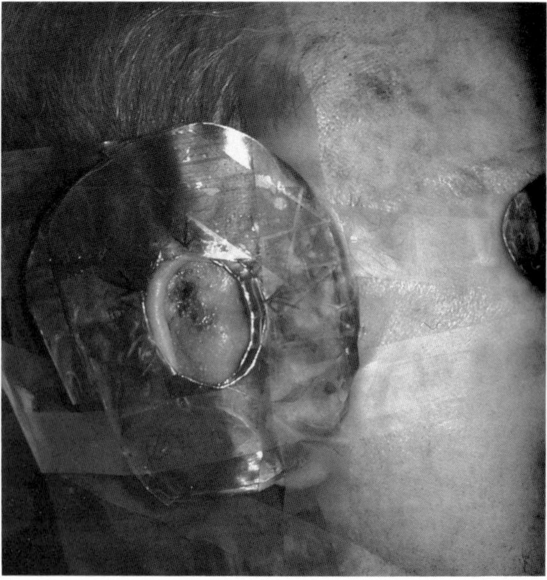

FIGURE 7.29. Overlay lead shield limits radiation to involved area.

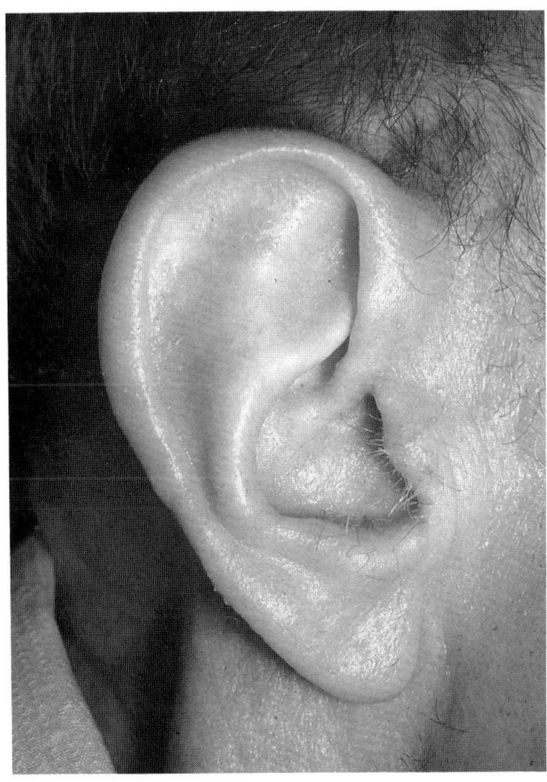

FIGURE 7.30. Good cosmetic result 5 years after treatment with 4400 cGy (43 kV; HVL 0.38 mm Al; D½ 6 mm) delivered in 400-cGy fractions over a 17-day period. (Reprinted by permission of the publisher from Ref. 89. Copyright 1983 by Elsevier Science Publishing Co., Inc.)

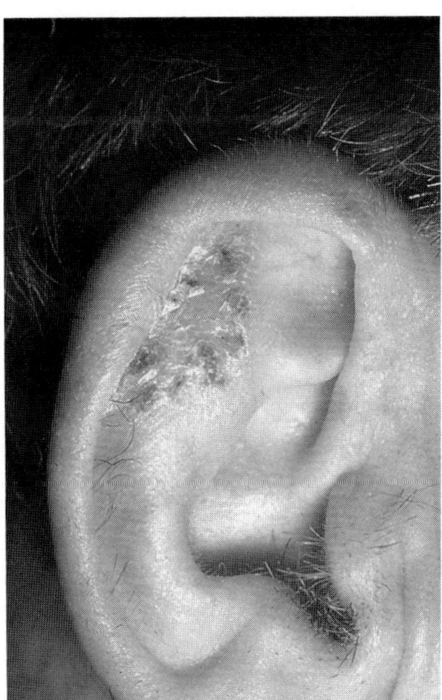

FIGURE 7.31. Crusted basal cell carcinoma that had recurred 3 times following curettage and electrodesiccation, measuring 2.5 × 1.5 cm. (From ref. 90.)

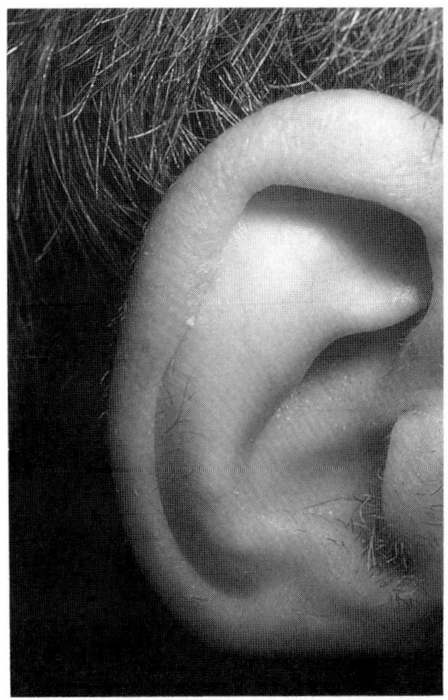

FIGURE 7.32. Good therapeutic and cosmetic results after radiotherapy with 5500 cGy (43 kV; HVL 0.38 mm Al; D½ 6 mm) delivered over a 2 week period. (From ref. 90.)

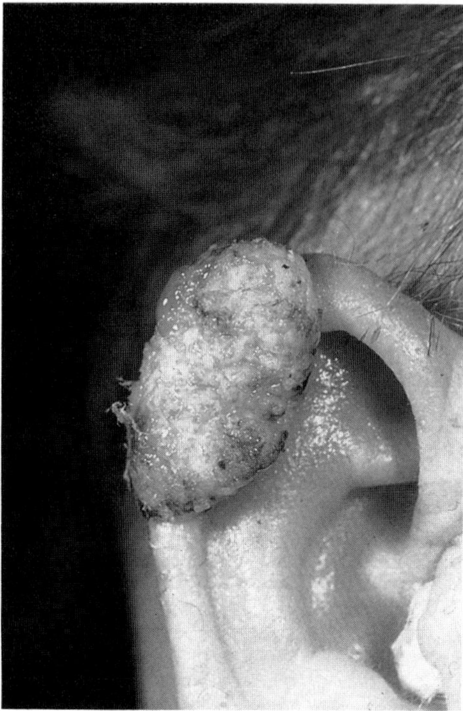

FIGURE 7.33. Exophytic, squamous cell carcinoma of the pinna measuring 3.8 cm. The patient refused surgery. Such a tumor could be "debulked" before beginning radiotherapy.

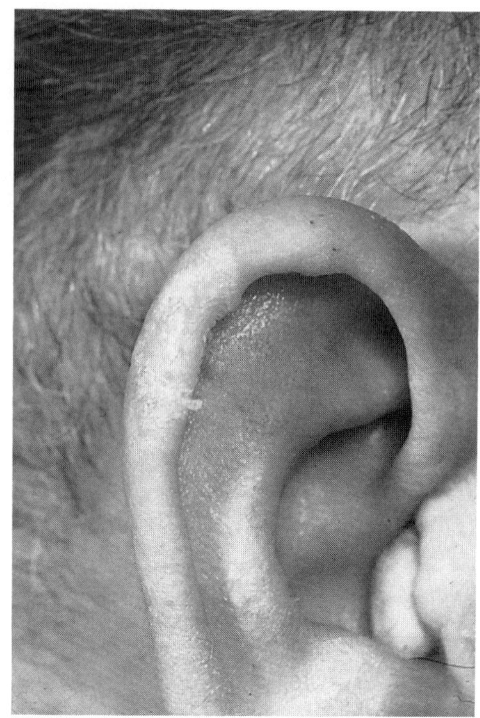

FIGURE 7.34. Complete resolution of the tumor 6 weeks after radiation therapy with a total dose of 5600 cGy given in fractions within 24 days (50 kV; HVL 1.4 mm Al; D½ 18 mm).

per week, up to a total of 4000 to 5000 cGy for most carcinomas of the ear. For larger tumors (>3 cm in diameter), individual fractions may be reduced to 250 to 350 cGy up to a total dose of 5000 to 6000 cGy (Figs. 7.33, 7.34, 7.37, 7.38). Some radiation oncologists use even smaller daily doses (200 cGy) over a period of 4 to 6 weeks, with a total dose of 5000 to 6000 cGy.[5,58,66]

Protection and Shielding

As in all tumors on the face, the eye region should be protected with lead eye shields during treatment. The importance of shielding the thyroid and gonads has been stressed in Chapter 5.

Because the pinna of the ear is a relatively thin structure, the exit dose is of greater importance than in other anatomic areas. Special shielding techniques (Figs. 7.28 and 7.29) are necessary to prevent undesirable side effects, such as temporary or permanent alopecia of the hairy scalp behind the ear.

Anterior Surface of Ear

A crescent-shaped lead shield is placed between the posterior surface of the ear and the head to minimize the exit dose (Fig. 7.28). The surrounding uninvolved skin of the anterior surface in the periphery of the tumor is protected with a sufficiently large lead cutout (Fig. 7.29). When indicated, a small lead shield can be inserted into the ear canal to protect the posterior aspect of the ear canal.

Posterior Surface of Ear and Retroauricular Sulcus

The ear is bent forward to expose the involved area, and lead shielding is applied to both surfaces

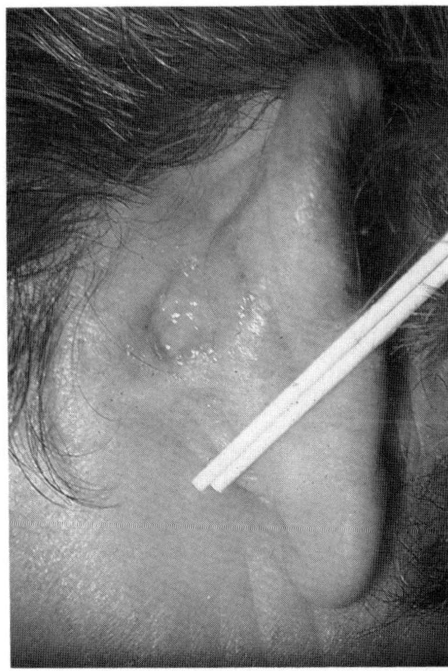

FIGURE 7.35. Erosive basal cell carcinoma, 2.8 × 1.5 cm, of the posterior auricular area with deep central ulceration. The tumor had recurred 1 year after primary excision and closure.

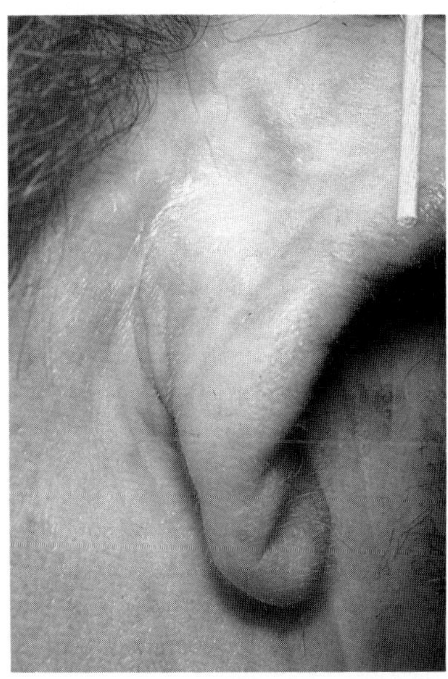

FIGURE 7.36. Excellent resolution of tumor 6 months after 5600 cGy of x rays (50 kV; HVL 0.75 mm Al; D½ 12 mm) delivered in 400-cGy fractions.

of the ear to prevent side effects from the exit dose. After the lead shield has been placed between the preauricular skin and the anterior auricular surface, the pinna is fixed with tape to assure as flat a surface as possible, and overlay shielding with a sufficiently large margin is then applied.

Radiation Reactions

Acute Radiation Reaction

The sequence of postradiation changes is not different from reactions in other skin areas. When more penetrating radiation is used on the anterior surface of the pinna, a mild erythematous reaction may appear on the posterior surface of the ear opposite the radiation field. This is followed by a mild scaling reaction for up to 2 weeks. As pointed out previously, care must be taken to protect the scalp from the exit dose to prevent temporary alopecia.

Chronic Radiation Sequelae

With the exception of some atrophic changes, telangiectasias, and occasional ivory-colored discolora-

tion of the radiation field, the ear does not have a strong tendency to develop unsightly radiation sequelae. A depressed scar or notching of the border of the ear is seen only in patients with large and/or deep carcinomas. Radiation chondritis or chondronecrosis is a rare side effect when modern radiation techniques are used. Permanent epilation of the treatment field is an unavoidable but cosmetically insignificant side effect of radiotherapy to the retroauricular fold.

Review of Recent Literature

The reports of the following authors include complicated carcinomas of the ear of all sizes, and therefore the incidence of recurrences and radiation side effects is higher than for the limited indications recommended by us.

Storck and colleagues[17] and Panizzon[14] treated 422 carcinomas of all sizes with satisfactory results. The recurrence rate of irradiated cancers of the helix, tragus, and posterior surface of the pinna was 10%, and 20% for the retroauricular sulcus. The authors warn against simple radiotherapy of carcinomas extending into the external auditory canal

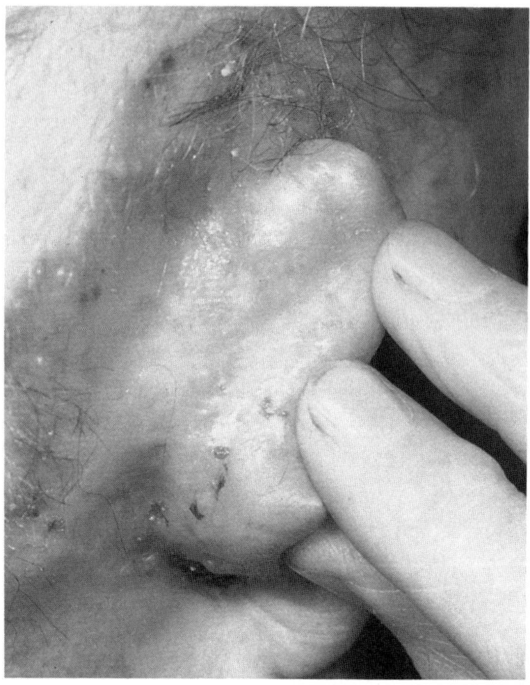

FIGURE 7.37. A very large but relatively superficial basal cell carcinoma of the posterior auricular area, retroauricular sulcus, and scalp in an elderly patient who refused surgery. (Reprinted by permission of the publisher from ref. 89. Copyright 1983 by Elsevier Science Publishing Co., Inc. From ref. 7, with permission.)

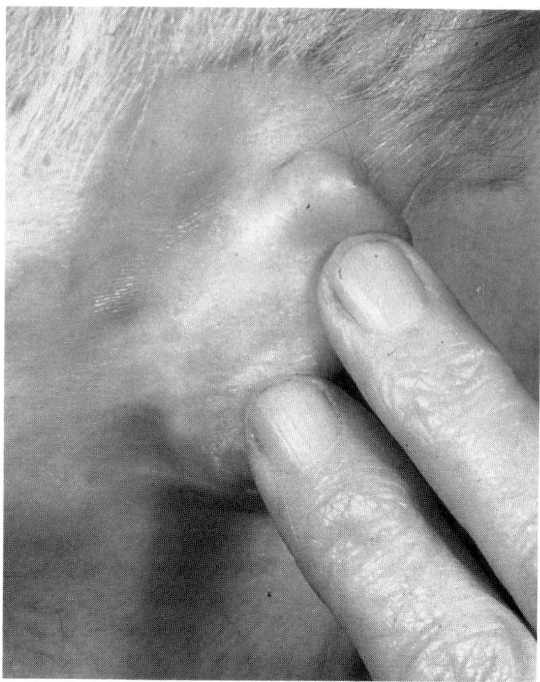

FIGURE 7.38. Appearance 8 months after radiotherapy with 5400 cGy administered in 300-cGy fractions over a 4 week period (43 kV; HVL 0.38 mm Al; D½ 6 mm). (Reprinted by permission of the publisher from ref. 89. Copyright 1983 by Elsevier Science Publishing Co., Inc. From ref. 7, with permission.)

and recommend combined radiation therapy and surgery for tumors that invade bone. Surgical treatment is preferred for carcinomas involving cartilage.

Del Regato and Vuksanovich[1] reported a cure rate of 91% in 11 previously untreated cases of carcinomas of ears. Twenty four recurrences after surgical and other treatments were irradiated in a radiation oncology department, with a re-recurrence rate of 13%. The authors consider radiation therapy the treatment of choice for most tumors. The only cases of radionecrosis occurred in patients irradiated for recurrences of cancers previously treated with radium. Chahbazian and Brown[57] recently confirmed these findings. Wiskemann and associates[6] treated 21 cases of carcinoma of the ear with soft x rays and obtained a cure rate of 86% with good cosmetic results. Two cases developed chondronecrosis.

Mustafa[35] analyzed the distribution of 192 carcinomas of the ear: 41.6% occurred on the helix, 17.5% on the antihelix, 14% on the concha, 10.3% in the retroauricular sulcus, 6.3% on the posterior surface of the ear, 4.7% on the tragus, and 3.6% on the lobule. For 94 patients with tumors smaller than 2.5 cm, the cure rate following contact therapy was 97%; for larger and recurrent tumors the cure rate was considerably lower. Several patients with squamous cell carcinomas developed metastases, and nine patients died of complications. Chondronecrosis occurred in 11 cases; of these, three were treated surgically and the remainder healed spontaneously.

Fiebelkorn and Gräfe[67] reported on 90 cases of carcinomas of ears and stated that they obtained good cosmetic results in small cancers that had not invaded cartilage (12% recurrence rate, mostly in the periphery of the field). Larger tumors with involvement of the cartilage or adjacent scalp were more resistant to treatment, and several patients died of metastatic squamous cell carcinoma.

Von Balogh and Schwarz[68] also stressed that carcinomas of the ear should not be considered harmless tumors. They treated 162 basal cell and 130 squamous cell carcinomas of all sizes in a radiotherapy department, including in their treatment schedules massive single doses that are now considered inadvisable. The total cure rate for all types of radiotherapy was only 76% for basal cell carcinomas and 71% for squamous cell carcinomas. The authors attributed these poor results to various factors, including type of tumor (squamous cell carcinomas have a worse prognosis than do basal cell carcinomas), size of tumor (more recurrences occur in tumors larger than 2 cm), location (tumors in the external auditory canal and retroauricular sulcus are more resistant to radiation), involvement of cartilage (poor prognosis), and presence of metastases.

Parker and Wildermuth[69] administered x-ray treatment to 39 of 77 patients with cutaneous cancers of the pinna and achieved a primary cure rate of 88%. The authors stressed that radiotherapy is a useful alternative in patients for whom surgical resection would be cosmetically objectionable.

Bart and co-workers[33] reported a 5-year cure rate of 92.3% for 33 carcinomas of the ear treated by the standardized x-ray technique of the New York Skin and Cancer Unit. Primary excision of nine basal cell carcinomas of the ear done at the same center showed a cure rate of 66.7%.[38]

Avila and colleagues[70] described 97 consecutive cases of carcinoma of the pinna (56 basal cell carcinomas, 30 squamous cell carcinomas): 50 patients were surgically treated and 45 were irradiated. Small and/or peripheral lesions were excised and the large and/or centrally located lesions were referred for irradiation. Analysis of the results showed no difference in rates of control of the tumors; the rates of complication were also comparable. Three cases of chondritis were observed after radiotherapy; all of these had received high doses. One case of chondritis was also seen after surgery. The primary cure rate after radiotherapy was 87%; radiotherapy was used in some patients for a second course with a 93% total cure rate.

Pless[71] treated 260 carcinomas of the ear by standard surgical techniques. The recurrence rate at 5 years was 18% for basal cell carcinomas and 15% for squamous cell carcinomas. Twenty percent of the squamous cell carcinomas showed regional lymph node metastases.

Carcinoma of the Lip

Squamous cell carcinoma is more common on the lower lip, whereas basal cell carcinoma is more common on the upper lip. Cancers of the lower lip are 8 times more common than cancers of the upper lip, and they occur 5 times more frequently in men than in women.[17] Even though most squamous cell carcinomas are well differentiated, easy to diagnose, and highly curable by irradiation or excision, they should never be considered harmless tumors. In a large series of cases, metastases were reported in 13% of patients, usually involving the submaxillary or submental nodes. Only one of 519 patients developed distant metastases.[66,72] More than 90% of metastases occur within the first 2 years, often during the first 6 months after initial surgery. Frequent follow-up is required during this period.[73] The rates of metastasis, recurrence, and mortality correlate to a significant degree with the microscopic differentiation and depth of invasion of the tumor. Metastases are significantly more frequent in large carcinomas of the lip than in smaller tumors (Jorgenson, 869 cases[73]). Tumors smaller than 1 cm in diameter rarely metastasize. Although it may be uncommon for a practicing dermatologist to observe a metastasis, referral hospitals report a higher rate. Basal cell carcinomas often develop in the skin of the upper lip and extend secondarily into the vermilion border of the lip.

Indications for Radiotherapy

Type of Carcinoma

Squamous cell carcinomas in various stages of differentiation are highly radiosensitive and respond well to treatment.[5,58,66,74,75] Basal cell carcinomas of the upper lip can be treated as effectively as other basal cell cancers of the facial region.[76]

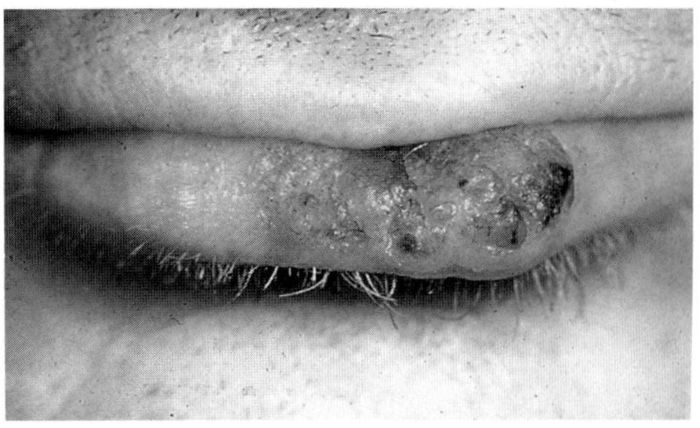

FIGURE 7.39. Crusted squamous-cell carcinoma of the lip measuring 2.2 cm. The patient refused surgery, which would have resulted in significant loss of lip tissue. (From ref. 90.)

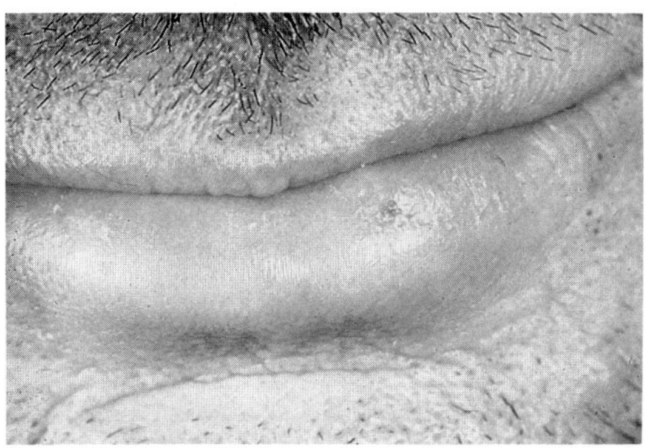

FIGURE 7.40. Result 2 months after 6000 cGy of x rays (50 kV; HVL 0.9 mm Al; D½ 15 mm) delivered over a 3 week period. (From ref. 90.)

Size of Tumor

Control of the primary tumor is rarely a problem in this accessible type of carcinoma. The choice of the therapeutic method depends largely on the size of the tumor. Well-defined tumors that are smaller than 1 cm are suitable for either surgery or radiotherapy. Surgical methods are favored for these small tumors in view of both the time needed for a course of radiotherapy and the potential later solar damage, particularly in younger patients.[77,78]

For somewhat larger lesions (1–2 cm, $T_1N_0M_0$) or even for some cancers up to 3 cm in diameter, where destruction of the lip by the tumor is minor but where surgical excision would necessitate more extensive plastic repair, radiotherapy is often preferred by dermatologists who are familiar with the good cosmetic and functional results obtainable with ionizing radiation[66] (Figs. 7.39 and 7.40). A recent comparison of 37 patients treated with either surgery or radiotherapy showed comparable cure rates but better functional results in irradiated patients, primarily due to the loss of sensation and elasticity following extensive surgery.[79]

Large (2 cm) or highly destructive tumors ($T_2N_0M_0$) can also be controlled by radiotherapy. However, primary resection is preferable in most of these cases because reconstructive surgery of irradiated lesions at a later stage will often be desirable for cosmetic reasons.

Location of Tumor

Most squamous cell carcinomas involve the central two-thirds of the lower lip. Radiotherapy is also effective in carcinomas involving the commissures of the lips, where surgical methods are often difficult. Treatment techniques are the same as for tumors in other locations. A sufficiently large border of normal-appearing lip must be included: it should be at least 0.5 to 1.0 cm wide in well-defined tumors, and up to 1.5 cm wide in tumors with indistinct borders. The inclusion of a large normal border is particularly important in the treatment of carcinomas recurring after surgery.

Recurrent Carcinomas

Carcinomas recurring after surgical treatment can be treated by radiotherapy.[66,75] The selection of a wider border is essential to effect a final cure.

Contraindications

Tumors larger than 2 cm are more suitable for primary resection because reconstructive surgery will often be required after radiotherapy. In the past, cancers recurring after radiotherapy were often treated with a second full course of radiation. This practice is discouraged in modern dermatologic therapy because of the danger of severe radiation sequelae.

Cancers with evident metastases can be successfully irradiated but are not suitable for office radiotherapy. These patients should be referred to radiation oncology departments.

Treatment Planning

Quality of Radiation

The selection of the proper radiation quality depends on the depth of the tumor, which can be determined by biopsy or by palpation. Since the thickness of the entire lip is known, it is rarely necessary to use radiation with a HVL higher than 1 or 2 mm Al (D½, 12–20 mm); in many early cases (i.e., most of those seen in office dermatology) a HVL of only 0.75 mm may be sufficient to permit adequate treatment of the entire tumor.

Dose

For carcinomas up to 3 cm, daily doses of 350 to 500 cGy can be used, up to a total dose of 5000 cGy. Other dose schedules are mentioned in Chapter 6.

Radiation Protection and Shielding

As in all types of radiotherapy of the head region, both eyes should be protected by external lead eye shields. Protection of the thyroid is also important in view of the anatomic proximity.[26] Shields for gonads are used routinely.

Since the exit dose can cause irritation of the gums and damage the teeth, a lead shield covered with a rubber finger cot is inserted between the buccal and gingival mucosa. An overlay lead shield is then firmly taped to the skin.[27] Similar protection techniques for radiation therapy of the upper lip are illustrated in Figure 7.41. At least 1 cm of apparently normal skin and/or mucous membrane should be included in the periphery of the treated field. For tumors extending to the buccal surface, the lip can be everted and taped into position to expose the tumor in such a way that the central beam will be perpendicular to the surface of the tumor. The lip can be packed forward by gauze inserted between the lip and gum. Large tumors involving the entire lip (both outer and inner surfaces) are best treated in radiation oncology departments.

For lesions up to 2 cm in size involving the skin below the vermilion border and extending posteriorly into the mucosa, a cross-fire technique may be used.[74] The first treatment (with 50% of the daily dose) is administered to the outer surface of the tumor at right angles to the teeth. A second treat-ment (with 50% of the daily dose) is then delivered to the buccal mucosa of the lip by everting the lip with a cotton roll and inserting a shield between the lip and the skin of the chin (in addition to the lead shield inserted between lip and teeth). The selection of a larger TSD (30 cm) is advisable.

Radiation Reactions

Acute Radiation Reaction

During the course of radiotherapy, the treated area tends to develop an erythematous, edematous, exudative, and crusted reaction that is usually more severe than in other body regions. The buccal mucosa affected by the exit dose develops an erosive reaction earlier than the treated skin region but also heals more quickly. The patient should be reassured that this mucositis is a normal and expected side effect of the treatment.

Undesirable reactions of the gingival mucosa can be completely prevented by the special shielding techniques already described.

Chronic Radiation Sequelae

The main advantage of radiotherapy also applies to tumors of the lip: the contour of the lip is not changed and no normal tissue is removed. For this reason the functional results of radiotherapy often surpass surgical results.[79] Late cosmetic results are also satisfactory. During the first 1 or 2 years after radiotherapy of relatively small lesions, the treated area is inconspicuous. Chronic radiodermatitis, manifested by atrophy, hypo- and hyperpigmentation, and telangiectasias, may appear in some patients at later stages, especially when additional solar damage is not prevented. The healed lip must be shielded from sunburn and irritation by smoking. Patients should be instructed to use effective sunscreen products on the lip and surrounding normal skin. They should also be informed that permanent alopecia will develop in the beard and mustache areas included in the treated field.

Review of Recent Literature

Landthaler and associates[80] recently described results of radiotherapy with soft x rays of 109 carcinomas of the lip in 107 patients (102 men, 5

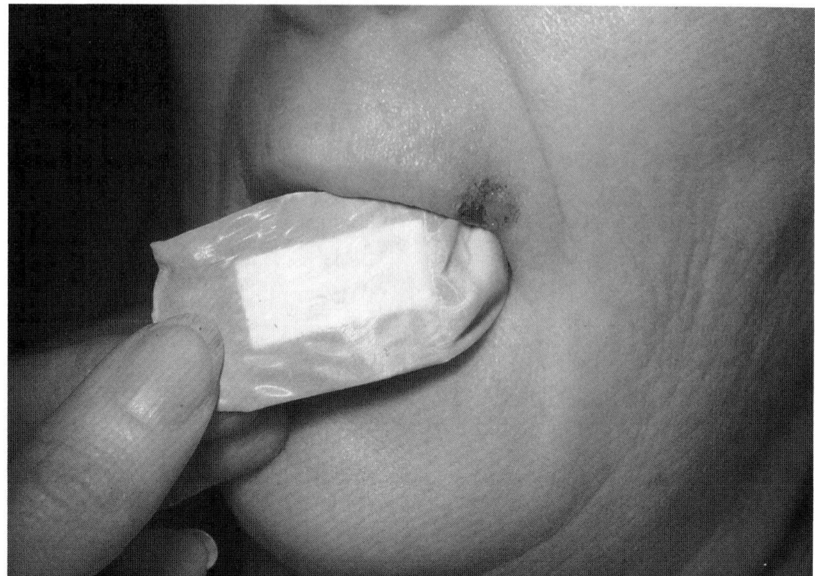

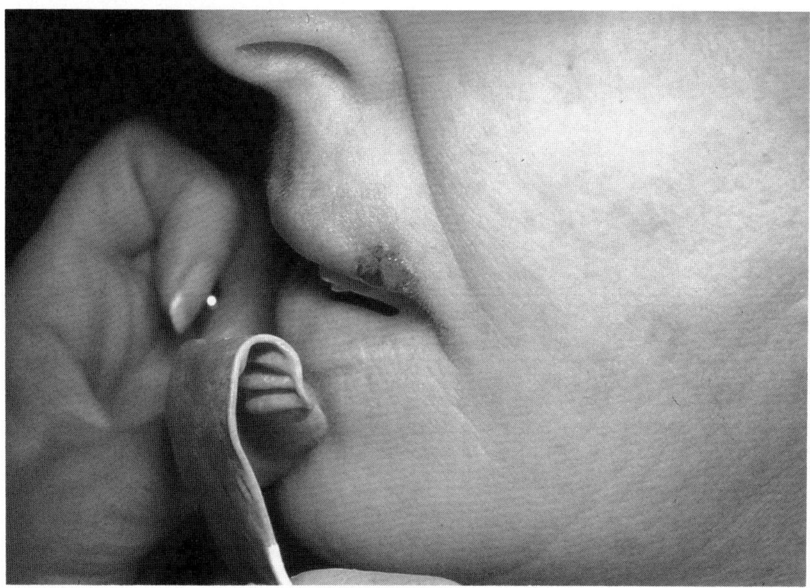

FIGURE 7.41. Radiation protection measures for a basal cell carcinoma of the left upper lip. A, A lead shield covered with a rubber finger cot is inserted between the buccal and gingival mucosa. B, A bent lead shield is applied to the lower lip.

women). Most tumors were smaller than 2 cm. Only patients without metastases were treated. The average HVL was 0.9 mm Al; deeper tumors were treated with a HVL of 1.4 mm Al. Most patients were followed for 5 years or longer. The cure rate was 92%, and all recurrent tumors were secondarily cured with other treatment modalities. Good functional results were noted in 88% of patients, and good cosmetic results were observed in 77%, even though most patients were treated

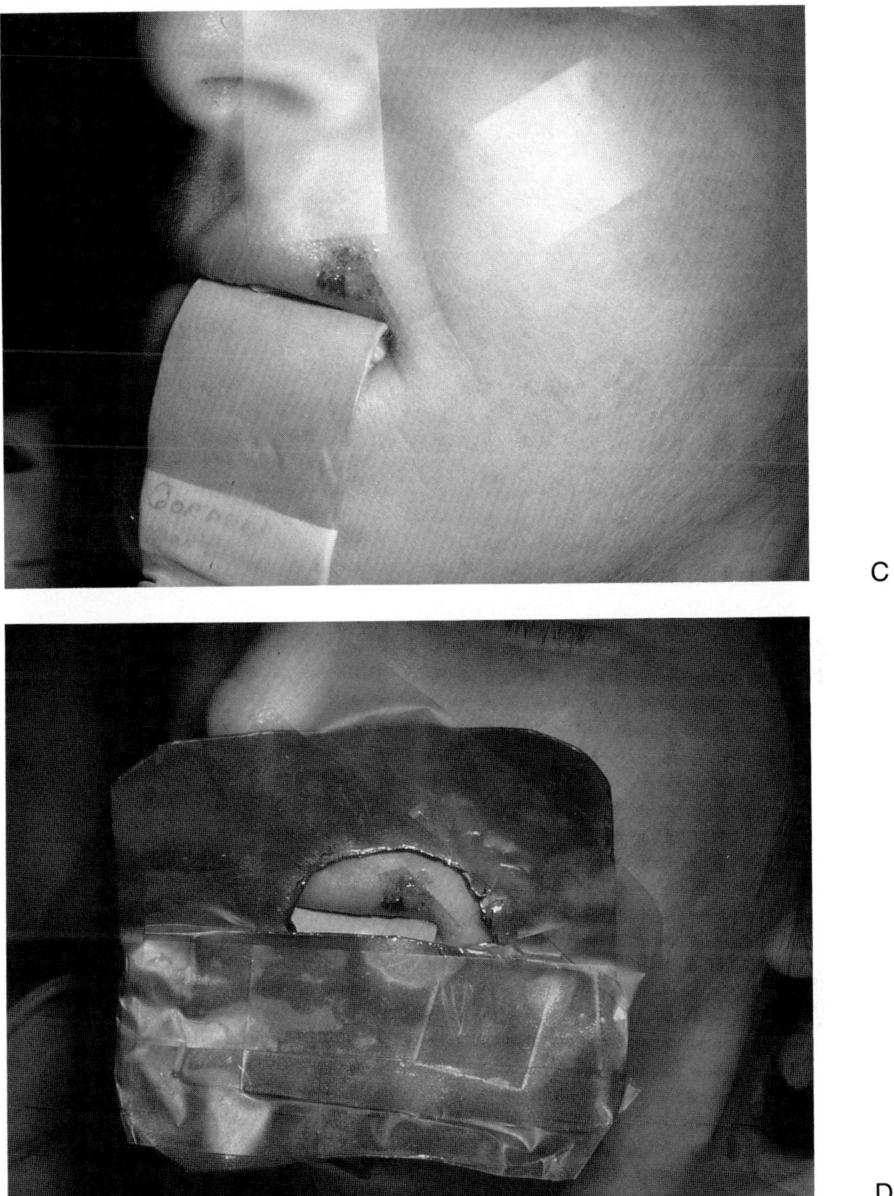

FIGURE 7.11. C, The lead shield in place. D, A lead overlay shield limits radiation to the involved area.

with relatively high total doses (6000–10,000 cGy) in fractions of 300 to 500 cGy. The authors advised continuing re-examinations for recurrences even after 5 years.

Szabo[81] treated 190 patients with carcinoma of the lip (156 squamous cell cancers, 14 with meta-
tases; 34 basal cell carcinomas). The recurrence rate for 142 squamous cell carcinomas of up to 2 cm in diameter without metastases was 4.2%. The tendency to recur was much higher for carcinomas 2 to 4 cm in diameter with metastases. Traenkle and associates[82] described results of radiotherapy with

approximately 5000 cGy in 158 cases of squamous cell carcinoma of the lip. Ninety four were smaller than 1 cm, 52 were 1 to 2 cm in diameter, and 12 were larger than 2 cm. The cure rate was 95% after 3 to 5 years. Eight recurrences were seen, four of them during the first 6 months after therapy. The percentage of failures and metastases (5%) increased with the size of the primary lesion. Von Essen[83] treated 131 carcinomas of lips and noted eight recurrences. Petrovich and colleagues[84] treated 250 patients with carcinoma of the lip in a radiation therapy department. The failure rate was 11%; 9% developed metastases to lymph nodes and 7% died. Wiskemann and associates[6] treated 74 carcinomas of lips with contact therapy or soft x rays and observed six recurrences. Tapley and Fletcher[37] used 7 to 11 MeV electron beam therapy on 14 patients with carcinoma of the lip. Additional treatment with interstitial radium or iridium implants or additional external beam radiotherapy was necessary in four patients; 11 of 14 patients (79%) were free of disease after 5 years. Ehring and Gattwinkel[76] followed 28 basal cell carcinomas of the upper lip for 5 to 22 years after x-ray treatment. No recurrences were observed in 19 tumors of up to 2 cm in diameter; two of nine carcinomas 2 to 3 cm in size and involving the nasolabial fold recurred. The authors emphasized the good cosmetic results even after total doses of 6000 to 7000 cGy.

Carcinoma of Other Regions

Scalp

Although good therapeutic x-ray therapy results have been reported following x-ray therapy,[85] surgical methods are preferred for carcinomas of the scalp.[24] Radiotherapy is always followed by permanent alopecia. Increased absorption of soft x rays in bone tissue (3 times higher than in skin) and increased backscatter also must be considered when radiotherapy is chosen in rare cases where surgery is not advisable. The dangers of very penetrating x-ray qualities (sometimes resulting in brain damage) have been described.[86] If the skin is movable over the skull and if x rays show the absence of bone involvement, small fractionated doses (250–300 cGy daily up to 4500–5000 cGy)

may be used for small (2–3 cm²) tumors with proper protection of the eye region. Soft radiation qualities (D½ 5–10 mm) are preferred. A promising alternative is the application of electron-beam therapy (see Chapter 11); because of the rapid fall-off of the administered dose and the lower absorption in bone, (compared to x rays) the possibility of bone and brain damage is markedly reduced. When bone is involved, office radiotherapy is obviously not recommended as a therapeutic alternative. The damages and complications of irradiation of large cancers of the scalp were reviewed by Howell and Riddell.[87]

Forehead

The limitations of x-ray therapy in the scalp region apply to a lesser degree to tumors of the forehead and temple.[75] Soft radiation qualities and smaller daily doses are recommended (Figs. 7.42 and 7.43). Electron beam treatment is highly suitable for lesions close to the bone.

Cheeks and Chin

Various surgical methods can be used effectively for the cheeks and chin. Radiotherapy serves as an alternative method in patients when surgery is associated with complications or for patients refusing surgical treatments.

The techniques, radiation qualities, and dose schedules are identical to those used in other facial areas. Figures 7.44 to 7.47 show radiotherapeutic results in the cheek and chin regions. Large tumors may leave slightly depressed scars, followed by telangiectases and atrophy at a later stage. These undesirable effects can be aggravated by excessive sun exposure.

Trunk

As mentioned already, the skin of the trunk has a greater tendency to develop unsightly radiation sequelae (telangiectases, pigmentary and sclerotic changes) than other anatomical locations.[89] Since most carcinomas of the trunk can be excised easily without complicated surgical procedures, surgery is the preferred modality for this region. A possible exception to this rule are larger superficial basal cell carcinomas of the back and chest, which

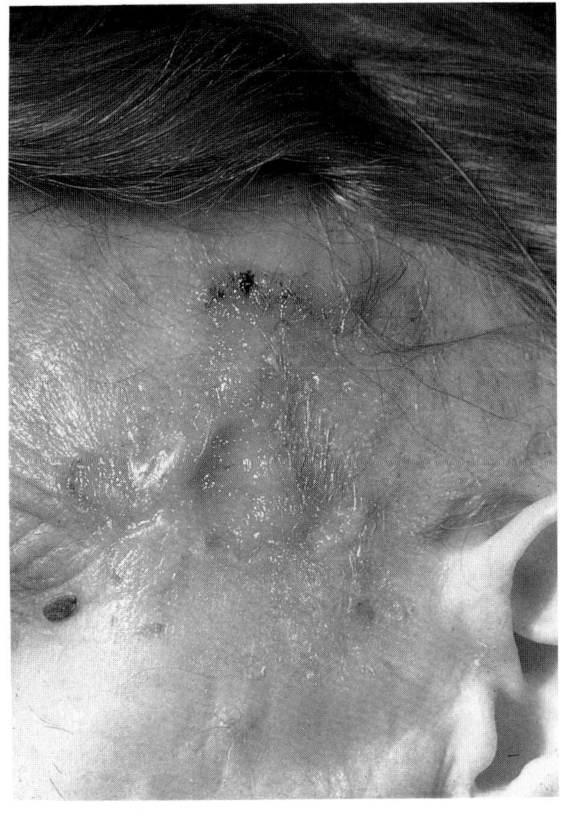

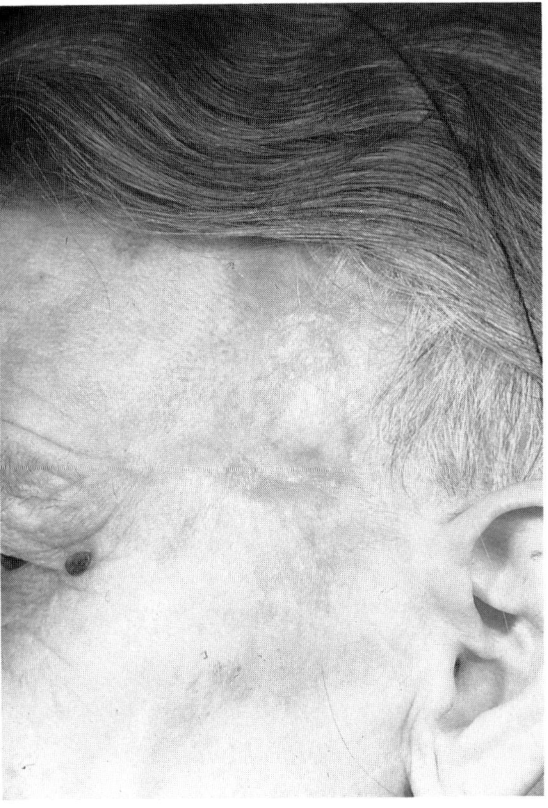

FIGURE 7.42. Large 8 × 10 cm recurrent basal cell carcinoma of left temple. Patient refused surgery.

FIGURE 7.43. Result 2 years after radiation therapy with 5000 cGy administered in daily 250-cGy fractions (HVL 0.75 mm Al; D½ 12 mm). Treated area slightly depressed and atrophic.

respond readily to grenz ray or soft x-ray qualities. Miescher[88] was the first to point out the increased tendency to telangiectases following radiotherapy of superficial basal cell carcinoma of the trunk. He published comparative investigations of various dose schedules that suggested that these late cosmetic effects can be reduced by lowering individual doses to 200 cGy. Since lower doses require more frequent office visits, he recommended other forms of therapy for routine treatments for these relatively benign tumors.

Extremities

Surgical methods are also recommended for most cancerous lesions of the extremities.[8,16,89,90] Squa-mous cell carcinomas are not uncommon over the dorsa of the hands where the skin is usually very thin, shows severe solar damage, and is close to the bone. Only in rare cases should soft radiation qualities in small fractions be used in this area. Electron-beam therapy has many advantages over x rays in this anatomical site (see Chapter 11) and is now considered preferable to the former use of radium molds and other radioisotypes. Because of circulation problems and the frequent presence of varicose veins, the healing process of the lower leg region following radiation therapy is even more impaired than on the upper extremities. In some cases, the normal radiation reaction can develop into an ulcer that may take several months to heal.

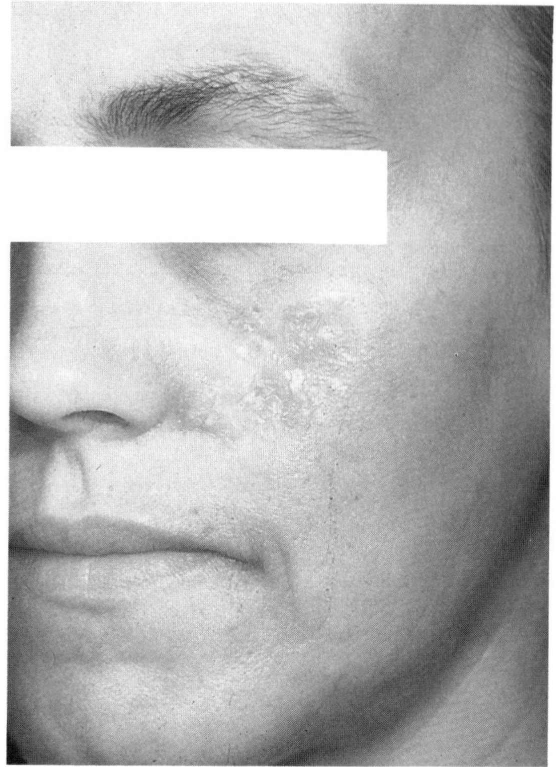

FIGURE 7.44. 6 × 6 cm basal cell carcinoma of cheek, referred by plastic surgeon.

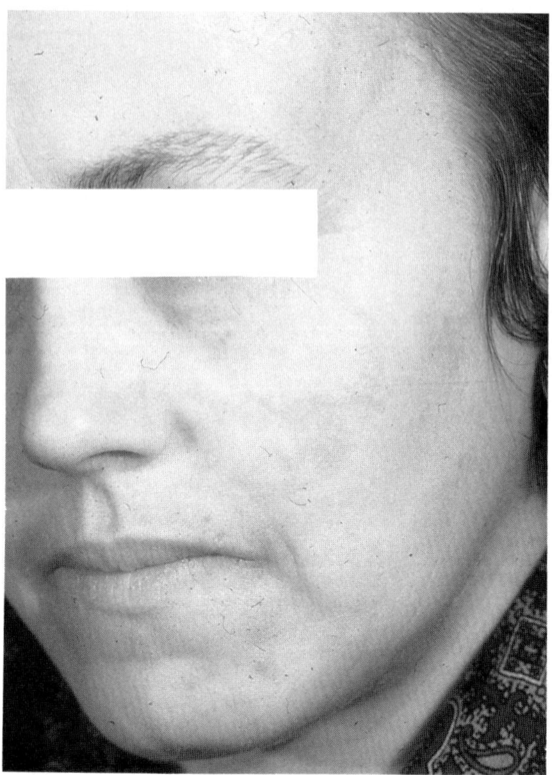

FIGURE 7.45. Cosmetic result 4 years after irradiation with 5200 cGy administered in 300-cGy daily fractions (HVL 0.75 mm; D½ 12 mm). Slight telangiectasia.

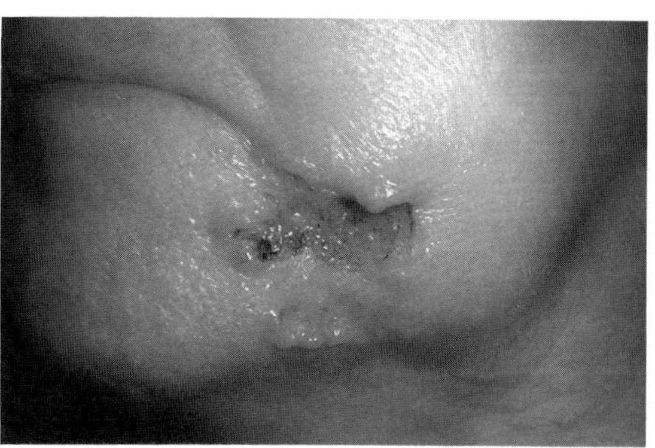

FIGURE 7.46. Large, deeply infiltrated 9 × 9 cm basal cell carcinoma of chin with central ulceration. Patient refused surgery because surgeon warned her that nerve damage might occur.

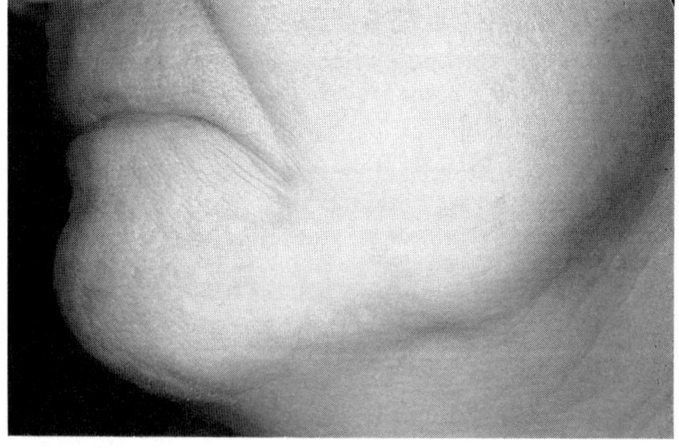

FIGURE 7.47. Result 7 years after radiation therapy with 5500 cGy in 300-cGy daily fractions (HVL 0.75 mm; D½ 12 mm). Slightly irregular scar with some telangiectases.

References

1. Del Regato JA, Vuksanovich M. Radiotherapy of carcinomas of the skin overlying cartilage of the nose and ear. *Radiology.* 1962;79:203–208.
2. Roenigk RK, Ratz JL, Bailin PL, et al. Trends in the presentation of basal cell carcinomas. *J Dermatol Surg Oncol.* 1986;12:860–865.
3. Knox JM, Treatment of skin cancer. *J Am Acad Dermatol.* 1985;3:859.
4. Jolly HW Jr. Superficial x-ray therapy in dermatology. *Int J Dermatol.* 1978;17:691–697.
5. Murphy W. X-ray therapy. In: Helm F, ed. *Cancer Dermatology.* Philadelphia, Penn: Lea & Febiger; 1979:322–324.
6. Wiskemann A, Lippert HD, Lotz GR. Röntgentherapie der Basaliome, spinozellulären Karzinome und Keratoakanthome. In: Braun-Falco O, Marghescu S, eds. *Fortschritte der Praktischen Dermatologie und Venerologie.* Berlin: Springer-Verlag; 1976.
7. Goldschmidt H. Radiotherapy of skin cancer. Modern indications and techniques. *Cutis.* 1976;17:253–261.
8. Proppe A. Spezielle röntgenbehandlung. In: Gottron HA, Schonfeld W, eds. *Dermatologie und Venerologie II/1.* Stuttgart: Georg Thieme Verlag; 1958:26–132.
9. Storck H. Radiotherapy of cutaneous cancers and some other malignancies. *J Dermatol Surg Oncol.* 1978;4:573–584.
10. Barton FE. Principles of nasal reconstruction. *J Dermatol Surg Oncol.* 1982;8:568–574.
11. Union Internationale Contre le Cancer (UICC): *TNM Classification of Malignant Tumors.* 3rd ed. Geneva: UICC; 1978:137–140.
12. Zacarian SA. Cryosurgery in dermatology. In: Goldschmidt H, ed. *Physical Modification in Dermatologic Therapy.* New York, NY: Springer-Verlag; 1978:270–282.
13. Wang CC. *Radiation Therapy for Head and Neck Neoplasms.* Boston, Mass: John Wright, PSG Inc; 1983.
14. Panizzon R. Die Strahlentherapie des Basalioms. In: Eichmann E, Schnyder UW, eds. *Das Basaliom. Der häufigste Tumor der Haut.* Berlin-New York: Springer-Verlag; 1980:103–112.
15. Kuflik EG. Treatment of basal and squamous cell carcinomas on the tip of the nose by cryosurgery. *J Dermatol Surg Oncol.* 1980;6:811–815.
16. Schirren CG. Die Röntgentherapie gutartiger and bösartiger Geschwulste der Haut. In: *Jadassohn (ed): Handbuch der Haut und Geschlechtskrankheiten.* Suppl Vol. V/2. Berlin: Springer-Verlag; 1959:289– 463.
17. Storck H, Ott F, Schwartz K. Haut. In Zuppinger A, Krokwski E, eds. *Handbuch der Medizinischen Radiologie.* Heidelberg: Springer-Verlag; 1972:17–160.
18. Braun-Falco O, Lukacs S, Goldschmidt H. *Dermatologic Radiotherapy.* New York: Springer-Verlag; 1976.
19. Wong CS, Cummings BJ. The place of radiation therapy in squamous cell carcinoma of the nasal vestibule. *Acta Oncol.* 1988;27:203–208.
20. Fitzpatrick PJ. Skin cancer of the head – treatment by radiotherapy. *J Otolaryngol.* 1984;13:261–266.
21. Mendenhall W, Parsons JT, Mendenhall NP, Million RR. T2–T4 carcinoma of the skin of the head and neck treated with radical irradiation. *Int J Radiat Biol Phys.* 1987;13(7):975–981.
22. Del Regato JA, Spjut HG. *Ackerman and Del Regato's Cancer: Diagnosis, Treatment and Prognosis.* 5th ed. St. Louis, Mo: CV Mosby Co, 1977.
23. Farina AT, Leider M. Treatment of complicated cutaneous malignant neoplasms by modern radiotherapy: principles, practice, and results. *J Dermatol Surg Oncol.* 1978;4:759–763.
24. Gladstein AH, Kopf AW, Bart RS. Radiotherapy of cutaneous malignancies. In: Goldschmidt H, ed. *Physical Modalities in Dermatologic Therapy.* New York, NY: Springer-Verlag; 1978.
25. Petrovich Z, Kmisk H, Langholz B, et al. Treatment results and patterns of failure in 646 patients with carcinomas of the eye lids, pinna and nose. *Am J Surg* 1987;154:447–450.
26. Goldschmidt H, Sherwin WK. Reactions to ionizing radiation. *J Am Acad Dermatol.* 1980;3:551–579.
27. Gladstein AH. Radiation protection. In: Goldschmidt H, ed. *Physical Modalities in Dermatologic Therapy.* New York, NY: Springer-Verlag; 1978.
28. Stein KM, Leyden JJ, Goldschmidt H. Localized acneiform eruption following cobalt irradiation. *Br J Dermatol.* 1972;87:274.
29. Engels EP, Leavell J, Mauyama Y. Radiogenic acne and comedones. *Radiol Clin Biol.* 1974;43:48.
30. Graul EH. Uber die Comedonereaktion nach Chaoulscher Nahbestrahlung. *Strahlentherapie.* 1953;91:410 415.
31. Vannicuwenhuyse JB, Duflos M. Nasolabial flaps for repair of defects of the upper lip and lateral aspects of the nose. *J Dermatol Surg Oncol.* 1982;8:351–355.
32. Rubisz-Brzezinska J, Musialowicz D, Zebracka T. Treatment of basal cell epitheliomas. *Dermatol Digest.* 1976;9:10–15.
33. Bart RS, Kopf AW, Petratos MA. X-ray therapy of skin cancer. Evaluation of a "standardized" method for treating basal cell epitheliomas. In: *Sixth*

National Cancer Conference; Proceedings of the American Cancer Society. Philadelphia, Penn: JB Lippincott; 1970:559–570.

34. Stoll HL Jr, Milgram H, Traenkle HL. Results of roentgen therapy of carcinoma of the nose. *Arch Dermatol.* 1964;90:577–580.

35. Mustafa E. Ergebnisse der Nase und der Ohrmuscheln. *Strahlentherapie.* 1966;131:505–519.

36. Fischbach AJ, Sause WT, Plenk HP. Radiotherapy of skin cancer. *West J Med.* 1980;133:379–382.

37. Tapley N duV, Fletcher GH. Applications of the electron beam in the treatment of cancer of the skin and lips. *Radiology.* 1973;109:424–428.

38. Bart RS, Schrager D, Kopf AW, et al. Scalpel excision of basal cell carcionomas. *Arch Dermatol.* 1978;114:739–742.

39. Collin JRO. Basal cell carcinoma in the eyelid region. *Br J Ophthalmol.* 1976;60:806–809.

40. Lederman J. Radiation treatment of cancer of the eyelids. *Br J Ophthalmol.* 1976;60:794–805.

41. Renfer H. Die Therapie der Hauttumoren im medialen Augenwinkel mit besonderer Berücksichtigung der Funktion der Tränenwege. *Strahlentherapie.* 1956;99:345–353.

42. Green R, Kopf AW, Bart RS. X-irradiation of basal cell epitheliomas of the eyelids and canthi. In: McCarthy WH, ed. *Proceedings of the International Cancer Conference.* VCN Blijt Publishers; 1972: 333–342.

43. Helm F. *Cancer Dermatology.* Philadelphia, Penn: Lea & Febiger; 1979.

44. Sullivan JJ. Eyelid surgery. *J Dermatol Surg Oncol.* 1980;6:905–909.

45. Dizon RV, Shannon GM, Siliquini JJ. Basal cell carcinoma recurrence: early diagnosis and surgical treatment. *Ophthalmol Surg.* 1977;8:31–39.

46. Zacarian SA. Cryosurgery of skin cancer: fundamentals of technique and application. *Cutis.* 1975;16:449–460.

47. Biro L, Price E. Basal cell carcinomas on eyelids: experience with cryosurgery. *J Dermatol Surg Oncol.* 1979;5:397–401.

48. Fraunfelder FT. Cryosurgery for malignancies of the eyelid. *Ophthalmology.* 1980;87:461–665.

49. Cottel WI, Proper S. Mohs surgery, fresh-tissue technique. *J Dermatol Surg Oncol.* 1982;8:576–587.

50. Gladstein AH. Efficacy, simplicity, and safety of x-ray therapy of basal cell carcinomas on periocular skin. *J Dermatol Surg Oncol.* 1978;4:586–593.

51. Henkind P, Friedman A. Cancer of the lids and ocular adnexa. In: Andrade R, Gumport SL, Popkin GL, et al, eds. *Cancer of the Skin.* Philadelphia, Penn: WB Saunders Co; 1976:1349.

52. Bart RS, Kopf AW. Tumor Conference #26: a bulky basal cell carcinoma of the lower eyelid. *J Dermatol Surg Oncol.* 1979;5:838–839.

53. Robins P, Bennett RG. *Current Concepts in The Management of Skin Cancer.* New York, NY: Clinicom; 1979.

54. Kopf AW, Grisewood EN, Bart RS, et al. X-irradiation of ocular tissues measured by thermoluminescence dosimetry. *J Invest Dermatol.* 1967;49:512–518.

55. Kopf AW, Allyn B, Andrade R, et al. Leukoplakia of the conjunctiva. *Arch Dermatol.* 1966;94:552–557.

56. Gladstein AH. Modification of eye shields for use in x-ray therapy of eyelid cancers. *Arch Dermatol.* 1974;110:793–794.

57. Chahbazian CM, Brown GS. Radiation therapy for carcinoma of the skin of the face and neck. *JAMA* 1980;244:1135–1137.

58. Del Regato JA, Spjut HJ. *Ackerman and Del Regato's Cancer: Diagnosis, Treatment, and Prognosis.* 5th ed. St. Louis, Mo: CV Mosby Co; 1977.

59. Fitzpatrick PJ, Jamieson DM, Thompson GA, et al. Tumors of the eyelids and their treatment by radiotherapy. *Therapeut Radiol.* 1972;104:661–665.

60. Saitmacher H, Kropp R. Die therapie des lidkarzinomas. *Strahlentherapie.* 1959;110:354–366.

61. Domonkos AN. Treatment of eyelid carcinomas. *Arch Dermatol.* 1965;91:364.

62. Elliott JA, Welton DG. Epithelioma: report on 1742 treated patients. *Arch Dermatol Syphilol.* 1946;53: 307–332.

63. Gage AA. Cryosurgery for cancer of the ear. *J Dermatol Surg Oncol.* 1977;3:417–421.

64. Bumsted RM, Ceilley RI. Stellate excision of malignancies on the auricles. *J Dermatol Surg Oncol.* 1980;6:33–35.

65. Tebetts JD. Auricular reconstruction: selected single-stage techniques. *J Dermatol Surg Oncol.* 1982;8: 557–566.

66. Moss T, Brand WM, Battifora H. *Radiation Oncology.* 5th ed. St. Louis, Mo: CV Mosby Co; 1979.

67. Fiebelkorn HJ, Grafe E. Uber die Behandlung der Ohrmuschelgeschwulste. *Strahlentherapie.* 1960; 111:525–531.

68. Von Balogh K, Schwarz K. Die Strahlentherapie der Neoplasien des Äusseren Ohrs. *Dermatologia.* 1968; 137:250–258.

69. Parker RG, Wildermuth O. Radiation therapy of lesions overlying cartilage. *Cancer.* 1962;15:57–65.

70. Avila J, Bosch A, Aristizabal S, et al. Carcinoma of the pinna. *Cancer.* 1977;40:2891–2895.

71. Pless J. Carcinoma of the external ear. *Scand J Plast Reconstr Surg.* 1976;10:147–151.

72. Gladstone WS, Keer HD. Epidermoid carcinoma of the lower lip: results of radium therapy of the local lesion. *Am J Roentgenol.* 1958;79:101–103.

73. Jorgensen F. Carcinoma of the lip. *Acta Radiol Ther (Stockh).* 1973;12:177–190.

74. Cipollaro AC, Crossland PM. *X-Rays and Radium in the Treatment of Diseases of the Skin.* 5th ed. Philadelphia, Penn: Lea & Febiger, 1967.

75. Murphy W. X-ray therapy. In: Helm F, ed. *Cancer Dermatology.* Philadelphia, Penn: Lea & Febiger; 1979.

76. Ehring E, Gattwinkel W. Die Strahlentherapie des Basalioms der Oberlippe. *Hautarzt.* 1974;25:368–372.

77. Davidson TM, Bartlow GA, Bone RC. Surgical excisions from and reconstructions of the oral lips. *J Dermatol Surg Oncol.* 1980;6:133–141.

78. Jemec BIE. A short review of some methods of excisions from and reconstructions of lower lips. *J Dermatol Surg Oncol.* 1981;7:576–580.

79. Stranc MD, Fogel M, Dische S. Comparison of lip function: surgery vs radiotherapy. *Br J Plast Surg.* 1987;40:598–604.

80. Landthaler M, Lukacs S, Braun-Falco O, et al. Röntgenweichstrahltherapie der Lippenkarzinome. *Hautarzt.* 1981;32:80–83.

81. Szabo P. Klinik und Röntgentherapie von Lippencarcinomen. *Hautarzt.* 1975;26:524–528.

82. Traenkle HL, Stoll HL Jr, Lonkar A. Results of roentgen therapy of carcinoma of the lip. *Arch Dermatol.* 1962;85:96–97.

83. von Essen CF. Roentgen therapy of skin and lip carcinoma: factors influencing success and failure. *Am J Roentgenol.* 1960;83:556–570.

84. Petrovich Z, Kuisk H, Tobochnik N. Carcinoma of the lip. *Arch Otolaryngol.* 1979;104:282–285 and 105:187–191.

85. Szabo P. Klinik und Röntgentherapie von Kopfhautkarzinomomen. *Z Hautkr.* 1978;53:449–452.

86. Lorenzo ND, Holletti A, Palma L. Late cerebral radionecrosis. *Surg Neurol.* 1978;10(5):281–290.

87. Howell JD, Riddell JM. Cancer of forehead and scalp. *JAMA.* 1954;154:13–20.

88. Miescher G. Erfolge der Karzinombehandlung an der dermatologischen Klinik Zürich. Einzeitige Höchstdosis und fraktionierte Behandlung. *Strahlentherapie.* 1934;49:65–81.

89. Goldschmidt H, Sherwin WK. Office radiotherapy of cutaneous carcinomas. *J Dermatol Surg Oncol.* 1983;9:31–76.

90. Goldschmidt H, Sherwin WK. Dermatologic radiation therapy. In: Moschella SC, Hurley HJ, eds. *Dermatology.* 2nd ed. Philadelphia, Penn: WB Saunders Co; 1985.

8

Radiation Therapy of Other Cutaneous Tumors

Herbert Goldschmidt

Keratoacanthoma

Most keratoacanthomas occur in elderly patients; they are believed to be benign epidermal neoplasms. Solitary keratoacanthomas are most common; multiple or eruptive lesions are seen only rarely. Most dermatologists agree that in the absence of functional or cosmetic complications, careful observation without active intervention is the best therapeutic approach for small keratoacanthomas. In most patients, spontaneous resolution with some formation of scar tissue is the usual course of events in the relatively common, small, solitary type of lesion.

Although radiotherapy is effective in most patients,[1-3] its use should be limited to exceptional cases, especially those where surgical management, cryosurgery, intralesional or systemic chemotherapy, or oral retinoid therapy would be difficult, complicated, or contraindicated. One of these exceptions is the "giant keratoacanthoma." This term is arbitrarily applied to rapidly growing tumors with a diameter larger than 2 cm. Radiation therapy may also be indicated in cases where the histopathologic picture can easily be confused with that of a squamous cell carcinoma because of the extensive pseudoepitheliomatous hyperplasia. Furthermore, the rare association of keratoacanthoma with squamous cell carcinoma and basal cell carcinoma[4] also can make it difficult to determine with certainty which type of tumor is present. Regardless of the fact that keratoacanthomas are considered benign tumors, they can be destructive and the microscopic features are generally not helpful in predicting whether a particular lesion will behave in a benign or aggressive fashion.[5] The most destructive type of these rapidly growing tumors occurs in the facial region, especially on the nose, ears, lips, and cheeks. Some of these growths also have a strong tendency to grow back rapidly following unsuccessful attempts at surgical removal.[6,7] In these giant keratoacanthomas, radiotherapy may often be the treatment of choice, particularly when continued growth is anticipated, or when the tumor encroaches upon vital structures or threatens cosmetically important areas.[8] In these instances, spontaneous resolution may occur only after the lesion has reached considerable size and has already caused extensive disfigurement.[9]

Our therapeutic approach for keratoacanthoma does not differ from the principles described for basal cell or squamous cell carcinomas (Figs. 8.1 to 8.6). Once the decision has been made to use radiotherapy, a full cancericidal course of radiation should be given.[2,8,10,11] In cases where there is doubt about the correct diagnosis (keratoacanthoma vs. squamous cell carcinoma), a full course of treatment assures proper treatment of a possible underlying squamous cell cancer. This possibility should always be included in the differential diagnosis, especially in view of the potential of rapidly growing large squamous cell carcinomas to form metastases.

Review of Recent Literature

The largest series of 55 patients with keratoacanthomas, most of the facial region, was reported by Caccialanza and Sopelama.[12] Most patients were treated with Chaoul contact x-ray therapy (60 kV), the remainder with soft x rays (50 kV, 1 mm

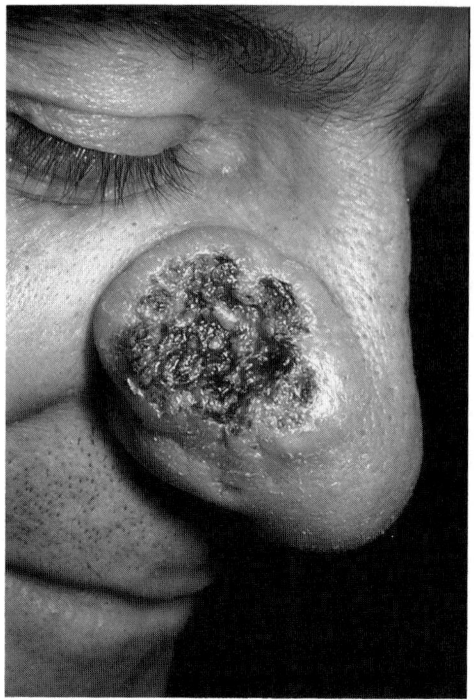

FIGURE 8.1. 3.8 × 3.2-cm keratoacanthoma of nose and cheek that recurred after surgical extirpation. The tumor is markedly raised and rapidly growing toward the orbital area. (Reprinted by permission of the publisher from ref. 44. Copyright 1983 by Elsevier Science Publishing Co., Inc.)

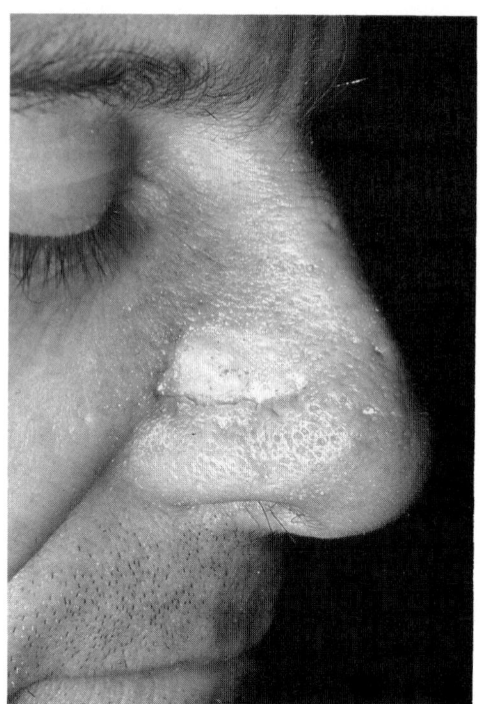

FIGURE 8.2. Appearance 3 months after treatment, showing a strong comedo reaction. The patient refused suggested minor cosmetic repair of residual depressed scar. (Reprinted by permission of the publisher from ref. 44. Copyright 1983 by Elsevier Science Publishing Co., Inc.)

Aluminum [Al] filtration). In 52 cases, the total dose delivered was 4000 cGy, administered in 2 weekly fractions of 400 cGy. Three cases with pronounced cellular atypia were treated with 2 weekly fractions of 500 cGy up to a total dose of 6000 cGy. One month after the last dose all lesions had disappeared. No recurrences were observed.

Brady and co-workers[13] irradiated 12 patients with keratoacanthoma without any recurrence.

Farina and colleagues[14] reported five cases of large, aggressive, and destructive keratoacanthomas of the facial area treated with total doses of 4500 to 5000 cGy administered in 10 to 20 fractions of orthovoltage x rays with a half-value layer (HVL) of 3 mm Al. They describe radiotherapy as a conservative, painless, and rational treatment and recommend x-ray therapy as the treatment of choice not only for large tumors but also for rapidly growing smaller lesions.

Kopf and Bart[10] also advise against lower doses in cases where there is any doubt about the diagnosis because cancerocidal doses will eradicate the tumor whether it is cancerous or pseudocarcinomatous. The response of 13 patients at the Massachusetts General Hospital was described by Shimm and his associates.[15] They found smaller total doses (2500 cGy administered in five fractions on consecutive days) of orthovoltage x rays or electrons effective in eradicating keratoacanthomas of various sizes. The time to regression was dose-dependent up to a time-dose-fractionation factor (TDF) of 50; increasing the dose beyond this level did not accelerate regression. Even lower doses were used by Epstein and Epstein[6] (500 cGy twice at a 4-day interval). Similar small doses were also suggested by Taylor[16] and Wallach (800–1500 cGy).[17] A split dose course is recommended by Koster and associates.[18] They administered a

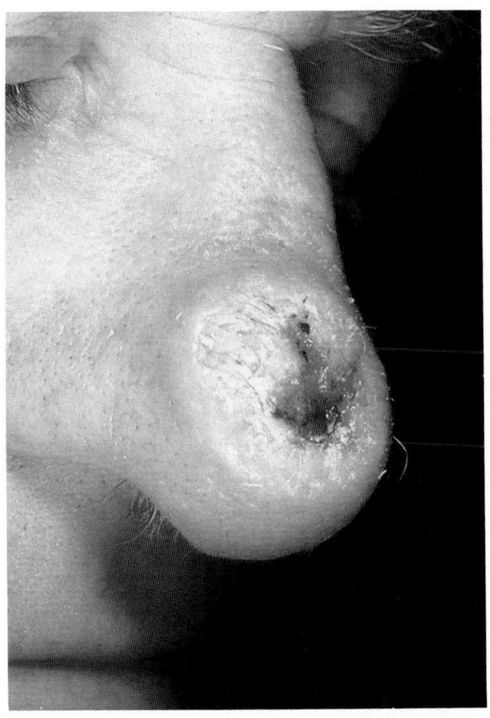

FIGURE 8.3. Recurrent rapidly growing 3.0 × 3.5 cm keratoacanthoma of the nose.

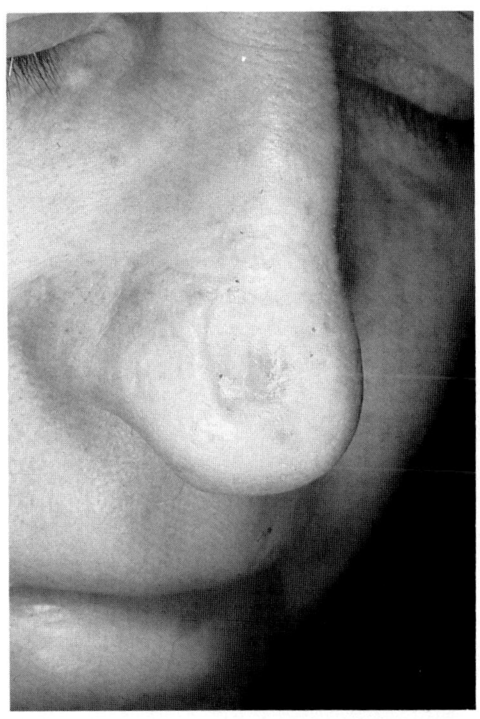

FIGURE 8.4. Result after radiotherapy with 5000 cGy in 350–400 cGy fractions over a period of 3 weeks (HVL 0.75 mm Al; D½ 12 mm).

course of 2400 cGy in daily fractions of 400 cGy and waited 2 weeks, assuming that this dose would cause involution of a keratoacanthoma. Without any visible regression they then continued therapy up to a full cancerocidal dose of approximately 5000 cGy, which would be sufficient to eradicate a squamous cell carcinoma.

Kaposi's Sarcoma

In the classic type of Kaposi's multiple idiopathic hemorrhagic sarcoma, the mere presence of a lesion is not sufficient reason for irradiation because it may remain stationary for years without any therapy. However, if the tumor is ulcerated, painful, infected, rapidly growing, or cosmetically disfiguring, x-ray therapy should be considered.[2]

Ionizing radiation therapy will often induce effective but slow resolution of lesions, often with residual pigmentation. Since the tumors are relatively radiosensitive, small doses of x rays were used in the past from time to time to keep recurrent tumors under control. For example, two doses of 800 to 1000 cGy (1600–2000 cGy) were administered for small lesions, and larger lesions received five to eight doses of 400 cGy (2000–3200 cGy) or five to six doses of 600 cGy (3000–3600 cGy) in two treatments weekly.[19] Because of their depth, most lesions require relatively penetrating radiation (half-value depth [D½] 5–20 mm), either by filtered superficial x rays, orthovoltage radiation, cobalt treatment, or electron-beam therapy.

The recurrence rate depends on many factors, yet there is evidence that, in contrast to older recommendations, higher total doses are more likely to control individual lesions for longer periods of time. A recent study by Cooper and co-workers[20] of 82 cases suggests that high total doses result in long-term local control of the disease. The authors advocate a dose of 3000 cGy in 10 fractions over 2 weeks; more than half of all lesions were free of disease for 10 years and longer. Tumors responding rapidly and completely several weeks after therapy were less likely to recur than slowly

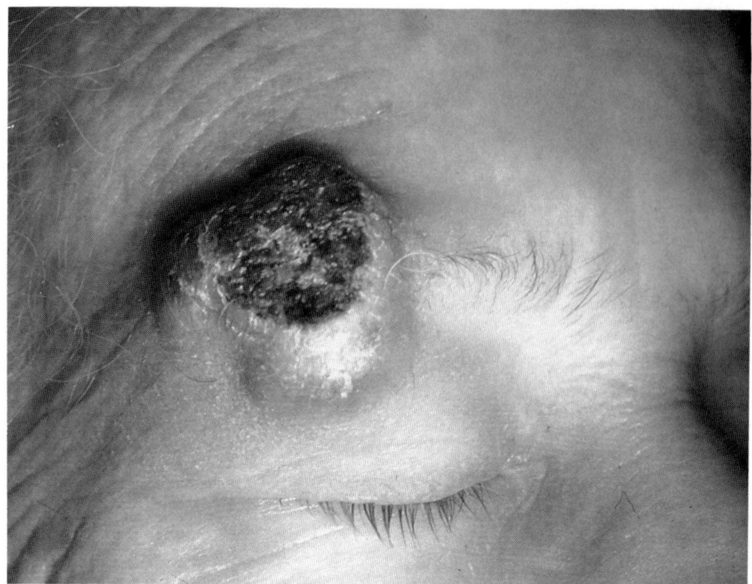

FIGURE 8.5. Rapidly enlarging, 4.0-cm markedly raised keratoacanthoma of the forehead and eyebrow that had recurred after surgical excision. The recurrent tumor is invading the orbital region. (Reprinted by permission of the publisher from ref. 44. Copyright 1983 by Elsevier Science Publishing Co., Inc.)

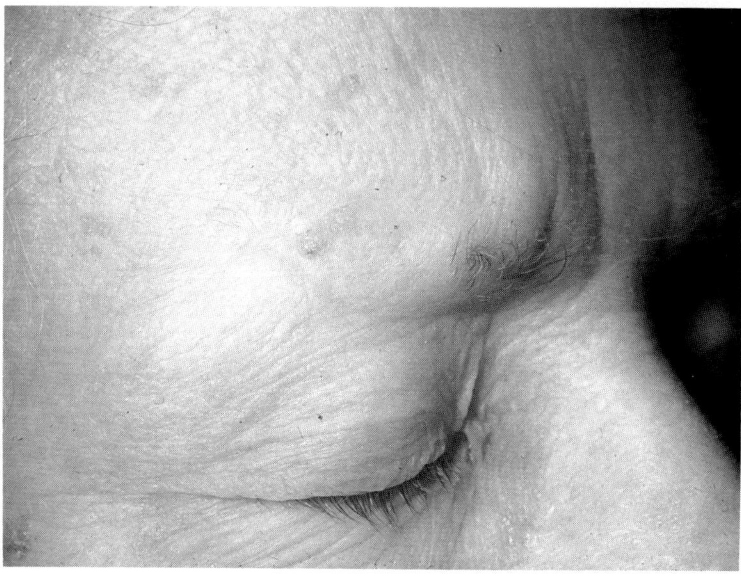

FIGURE 8.6. Appearance of the area 3 months after radiotherapy with 4800 cGy of x rays (50 kV; HVL 0.75 mm Al; D½ 12 mm) delivered in 12 fractions over a 3-week period. Permanent loss of eyebrow. (Reprinted by permission of the publisher from ref. 44. Copyright 1983 by Elsevier Science Publishing Co., Inc.)

resolving lesions without complete resolution. Caution is advisable in treating acral areas of the lower leg; cumulative doses exceeding 2000 to 3000 cGy may cause considerable radiation sequelae, in rare instances even chronic radiation ulcers.

More recently, an extended field technique (at least half of a limb with a 15-cm margin) with only one single dose of 800 cGy has been recommended for large or multiple smaller lesions on the extremities. This treatment is administered by a parallel anterior and posterior opposing pair of fields on megavoltage equipment.[21] Prophylactic radiotherapy of Kaposi's sarcoma was discussed by Borok and colleagues.[22]

Review of Recent Literature

Hamilton and associates[23] reviewed 27 cases treated by local field radiotherapy with complete remission in 17 patients; six have remained relapse-free.

Treatment varied from a single treatment of 300 to 800 cGy to schedules of 3500 cGy administered in five fractions. Ten patients did not achieve complete remission and showed continuously active Kaposi's sarcoma, which was directly responsible for death in four patients. Fifty six patients received extended field therapy, usually with a single fraction of 800 cGy megavoltage, γ-ray, or photon therapy; 38 achieved complete remission and 24 have remained relapse-free for a median duration of 3 years. Eighteen patients never achieved complete remission; 11 of these have died, five due to sarcoma. The authors concluded that extended field therapy is preferable in patients with multiple lesions. Lo and colleagues[24] treated 60 patients and found single doses of 800 to 1200 cGy most effective for small tumors. No significant difference in tumor response was found when an adequate dose was delivered with megavoltage electrons, photons, or a combination of both.

Nisce and co-workers[25] describe results of total and subtotal skin electron-beam therapy (3.5 MeV) for Kaposi's sarcoma. They achieved a complete response in 17 of 20 patients (85%) following once-weekly doses of 400 cGy for 6 to 8 weeks. No relapses were seen over a median period of 48 months.

Epidemic Kaposi's Sarcoma (Acquired Immunodeficiency Syndrome)

Local irradiation of lesions of acquired immunodeficiency syndrome (AIDS)-related Kaposi's sarcoma is an effective palliative treatment in patients with substantial cosmetic disfigurement and for painful, edematous, or ulcerated lesions. Compared to other forms of treatment, local radiotherapy has few side effects; in contrast to many systemic therapies, it does not cause immunosuppression and therefore does not have any potential negative effects on the course of the disease.

Effective control of the lesions can often be achieved with relatively small doses. Most experts agree that there is no major difference in radiosensitivity between epidemic Kaposi's sarcoma and classic Kaposi's sarcoma. This also applies to the management of Kaposi's sarcoma related to

immunosuppressive drugs.[26] Harwood and co-workers[27] found lesions in immunosuppressed kidney transplant patients more resistant to radiotherapy than other types of Kaposi's sarcoma.

Dose recommendations vary considerably; on an average, 300 cGy administered twice a week 3 to 6 times seem to be effective for most patients; doses exceeding 3000 cGy are rarely needed. The D½ depends on the depth of the tumor (D½, 5–20 mm); radiation oncologists prefer 100-kV x rays, orthovoltage, or megavoltage radiation.

Review of Recent Literature

Cooper and colleagues[28] reported initial observations on the effect of kilovoltage and/or megavoltage radiation of 17 lesions of Kaposi's sarcoma in various body areas, particularly on the lower extremities. Nine lesions regressed completely, and three others healed with marked residual hyperpigmentation. The remaining patients showed partial remission. Daily doses of 300 cGy were administered with total doses between 1800 and 3000 cGy. Some lesions resolved during treatment but most required several weeks or months for maximum clinical response.

Reed[29] reported an overall initial response rate of 90% in 74 patients with 172 sarcomas. Most patients received 800 to 3000 cGy in 1 to 15 days. Seventy eight of the lesions were controlled for more than 3 months. At this time 26 patients were alive with their disease, 41 had died of opportunistic infections, and four patients had developed secondary malignancies. About half of the patients had been referred because of pain, about one-fifth for edema (including severe facial edema), and an equal proportion for cosmetic reasons. Radiation therapy was generally effective in reducing pain, flattening nodular lesions, and decreasing wound breakdown; pigmentation remained for 3 to 6 months.

Groopman[30] recommends radiotherapy for large lesions of epidemic Kaposi's sarcoma causing distal edema in the lower extremities and for cosmetically disfiguring lesions. He also treats lesions around the orbit but cautions against radiation of the oral cavity because of the resulting significant sloughing of the palatal mucosa.

Harris and Reed[31] confirmed that the radiation doses required to control epidemic Kaposi's sarcoma are similar to those used in classic Kaposi's sarcoma.

They analyzed the charts of 32 patients and concluded that either single doses of 800 cGy or the equivalent in fractionated doses can produce short-term regression. They advocated fractionating treatment of foot, eye, or oral cavity lesions over 2 to 4 weeks to reduce morbidity, reserving single high-dose therapy for lesions on arms and legs.

Various dosage schedules for epidemic Kaposi's sarcoma were reviewed by Hill,[32] who concluded that radiotherapy can improve the quality of life in patients with lesions that are painful or functionally disturbing.

Significant palliation with relatively low doses (10 fractions of 200 cGy) was observed by Nisce and Safai[33] in a series of 38 patients treated with electron-beam therapy.

Nobler and co-workers[34] irradiated 33 patients with cutaneous and systemic lesions of AIDS. Twelve cutaneous tumors responded to daily doses of 200 to 400 cGy up to a total dose of 1200 to 2400 cGy. Due to systemic problems, the average survival rate was only 8.7 months.

In the first series reported from Britain, Spittle[35] recommended a single fraction irradiation technique as an effective palliative treatment with minimal side effects and without any risk of causing immunosuppression. Eighteen patients were treated with a good clinical response; small lesions of the face received a single dose of 800 cGy, larger lesions in other areas were treated with one to four doses of 400 cGy. The author emphasizes the importance of protective clothing for the staff, especially for bleeding, ulcerated lesions of the feet and for intraoral lesions.

Hommel and colleagues[36] reported good results in patients with Kaposi's sarcoma of the head and neck area.

Bowen's Disease

The lesions present in Bowen's disease are considered precancerous tumors or early cutaneous neoplasms. Since other effective therapeutic measures are available, radiotherapy is rarely indicated even though the lesions are radiosensitive. Erythroplasia of Queyrat resembles Bowen's disease closely but does not respond as well to radiation therapy.[37]

Grenz rays or soft x rays can be used for large lesions or in special anatomical areas where surgery may be difficult (e.g., eyelids, fingers, penis, vulva[38]).

Review of Recent Literature

Stevens and colleagues[39] treated 19 histologically confirmed lesions of Bowen's disease and measured the total thickness of the lesions. They stress the safety of ultrasoft grenz-ray qualities (HVL 0.032 mm Al; D½, 0.5–1.4 mm tissue) used with individual doses of 500 cGy 3 times a week up to a total dose of 5000 cGy for selected patients who refuse surgery, for lesions that are extensive, or where surgery might lead to severe scarring, mutilation, and/or keloid formation. They also emphasize the usefulness of grenz rays for lesions of Bowen's disease involving the fingers. Slightly deeper soft x-ray qualities were recommended by several authors.

Hauss and Proppe[40] described good therapeutic results in 30 patients with 5000 to 6000 cGy of a very soft type of radiation (HVL 0.15 mm Al). Blank and Schnyder[41] reported excellent results after treatment of 77 lesions with a cumulative dosage of 3200 to 5000 cGy and a D½ of 3 to 7 mm. Only two recurrences were observed several months later.

Schoeffinius and co-workers[37] also applied soft x rays (0.2 mm Al HVL) in 200 to 500 cGy daily fractions with a total of 4000 to 6000 cGy in 33 patients; no relapses were seen.

Panizzon[42] reported no recurrences after 3 years' observation in 38 patients with 45 large lesions of Bowen's disease (9% with erythroplasia) treated with 400 cGy doses of soft x rays, (D½, 0.2–1.7 mm) administered twice a week, at least 10 times.

Cutaneous Lymphomas (Mycosis Fungoides)

Localized Lesions

X-ray therapy is often the treatment of choice for localized lesions of mycosis fungoides and other cutaneous lymphomas. Early plaques and tumors are highly radiosensitive and respond to low doses of ionizing radiation.[43] Like other therapeutic modalities, radiation treatment is only palliative. Recent investigations have shown that the survival rate of patients treated early with ionizing radiation is not lower or higher than that of patients given cytostatic drugs, antimetabolites, or other modalities. Moreover, cutaneous radiation therapy has the added advantage of producing systemic side effects only in rare instances. Systemic drug therapy is preferred when internal organs are involved.

Radiation therapy is given with a D½ matching the depth of the lesion, in small doses of 50 to 150 cGy at weekly intervals or 3 times weekly until the lesion shows early involution. In many cases, satisfactory therapeutic responses can be observed after a total dose of only 200 to 500 cGy. Large tumor doses are definitely not required.[44] Recurrent lesions may be treated repeatedly with caution; the normal cumulative limit of 1000 cGy does not apply to mycosis fungoides because it is a potentially lethal disease in which cosmetic considerations are not essential. For widespread involvement, electron-beam treatment or teleroentgentherapy are indicated.

Widespread Lesions

Total Skin Electron Irradiation

Electron beam therapy of widespread cutaneous lymphomas is discussed in detail in Chapter 11.

Teleroentgen Therapy with Soft X Rays

Although teleroentgen therapy with soft x rays has now been largely superseded by electron-beam therapy, which is more effective because of its deeper penetration into the skin (average: 1 cm), it is a useful and relatively simple technique for the treatment of widespread superficial dermatoses in hospitals and offices where elaborate electron-beam therapy units arc not available. "Teleroentgen therapy" denotes radiation techniques that have a target-skin distance long enough to produce effective whole-body radiation. A distance of 2 m is usually sufficient to permit radiation of the entire body surface. Total-body "spray" irradiation with highly penetrating x rays (1 mm Cu HVL) was used in leukemias and Hodgkin's disease. Since at 10-cm tissue depth only 50% of this radiation is absorbed, even low doses (5 to 15 cGy), given several times, invariably cause depression of the hematopoietic system. An entirely different and safe technique was proposed by Schirrcn (1955),[45] who used soft x rays for generalized dermatoses. Hematologic or other side effects have not been observed because of the low half-value depth; 50% of the surface dose is absorbed at a depth of only 2 mm. This limited penetration makes teleroentgen therapy with soft x rays well suited for most generalized superficial skin disorders. Long-term results of teleroentgen therapy in mycosis fungoides were reviewed by Goldschmidt and co-workers.[46] Wiskemann and Buck[47] treated eight body regions in 98 patients at a distance of 1.2 m with single doses of 300 cGy administered at 3-week intervals; total doses ranged from 300 to 1500 cGy.

Any high-output beryllium window unit (preferably at 25 mA or higher; kilovoltage at least 50kV) can be utilized for this technique. Beryllium window machines operating at less than 10 mA or glass window machines are less satisfactory because of the limited dose at a distance of 2 m and the resulting very long exposure times.

The primary indication for teleroentgen therapy is widespread mycosis fungoides in all stages (with the exception of markedly raised tumors) and other superficially located cutaneous lymphomas. Doses of 50 to 100 cGy are given daily (or three times a week) to the anterior, posterior, and lateral surfaces up to a total of 500 to 1000 cGy per course, with the eyes and gonads shielded. Pruritus is often alleviated after only two or three treatments; clinically visible manifestations usually disappear 2 to 4 weeks after the last treatment. Relapses are as frequent as in other forms of therapy; remissions may last from 3 to 12 months. Widespread mycosis fungoides with a limited number of raised lesions can be treated with teleroentgen therapy followed by low doses of more penetrating x rays to residual tumors. (When numerous elevated tumors are present, teleroentgen therapy is not suitable because of its limited penetration. In these cases, electron beam therapy is more effective; it can be adjusted to greater depths than teleroentgen therapy and is therefore useful in all stages of mycosis fungoides.) In lymphomas, repeated courses are possible, but early radiodermatitis (telangiectases) should be expected several years later when more than 2000 cGy are administered. At 2-m distance, the half-value layer is 0.1 to 0.2 mm Al and the half-value depth is only 2 mm when no additional filtration is used. Beryllium units at 50 kV and 25 mA yield a dose rate of 20 cGy per minute at a target skin distance of 2 m; at this TSD the major portion of the long wavelength radiation is absorbed by air.

References

1. Wiskemann A, Lippert HD, Lotz GR. Röntgentherapie der Basaliome, spinozellulären Karzinome und Keratoakanthome. In: Braun-Falco O, Marghescu S, eds. *Fortschritte der Praktischen Dermatologie und Venerologie*. Berlin: Springer-Verlag; 1976.

2. Gladstein AH, Kopf AW, Bart RS. Radiotherapy of cutaneous malignancies. In: Goldschmidt H, ed. *Physical Modalities in Dermatologic Therapy*. New York, NY: Springer-Verlag; 1978.

3. Braun-Falco O, Lukacs S, Goldschmidt H. *Dermatologic Radiotherapy*. New York, NY: Springer-Verlag; 1976.

4. Burge KM, Winkelmann RH. Keratoacanthoma; association with basal and squamous cell carcinoma. *Arch Dermatol*. 1969;100:306–310.

5. Kingman J, Callen JP. Keratoacanthoma: a clinical study. *Arch Dermatol*. 1984;120:736–740.

6. Epstein EH Jr, Epstein EH. Keratoacanthoma recurrent after surgical excision. *J Dermatol Surg Oncol*. 1978;4:524–525.

7. Bart RS, Popkin GL, Kopf AW, et al. Giant keratoacanthoma: a problem in diagnosis and management. *J Dermatol Surg Oncol*. 1975;1:49–55.

8. von Essen CF. Skin and lip. In: Fletcher S, ed. *Textbook of Radiotherapy*. 3rd ed. Philadelphia, Penn: Lea & Febiger; 1980:271–285.

9. Wolinsky S, Sivers DN, Kohn SR, et al. Spontaneous regression of a giant keratoacanthoma: photographic documentation and histopathologic correlation. *J Dermatol Surg Oncol*. 1981;7:897–901.

10. Kopf AW, Bart RS. Giant keratoacanthoma. *J Dermatol Surg Oncol*. 1978;4:444–445.

11. Goldschmidt H, Sherwin WK. Office radiotherapy of cutaneous carcinomas. *J Dermatol Surg Oncol*. 1983;9:660–682.

12. Caccialanza M, Sopelama N. Radiation therapy of keratoacanthomas: results in 55 patients. *Int J Radiat Oncol Biol Phys*. 1988;16:475–477.

13. Brady LW, Binnick SA, Fitzpatrick PJ. Skin cancer. In: Perez CA, Brady LW, eds. *Principles and Practice of Radiation Oncology*. Philadelphia, Penn: JB Lippincott; 1987:372–394.

14. Farina AT, Leider M, Newall C, et al. Radiotherapy for aggressive and destructive keratoacanthomas. *J Dermatol Surg Oncol*. 1977;3:177–180.

15. Shimm DS, Duttenhaver JR, Ducette J, et al. Radiation therapy of keratoacanthoma. *Int J Radiat Oncol Biol Phys*. 1983;9:759–761.

16. Taylor JH. Keratoacanthoma. *Dermatology*. Nov 1979;27–37.

17. Wallach EA. X-ray may be choice for keratoacanthomas. *Dermatol News*. 1987;20(7):1–6.

18. Koster W, Nasemann T, Reimlinger S, Wiskemann A. Röntgendifferentialtherapie des Keratoacanthomas. *Z Hautkr* 1985;60:215–218.

19. Storck H, Ott F, Schwarz K. Haut. In Zuppinger A, Krokowski E, eds. *Handbuch der Medizinischen Radiologie*. Heidelberg: Springer-Verlag; 1972:17–160.

20. Cooper JS, Sacco J, Newall J, et al. The duration of local control of classic (non-AIDS–associated) Kaposi's sarcoma by radiotherapy. *J Am Acad Dermatol*. 1988;19:59–66.

21. Harwood AR, Kaposi's sarcoma: an update on the results of extended field therapy. *Arch Dermatol*. 1981;117:775–778.

22. Borok T, Farina AT, Leider M. Radiotherapy for Kaposi's sarcoma. *J Dermatol Surg Oncol*. 1979; 5:39–42.

23. Hamilton CR, Cummings BJ, Harwood AR. Radiotherapy of Kaposi's sarcoma. *Int J Radiat Oncol Biol Phys*. 1986;12:1931–1935.

24. Lo TMC, Salzman FA, Smedal MI, Wright KA. Radiotherapy for Kaposi's sarcoma. *Cancer* 1980; 45:684–691.

25. Nisce LZ, Safai B, Poussin-Rosillo H. Once weekly total and subtotal skin electron beam therapy for Kaposi's sarcoma. *Cancer*. 1981;47:640–644.

26. El Akkad S, Bull CA, El Senoussi M, et al. Kaposi's sarcoma and its management by radiotherapy. *Arch Dermatol*. 1986;122:1296–1399.

27. Harwood AR, Osaba D, Hofstader SL. Kaposi's sarcoma in recipients of renal transplants. *Am J Med*. 1979;67:759–765.

28. Cooper JS, Fried PR, Laubenstein LJ. Initial observations on the effect of radiotherapy on epidemic Kaposi's sarcoma. *JAMA*. 1984;252:934–935.

29. Reed TA. Radiotherapy found effective for Kaposi's sarcoma. *Skin Allergy News*. June 1985;16:12.

30. Groopman JE. Therapy of epidemic Kaposi's sarcoma. *Semin Hematol*. 1986;23:14–19.

31. Harris JW, Reed TA. Kaposi's sarcoma in AIDS: the role of radiation therapy. *Front Radiat Ther Oncol*. 1985;19:126–132.

32. Hill DR. The role of radiotherapy for epidemic Kaposi's sarcoma. *Semin Oncol*. 1987;14(no 2, suppl 3):19–22.

33. Nisce LA, Safai B. Radiation therapy of Kaposi's sarcoma in AIDS. *Front Radiat Ther Oncol*. 1985; 19:133–137.

34. Nobler MP, Leddy ME, Huh SH. The impact of palliative irradiation on the management of patients with acquired immune deficiency syndrome. *J Clin Oncol*. 1987;5:107–112.

35. Spittle M. A simple and effective treatment for AIDS-related Kaposi's sarcoma. *Brit Med J*. 1987; 295:248–249.

36. Hommel D, Brown M, Kinzie J. Response to radiotherapy of head and neck tumors in AIDS patients. *Am J Surg*. 1987;154:443–446.

37. Schoeffinius H, Lucacs S, Braun-Falco O. Zur Behandlung von Morbus Bowen, Bowen-Carcinoma und Erythroplasie von Queyrat. *Hautarzt*. 1974;25:489–494.

38. Lewis HM. Grenz-ray therapy: regimens and results. In: Goldschmidt H, ed. *Physical Modalities in Dermatologic Therapy*. New York, NY: Springer-Verlag; 1978.

39. Stevens DM, Kopf AW, Gladstein A, Bart RS. Treatment of Bowen's disease with grenz rays. *Int J Dermatol*. 1977;16:329–339.

40. Hauss H, Proppe A. Radiotherapy of lentigo maligna and Bowen's disease. In: Goldschmidt H, ed. *Physical Modalities in Dermatologic Therapy*. New York, NY: Springer Verlag; 1978.

41. Blank AA, Schnyder UW. Soft x-ray therapy in Bowen's disease and erythroplasia of Queyrat. *Dermatologica*. 1985;171(2):89–94.

42. Panizzon R. Modern radiotherapy of skin neoplasms. In: Kukita A, Seiji M, eds. *Proceedings of the XVI International Congress of Dermatology, Tokyo 1982*. Tokyo: University of Tokyo Press; 1983:482–484.

43. Hollander MB. *Ultrasoft X-Rays*. Baltimore, Md: Williams & Wilkins; 1968.

44. Goldschmidt H, Sherwin WK. Office radiotherapy of cutaneous carcinomas. *J Dermatol Surg Oncol*. 1983;9:31–76.

45. Schirren CG. Roentgen irradiation at a distance using soft radiation at a distance, using soft radiation from beryllium-window tubes. *J Invest Dermatol*. 1955;24:463–467.

46. Goldschmidt H, Lukacs S, Schoefinius HH. Teleroentgen therapy of mycosis fungoides. *J Dermatol Surg Oncol*. 1978;4:600–605.

47. Wiskemann A, Buck C. Radiotherapy of mycosis fungoides: Twenty years of experience with teleroentgen and low-voltage x-ray therapy. *J Dermatol Surg Oncol*. 1978;4:606–610.

9

Radiation Therapy of Melanomas

Renato G. Panizzon

General Considerations

Although surgery is by far the most common form of treatment for most cutaneous melanomas, there are some limited indications for radiation therapy. Irradiation has a definitive role in the treatment of lentigo maligna (LM), especially with grenz rays. For lentigo maligna melanomas (LMM), more penetrating soft x rays show great promise as a curative treatment modality.[1-3] Therapeutic trials with radiotherapy of inoperable nonlentiginous melanomas and of metastatic lesions to skin or lymph nodes have shown that these lesions are less responsive to ionizing radiation. The results of numerous clinical investigations favor techniques that utilize high doses per fraction (the term "high dose" fraction is used in this connection, in contrast to the low standard 200-cGy fractions used in radiation oncology). In patients treated with curative intent, either definitively or adjunctively, the difference between high-dose fractions and low-dose fractions may be decisive. More prospective trials are needed to test the reported greater efficacy of high doses. Late complications associated with high dose per fraction irradiation are not a relevant risk in patients with metastatic melanoma where survival is generally limited. The use of high doses per fraction is not really new; radiotherapy of melanoma has a long tradition in our institution since Miescher first introduced it several decades ago.[3]

In a retrospective study Panizzon[29] reported that 60 patients with LM and 54 patients with LMM were controlled by either radiation therapy or surgery. Fifty six patients (47 LM and 9 LMM) had been irradiated; no recurrences were seen in either group after a mean follow-up time of 9.3 years. Conversely, 58 patients (13 LM and 45 LMM) were treated surgically; in the LM group there were two recurrences (18.2%) and seven (15.6%) in the LMM group, after a mean follow-up time of 4.8 years. The irradiated group and the surgically treated group of LMM were compared for tumor thickness and tumor levels and no statistically significant differences between the two treatment modalities were found. In our opinion, radiotherapy is the preferred modality in older patients with large lesions, particularly in the facial area, because it is easily accepted by the patient and gives excellent cosmetic results.

Experimental Findings

Barranco[4] and Dewey[5] carried out in vitro studies and found that melanoma is not quite as radioresistant as was previously thought. Wheldon[6] subsequently made the following observations:

1. The optimal single dose is directly proportional to D_0 (see Chapter 2)
2. The optimal time interval between the fractions is directly proportional to the doubling time of the tumor
3. Time and dose increase with the extrapolation number (n, see Chapter 2). The usefulness of higher dose fractions was also demonstrated in experiments with human EE melanomas and NA-II melanomas, which were implanted in athymic mice and then irradiated in vivo.[7] It could be shown that the re-oxygenation of the

TABLE 9.1. Possible reasons for the reduced radiosensitivity of melanomas.

High percentage of nonproliferating cells
High percentage of hypoxic cells
High probability of potentially lethal repair
Subpopulations of cells with different radiosensitivity in the "shoulder" region of the survival curve
Synthesis of prostaglandins (radioprotectors) in the tumor cells
Melanin is a scavenger of "radicals"

tumor is increased when higher single doses are administered, whereas hypoxia continues with daily low doses. This may explain the reduced radiosensitivity of melanomas.[8] Another helpful model for the investigation of radiosensitivity of melanomas is the spheroid culture model.[9] With this method it was shown that the growth of C-32 melanoma cells could only be stopped with a daily minimal single dose of 350 cGy.[10] However, despite these encouraging reports, there is no doubt that melanomas are neoplasms with reduced radiosensitivity; this is especially true for nonlentiginous melanomas. Possible reasons for the reduced radiosensitivity are shown in Table 9.1.

During the last few years considerable progress has been made to improve the results of radiotherapy of melanomas; the most promising approaches are listed in Table 9.2.

Review of the Literature

Even though the use of higher individual doses is often considered a new approach in the management of melanomas, the high dose per fraction therapy was already mentioned in the past.[3] In the 1970s Sealy and colleagues[17] tried to irradiate

TABLE 9.2. Measures to improve the efficacy of radiotherapy of melanomas.

Multiple fractions per day (hyperfractionation[11])
X rays of high LET
Additional use of radiosensitizers or antimetabolites[12,13]
Additional use of hyperthermia[14,15]
Thermal neutron capture therapy[16]

TABLE 9.3. Response rates of melanomas by fraction size: review of the literature.[a]

Authors	Fraction size (cGy)	Response (n)	Response rate (%)
Sealy et al., 1974[17]	450–500	13/24	54
Habermalz et al., 1976[18]	<400	2/15	13
	≥400	36/42	86
Hornsey et al., 1978[19]	<400	37/57	65
	≥400	30/37	81
Strauss et al., 1981 (cited in 3)	<400	15/39	38
	≥400	36/44	82
Katz, 1981 (cited in 3)	<400	5/19	26
	≥400	24/34	71
Lobo et al., 1981 (cited in 3)	180–300	47/69	68
Trott et al., 1981 (cited in 3)	<400	16/34	47
	≥400	4/14	40
Doss et al., 1982[20]	200–400	9/32	25
	400–800	6/9	67
Adam et al., 1982 (cited in 3)	600	19/24	79
Johanson et al., 1983[21]	800	17/32	53
Overgaard et al., 1986[22]	<400	5/13	38
	≥400	124/145	86
Konefal et al., 1987[23]	≤500	4/43	9
	≥500	12/24	50
Rounsaville et al., 1988[24]	<400	5/13	38[b]
	≥400	21/38	55[b]

[a] From ref. 24, with permission of S. Karger AG, Basel.
[b] Excluding bone and brain lesions.

melanomas with 400 to 500 cGy 2 times per week, and they thought that this type of fractionation was more responsible for the remission of treated melanomas than the concomitant use of hyperbaric oxygen.[17] Habermalz and Fischer later proposed single doses of more than 600 cGy applied 1 to 3 times per week.[18] Among other suggestions was the recommendation to apply at least 300 cGy 5 times per week.[19] In the 1980s several authors proposed minimum doses of 400 cGy, and single doses as high as 800 cGy (see Table 9.3). A possible correlation between large fractions and short overall

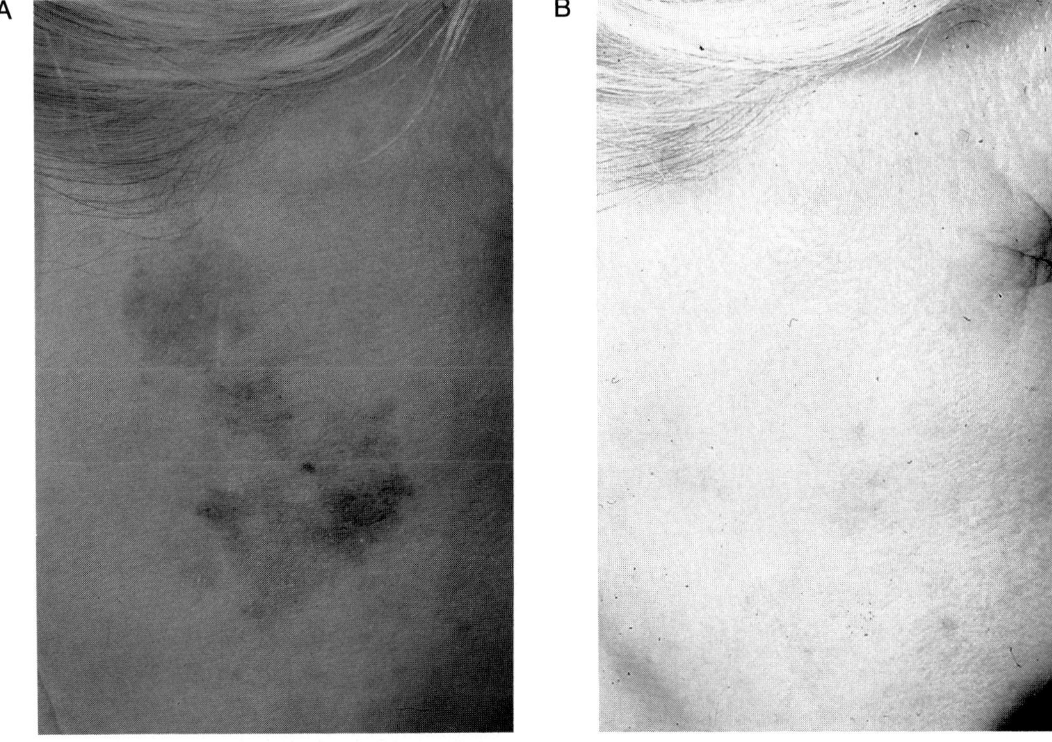

FIGURE 9.1. A, LMM on the right cheek in a 77-year-old female patient. B, Same patient 17 months after radiotherapy of 9 × 600 cGy, 20 kV, 0.4 mm Al filter, twice weekly. For details, see dose recommendations.

times also must be considered. For this reason it is difficult to distinguish between which is of greater importance: the larger fraction size or the short overall time. Doss and Mernula[20] showed that fraction size is in fact more important than time or total dose.

Lentigo Maligna Melanoma

As mentioned already, good curative results can be obtained in the treatment of lentigo maligna melanoma (LMM) or lentigo maligna (LM—the precursor lesion). This was also confirmed by other authors in hundreds of irradiated cases.[25-29] In our studies the cure rate in LM was 100% in 104 patients after a mean follow-up of 7.3 years (see Fig. 9.1). In LMM two recurrences occurred after a mean follow-up of 8.0 years in 18 patients. The cure rate was 89%.[29]

Ionizing radiation has rarely been used for LMM in U.S. centers since three cases of metastatic malignant melanoma in a series of 16 patients

treated with radiation were reported by Kopf and co-workers.[30] A careful evaluation of their cases shows that five of their LM and three of their LMM patients were treated repeatedly with other treatment modalities before radiotherapy; this might have been the cause of their unfavorable results. Our dose recommendations for LM and LMM are given in Tables 9-4 and 9-5, respectively.

Superficial Spreading Melanoma

Six patients with superficial spreading melanoma (SMM) were successfully treated with radiotherapy

TABLE 9.4. Dose recommendations for LM.

D½	0.1–1.0 mm
kV	5–19 (grenz)
Filter	1.0 mm cellon or Be
HVL	0.02–0.2 mm Al
Single dose	1000 or 2000 cGy
Total dose	10,000–12,000 cGy
Interval	3–6 days

TABLE 9.5. Dose recommendations for LMM.

D½	1–15 mm
kV	20–50 or more
Filter	0.4–2.0 mm Al
HVL	0.2–1.6 mm Al
Single dose	600 cGy
Total dose	4200–5400 cGy
Interval	3–6 days

by Harwood and Cummings.[31] The same authors suggested further investigations of the therapeutic effect of radiation on difficult tumors in the head and neck region and for melanomas where microscopic margins were incomplete after surgical excision.

Nodular Melanomas

Some nodular melanomas (NM) of the head and neck area respond to radiotherapy when single doses of at least 400 cGy are used.[18] Johanson et al. showed promising preliminary results with even higher single fractions.[21] It has also been emphasized that even NMs arising de novo are not radioresistant.[32]

Metastatic Melanoma

Palliative radiotherapy is used in some patients for melanomas metastatic to the skin,[33] and particularly for metastases of the lymph nodes, the brain, and the bones.

References

1. Cooper JS. Radiotherapy of malignant melanoma. *Dermatol Clin.* 1985;3:341–350.
2. Goldschmidt H. Ionizing radiation therapy. In: Domonkos AN, Arnold HL, Odom RB, eds. *Andrew's Diseases of the Skin.* Philadelphia, Penn: WB Saunders; 1990.
3. Panizzon R. Die Radiotherapie des malignen Melanoms der Haut—eine Renaissance? *Hautarzt.* 1986; 37:481–484.
4. Barranco SC, Romsdahl MM, Humphrey RM. The radiation response of human malignant melanoma cells grown in vitro. *Cancer Res.* 1971;31:830–833.
5. Dewey DL. The radiosensitivity of melanoma cells in culture. *Br J Radiol.* 1971;44:816–817.
6. Wheldon TE. Optimal fractionation for the radiotherapy of tumor cells possessing wide-shouldered survival curves. *Br J Radiol.* 1979;52:417–418.
7. Rofstad EK, Brustad T. Broad-shouldered survival curves of a human melanoma xenograft. *Acta Radiol (Oncol).* 1981;20:261–265.
8. Pourreau-Schneider N, Malaise EP. Relationship between surviving fractions using the colony method, the LD 50, and the growth delay after irradiation of human melanoma cells grown as multicellular spheroids. *Radiat Res.* 1981;85:321–332.
9. Sutherland RM, Inch WR, McCredie JA, et al. A multi-component radiation survival curve using an in vitro tumour model. *Int J Radiat Biol.* 1970;18: 491–495.
10. Yuhas JM, Blake S, Weichselbaum RR. Quantitation of the response of human tumour spheroids to daily radiation exposures. *Int J Radiat Oncol Biol Phys.* 1984;10:2323–2327.
11. von Rottkay P. Strahlentherapie bei Malignen Melanomen mit akzelerierter Fraktionierung. *Strahlenther Onkol.* 1987;163:139–143.
12. Klausner JM, Gutman M, Rozin RR, et al. Conventional fractionation radiotherapy combined with 5-fluorouracil for metastatic malignant melanoma. *Am J Clin Oncol.* 1987;10:448–450.
13. Dische S. Radiotherapy using the hypoxic cell sensitizer Ro 03-8799 in malignant melanoma. *Radiother Oncol.* 1987;10:111–116.
14. Arcangeli G, Benassi M, Cividalli A, et al. Radiotherapy and hyperthermia. *Cancer.* 1987;60:950–956.
15. Mameghan H, Knittel T. Response of melanoma to heat and radiation therapy. *Med J Aust.* 1988;149: 474–481.
16. Mishima Y, Ichihashi M, Tsuji M, et al. Treatment of malignant melanoma by selective thermal neutron capture therapy using melanoma-seeking compound. *J Invest Dermatol.* 1989;92(suppl):321s–325s.
17. Sealy R, Hockly J, Shepstone B. The treatment of malignant melanoma with cobalt and hyperbaric oxygen. *Clin Radiol.* 1974;25:211–215.
18. Habermalz HJ, Fischer JJ. Radiation therapy of malignant melanoma. Experience with high individual treatment doses. *Cancer.* 1976;38:2258–2262.
19. Hornsey S. The relationship between total dose, number of fractions and fraction size in the response of malignant melanoma in patients. *Br J Radiol.* 1978;51:905–909.
20. Doss LL, Memula N. The radioresponsiveness of melanoma. *Int J Radiat Oncol Biol Phys.* 1982;8: 1131–1134.
21. Johanson CR, Harwood AR, Cummings BJ, et al. 0-7-21 radiotherapy in nodular melanoma. *Cancer.* 1983;51:226–232.
22. Overgaard J, Overgaard M, Hansen PV, et al. Some factors of importance in the radiation treatment of

malignant melanoma. *Radiother Oncol.* 1986;5: 183–192.

23. Konefal JB, Emami B, Pilepich MV. Malignant melanoma: analysis of dose fractionation in radiation therapy. *Radiology.* 1987;164:607–610.

24. Rounsaville MC, Cantril St, Fontanesi J, et al. Radiotherapy in the management of cutaneous melanoma. Effect of time, dose, and fractionation. *Front Radiat Ther Oncol.* 1988;22:62–78.

25. Braun-Falco O, Lukacs S, Schoefinius HH. Zur Behandlung der melanosis circumscripta praecancerosa dubreuilh. *Hautarzt.* 1975;26:207–210.

26. Storck H. Treatment of melanotic freckles by radiotherapy. *J Dermatol Surg Oncol.* 1977;3:292–294.

27. Hauss H, Proppe A, Goldschmidt H. Radiotherapy of Lentigo maligna and Bowen's disease. In: Goldschmidt H, ed. *Physical Modalities in Dermatologic therapy.* New York, NY: Springer-Verlag; 1978:122–129.

28. Harwood AR. Conventional radiotherapy in the treatment of lentigo maligna and lentigo maligna melanoma. *J Am Acad Dermatol.* 1982;6:310–316.

29. Panizzon R. Radiotherapy of lentigo maligna and lentigo maligna-melanoma. In: Orfanos CE, Stadler R, Gollnick H, eds. *Dermatology in Five Continents.* Berlin: Springer-Verlag; 1988:930–932.

30. Kopf AF, Bart RS, Gladstein AH. Treatment of melanotic freckle with x-rays. *Arch Dermatol.* 1976; 112:801–807.

31. Harwood AR, Cummings BJ. Radiotherapy for malignant melanoma: a reappraisal. *Cancer Treat Rev.* 1981;8:271–282.

32. Haarwood AR. Conventional radiotherapy in the treatment of lentigo maligna and lentigo maligna melanoma. *J Am Acad Dermatol.* 1982;6:310–316.

33. Salmi R, Holsti P. Effects of roentgen irradiation on human melanoma metastases in the skin. *Acta Oncol.* 1987;26:37–40.

10

Radiation Therapy of Benign Tumors, Hyperplasias, and Dermatoses

Renato G. Panizzon

General Considerations

While modern indications for radiotherapy of skin cancers are well established, the use of ionizing radiation for benign skin diseases has decreased considerably as new and better systemic and local treatments have become available. In some diseases, ionizing radiation is a useful therapeutic alternative (e.g., for keloids or lymphocytoma cutis); in certain dermatoses (e.g., eczema) radiotherapy should be applied only after other therapeutic methods have failed or when active treatment seems essential for the well-being of the patient. Improved x-ray technology, accurate dosimetry, and strict adherence to safety rules have reduced cutaneous and noncutaneous side effects to a minimum.[1-4] The use of x rays for benign diseases in all medical specialties has recently been evaluated by the National Academy of Sciences. These recommendations are now endorsed by the Food and Drug Administration (FDA) (see Table 10.1[1]). The following discussion of radiation techniques for benign skin conditions is based on the assumption that the abovementioned criteria have been fulfilled, routine ways of therapy for these conditions have been found ineffective, contraindications to radiation therapy do not exist, the x-ray unit is calibrated regularly, and proper radiation protection is used.

Grenz-ray treatment (5–20 kV) is preferred for the treatment of very superficial skin conditions (see Chapter 12).

Soft and superficial x rays (20–100 kV) are more suitable for thick lesions, especially on the palms or soles. These x-ray qualities are appropriate for the treatment of lymphocytoma cutis, keloids, some recalcitrant eczematous disorders, and other resistant or recurrent dermatoses. It has been recommended to limit the total dose for soft x rays to 1200 cGy,[3,4] and for grenz rays to 5000 cGy.[5] Lindelöf and colleagues[6] conducted a large-scale investigation of grenz-ray therapy and concluded that even doses up to 10,000 cGy per lifetime and area are not associated with any significant side effects.[6] Superficial radiotherapy is a safe form of therapy provided that appropriate safety guidelines are adhered to, and that the prescribing physician has received adequate training.[7] In addition to the recommendations of the FDA, the following rules for the irradiation of benign skin diseases are emphasized in our department in Zürich:

The diagnosis must be clearly established (if possible by biopsy)

Radiotherapy should start at the most suitable time (e.g., in keloids)

There should be a reasonable expectation that radiotherapy would lead to an improvement

All patients should be questioned about previous irradiations

No area of the skin should be subjected to more than 1200 cGy of soft or superficial x rays per lifetime

No local treatment should be applied prior to radiotherapy to avoid irritating effects (e.g., 5-fluorouracil) or a reduction of the x-ray effect (e.g., zinc preparations)

"""

TABLE 10.1. FDA recommendations on ionizing radiation therapy of benign diseases.[a]

1. The potential risk of treatment with any form of radiation of a benign, non–life-threatening disease must be recognized. Ionizing radiation therapy may be considered if other safer methods have not succeeded in alleviating the condition and if the consequences of no further treatment are unacceptable
2. It must remain the prerogative of the physician to have available for use any form of therapy–radiation, drugs, or others—in which the benefits accruing to the patient from its use are considered to outweigh the risks inherent in its use
3. Infants and children should be treated with ionizing radiation only in exceptional cases
4. Direct irradiation of the skin areas overlying organs that are particularly prone to late effects, e.g., thyroid, eye, gonads, bone marrow, and breast, should be avoided
5. Medical practitioners using ionizing radiation should be adequately trained in both the practical and theoretical aspects of radiation therapy and protection
6. Meticulous radiation protection techniques should be used in all instances
7. The less penetrating x-ray qualities, e.g., grenz rays, offer a wider margin of safety
8. Laboratory and epidemiologic studies should be initiated and/or continued to fill the gaps in our knowledge of the effects of ionizing radiation at the doses used in the past and currently

[a] Reprinted by permission of the publisher from ref. 1. Copyright 1978 by Elsevier Science Publishing Co., Inc.

Lymphocytoma Cutis

Lymphocytoma cutis is a pseudolymphoma that occurs as a localized or disseminated type. Because there are different etiologic agents, a therapeutic trial with antibiotics may not induce quick resolution of the lesion. The localized and circumscribed type responds well to small doses of x rays. Early lesions are more radiosensitive than older lesions (Fig. 10.1.).

Review of Recent Literature

There are dose recommendations of 75 to 100 cGy weekly,[8] 2 times 100 cGy,[9] a single treatment of 150 to 200 cGy,[10] and single doses of 300 cGy at 3- to 4-week intervals up to a total of 1200 cGy.[8] Some authors suggest higher single doses of 500 cGy up to a total dose of 2500 cGy.[11] Multiple lesions in the face were treated with 1500 cGy in five fractions over a period of 5 to 7 days with excellent cosmetic

TABLE 10.2. Dose recommendations for lymphocytomas.

D½	1–15 mm
kV	20–50 or more
Filter	0.4–2.0 mm Al
HVL	0.2–1.6 mm Al
Single dose	100–200 cGy
Total dose	200–1200 cGy
Interval	4–7 days

results.[12] Goldschmidt and Sherwin recommend doses of 150 to 250 cGy, given at 1- to 3-week intervals in one to three sessions.[13] Our treatment schedule is shown in Table 10.2.

Keloid

In keloids, an active dynamic pathophysiologic process is associated with significant morbidity, such as stiffness, contraction, progressive growth, necrosis, and hyperesthesia. Large keloids on exposed body sites can result in isolation, discrimination, and restricted life style of the patient.

The popularity and enthusiasm for radiotherapy of keloids has varied. Recent reports stress the efficacy of postexcisional irradiation. This recommendation is based on the studies of several authors who have shown that the recurrence rate after keloid irradiation is much lower if radiation is administered following excision (25%–36%) than without prior excision (63%–74%).[14]

Review of Recent Literature

Radiotherapy is not always considered the treatment of first choice in primary keloids; however, radiotherapy can be administered alone or combined with other treatment modalities.[9,15] In such

TABLE 10.3. Dose recommendations for keloids.

D½	1–15 mm
kV	20–50 or more
Filter	0.4–2.0 mm Al
HVL	0.2–1.6 mm Al
Single dose	100–200 cGy
Total dose	400–1200 cGy
Interval	2–4 days

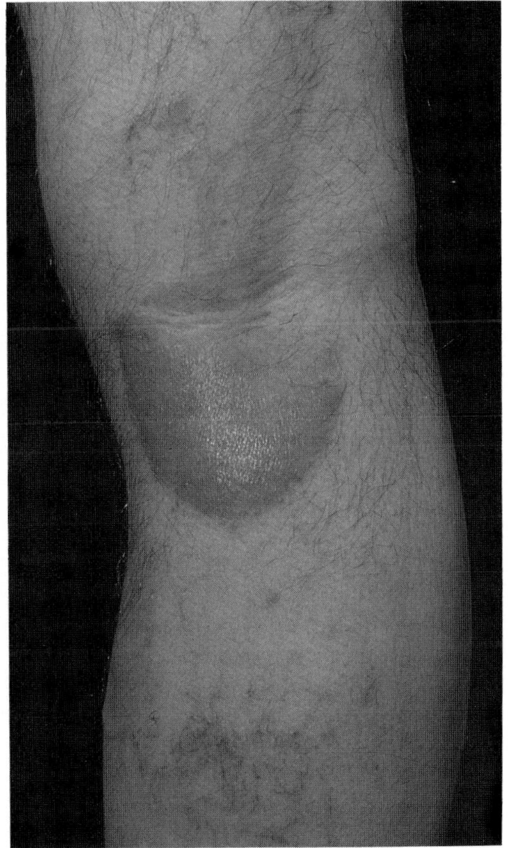
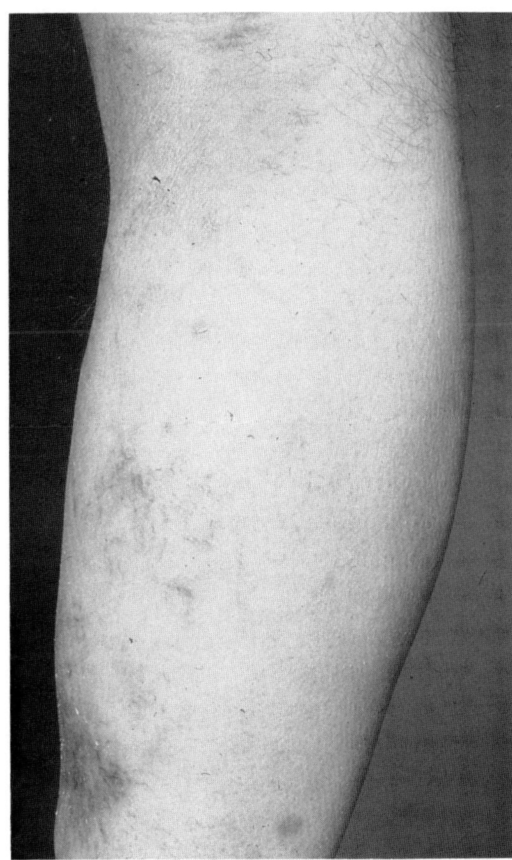

FIGURE 10.1. A, Lymphocytoma in the right popliteal area of a 72-year-old male patient. B, Same patient 6 months after radiotherapy with 4 × 200 cGy, 40 kV, 1.0 mm Al, every 4 days.

cases, the response is better if the keloid is treated at the earliest possible time. A study in our department has shown that radiation is much less effective in keloids older than 6 months.[16] Enhamre and Hammar[17] and Borok[14] found no correlation between therapeutic results and the time interval between excision and irradiation, reporting a 88% and a 99% favorable result, respectively. Borok used 1200 cGy in three fractions over 1 week.[14] Inalsingh[18] described impressive results and reemphasized the important role of radiation in the treatment of keloids.

In recent years various authors have suggested total doses ranging between 200 and 2000 cGy, administered over 1 to 2 weeks.[14,19-21] A minimum isoeffect time-dose line for postoperative keloid control was seen with 900 to 1000 cGy delivered over 1 week, or 1500 cGy over 2 weeks. A similar postoperative threshold dose of 1200 to 1600 cGy was confirmed by Edsmyr and colleagues.[22] Higher total doses[23] are more prone to induce telangiectases. Our dose recommendations for keloids are listed in Table 10.3.

Eczema/Dermatitis

General Considerations

As the frequency of use of x rays for benign dermatoses has decreased, the order of frequency of its use has also changed. In an earlier survey, acne, warts, and hidradenitis were more often irradiated than eczematous conditions.[24] In contrast, the emphasis in recent years has been on the use of superficial x rays for eczemas.[25] If superficial x rays are used, the least penetrating x rays should be preferred; in most cases, grenz rays (see Chapter 12) are suitable. However, in some chronic, long-standing eczematous conditions, especially of the palms and soles, more penetrating radiation qualities (>20 kV) are more effective.[26]

Experimental Studies

An investigation of the effect of different doses of soft x rays in eczemas was undertaken by Goldschmidt and colleagues.[27] They showed that small single doses (40 cGy or lower) are less effective because repeated treatments are necessary to compensate for the reduced effect of smaller doses. There were no significant differences between single doses of 60, 80, or 100 cGy. Pathogenetically, the effect of soft x rays on eczematous lesions is probably related to a decrease of epidermal Langerhans' cells after irradiation.[28]

Review of Recent Literature

Earlier reports showed a favorable response rate for hyperkeratotic eczemas and chronic lichenified eczemas. Weekly doses of 75 to 100 cGy were administered at weekly intervals over a period of 3 to 4 weeks.[2,8] Other suggestions were doses of 50 to 75 cGy once per week or every 2 weeks for two to three exposures.[9] In a recent investigation, 24 patients with chronic symmetrical constitutional eczema of the hands were treated with superficial x-ray therapy applying three fractions of 100 cGy in intervals of 21 days to one hand; the other hand received a placebo treatment. A significantly better therapeutic result was recorded on the hand that received active x-ray treatment.[25] The same authors also investigated in a double-blind trial the difference between superficial x-ray therapy and grenz-ray therapy, and found that a total dose of 300 cGy of conventional superficial x rays was superior to 900 cGy of grenz rays. The doses were administered in three fractions with a 21-day interval.[26] In atopic (constitutional) eczema, ionizing radiation is rarely advisable because of its high tendency to recur. Lichen simplex chronicus often responds quickly to radiation therapy; the

TABLE 10.4. Dose recommendations for chronic eczemas.

D½	1–3.0 mm
kV	20 or 30
Filter	0.4 or 0.5 mm Al
HVL	0.2 or 0.3 mm Al
Single dose	50–100 cGy
Total dose	300–1200 cGy
Interval	3–6 days

antipruritic effect of radiation in this dermatosis is striking.

Recent surveys indicate that the group of eczematous disorders constitute the most frequent indication for radiotherapy of benign lesions, especially in older patients with contraindications to systemic steroids or to the continued use of topical steroids.[29] Our dose recommendations are listed in Table 10.4. In general, a course of treatment consists of three to four treatments at 1- to 2-week intervals. A second or third course of therapy may be given 6 to 12 months after the preceding course.

Psoriasis

General Considerations

Once a widely used treatment modality, x-ray therapy is used only as a last resort in recalcitrant localized lesions. In view of the tendency of psoriasis to recur, x-ray therapy should be limited to severe cases. If properly used, radiation therapy is not associated with any major side effect and it remains to be seen whether antimetabolites or long-range psoralen-ultraviolet A (PUVA) treatments will show fewer sequelae than judiciously used x-ray therapy. Previous x-ray treatments are now considered a contraindication to PUVA therapy in view of the potential increase in the frequency of treatment-related skin cancers. Harber[30] has shown that there was no difference between conventional superficial therapy and grenz rays in more than 70% of the patients. Other authors found that the effect of superficial x rays were longer lasting than grenz rays.[31]

Current limited indications include psoriasis of the palms, soles, and nails, or scalp lesions. The latter are mostly treated by grenz rays (see Chapter 12). Palmoplantar pustular psoriasis is not considered a good indication for radiotherapy.[32]

A

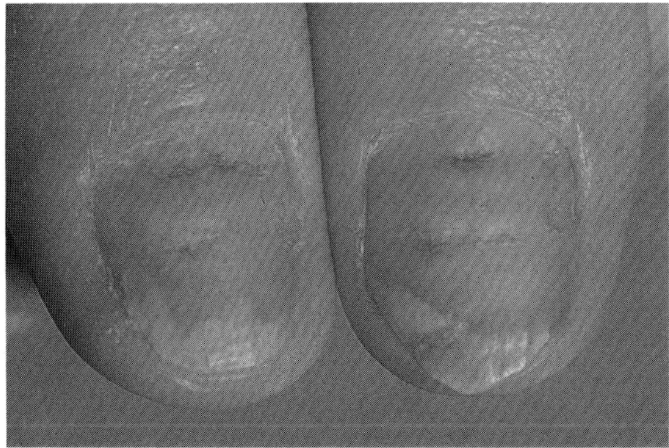

B

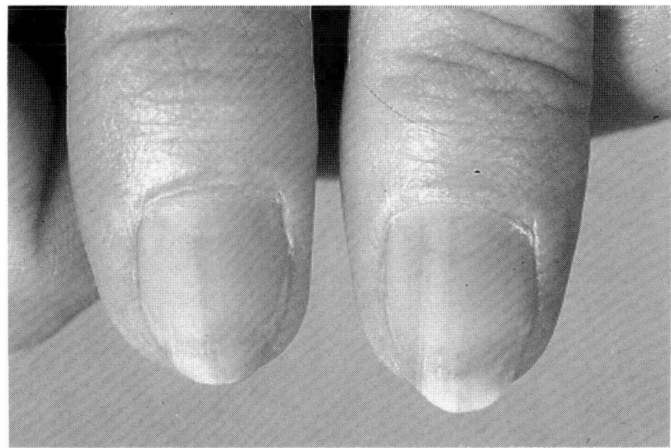

FIGURE 10.2. A, Psoriatic thumbnails in a 46-year-old female patient. B, Same patient 10 months after radiotherapy of 6 × 100 cGy, 30 kV, 0.5 mm Al, once per week.

TABLE 10.5. Dose recommendations for psoriasis of the nails.

D½	1–5 mm
kV	20 or 30
Filter	0.4 or 0.5 mm Al
HVL	0.2 or 0.3 mm Al
Single dose	100 cGy
Total dose	300–1200 cGy
Interval	4–7 days

several months.[36] Kouskoukis and colleagues[37] suggested 100 cGy at weekly intervals up to a total dose of 400 to 500 cGy with remissions lasting for months or years. In accordance with other reports in the literature, we recommend the dose schedule described in Table 10.5. Results are illustrated in Fig. 10.2.

Other Rare Indications for Radiotherapy

Lichen Planus

Severely pruritic and refractory cases of the verrucous form of lichen planus, particularly on the legs, may be considered for radiotherapy.[3,8,9] A sufficiently deep half-value depth must be selected, and one must be aware of temporary, occasionally long-lasting, hyperpigmentations.[2] Along with most other authors, we recommend the same dosages suggested for psoriasis (see Table 10.5).

Review of Recent Literature

Before irradiating psoriatic nails, it is important to estimate the nail thickness and to know the transmission of x rays through normal and diseased nails. Although grenz rays may be tried in psoriatic nails of normal thickness,[33] it has been shown that they are less effective in diseased nails, because they are thickened.[34] Since most psoriatic nails are relatively thick, we prefer soft x rays. Good responses were reported in 50% of irradiated patients, treated with three doses of 100 to 150 cGy at weekly intervals; the fingernails, nail matrix, and periungual area were included in the irradiated field.[8,35] Finnerty described three patients treated with six to eight doses of 50 to 75 cGy with total doses of approximately 400 to 600 cGy: all treated nails cleared after

Acne

Acne used to be the most common indication for dermatologic radiotherapy in the United States; therapy usually consisted of 6 to 8 weekly treatments of 60 to 80 cGy. Injudicious use of x rays with repeated courses of treatment leading to excessive total doses was the cause of many cases of chronic radiodermatitis and radiogenic carcinomas. Because of the introduction of systemic retinoids for severe forms of acne, radiation therapy is now used only in exceptional cases with contraindications to the use of retinoids. It is important to realize that doses of at least 500 cGy are necessary to obtain the desired therapeutic effect in acne.[2] A recent report indicates that it is possible to reduce sebum secretion temporarily with only three sessions of 50 cGy administered once a week.[38] In Zürich soft x-ray therapy is administered only in rare cases, usually in the back area. The doses applied are the same as for eczema (see Table 10.4), usually not exceeding a total dose of 500 cGy.

Hemangiomas

Strawberry angiomas disappear spontaneously during the first 5 years of life without any form of treatment. For exceptional hemangiomas involving locations close to vital organs or associated with rapid growth or thrombocytopenia (Kasabach-Merritt syndrome), and for hemangiomas not responding to oral corticosteroids, doses of 200 cGy in one to three sessions may be helpful.[9] Absolute contraindications prevail in locations over radiosensitive tissues. In one study, no difference was found between irradiated and placebo-irradiated hemangiomas.[39]

Verrucae

Because there is a variety of effective treatment modalities available, we have discontinued using radiotherapy of warts in our department. In some patients, the required doses may lead to sequelae.[40]

Hidradenitis Suppurativa

The chronic type of hidradenitis suppurativa is difficult to treat. In selected cases a combination of radiation therapy with other treatment modalities is possible. Seventy five to 100 cGy administered in four to six doses at weekly intervals, or 100 cGy 3 times at 3-week intervals, are often effective.[4] The acute painful type and the chronic type of hidradenitis require different techniques and different individual doses. (See Tables 10.6 and 10.7).

TABLE 10.6. Dose recommendations for painful parony-chia/hidradenitis/leg ulcers.

D½	1–15 mm
kV	20–50 or more
Filter	0.4–2.0 mm Al
HVL	0.2–1.6 mm Al
Single dose	20 cGy
Total dose	60–200 cGy (1st series)
Interval	daily

TABLE 10.7. Dose recommendations for chronic parony-chia.

D½	1–5 mm
kV	20 or 30
Filter	0.4 or 0.5 mm Al
HVL	0.2 or 0.3 mm Al
Single dose	50–100 cGy
Total dose	200–1200 cGy
Interval	3–6 days

Paronychia

As in hidradenitis suppurativa, we must distinguish between acute and chronic forms of paronychia. X irradiation is indicated only in exceptional cases, usually in combination with antibiotics and other treatment modalities. Paronychia is often multifactorial and even with proper local treatment, this disease may be resistant to treatment and cause considerable tenderness and discomfort. The dose schedules are similar to hidradenitis.[2,4,9] For painful lesions we prefer low single doses, which are usually sufficient to relieve symptoms quickly[41] (see Table 10.6); for more chronic inflammatory forms of paronychia, single doses of 50 to 100 cGy, once or twice weekly, in one to four sessions are recommended (see Table 10.7). We also consider low doses of x rays an excellent adjunctive treatment for painful leg ulcers.[42]

References

1. Goldschmidt H. FDA recommendations on radiotherapy of benign diseases. *J Dermatol Surg Oncol.* 1978;4:619–620.
2. Goldschmidt H, Sherwin WK. Radiation therapy of benign skin disorders. In: Moschella SL, Hurley HJ, eds. *Dermatology*, 2nd ed. Philadelphia, Penn: WB Saunders Co; 1985:2075–2078.
3. Rowell N. Adverse effects of superficial x-ray therapy and recommendations for safe use in benign dermatoses. *J Dermatol Surg Oncol.* 1978;4:630–634.
4. Rowell NR. Ionizing radiation in benign dermatoses. In: Rook AJ, ed. *Recent Advances in Dermatology, No. 4.* Edinburgh: Churchill Livingstone; 1977: 329–350.
5. Goldschmidt H. Ionizing radiation therapy. In: Arnold H, ed. *Andrews' Diseases of the Skin.* Philadelphia, Penn: WB Saunders Co; in press.

6. Lindelöf B, Eklund G. Incidence of malignant skin tumors in 14,140 patients after grenz-ray treatment for benign skin disorders. *Arch Dermatol.* 1986;122:1391–1395.

7. Sheehan-Dare RA, Goodfield MJD, Rowell NR. Superficial radiotherapy for benign dermatoses. *Br J Dermatol.* 1989;121(suppl):62–63.

8. Lukacs S, Braun-Falco O, Goldschmidt H. Radiotherapy of benign dermatoses: indications, practice, and results. *J Dermatol Surg Oncol.* 1978;4:620–625.

9. Jolly HW. Superficial x-ray therapy in dermatology 1978. *Int J Dermatol.* 1978;17:691–697.

10. Everett MA. Superficial x-ray for benign lesions termed useful adjunctive measure. *Dermatol Pract.* 1975;March-April:6–9.

11. Gilkes JJH, Munro DD. Lymphocytoma cutis. *Br J Clin Pract.* 1974;28:157–162.

12. Olson LE, Wilson JF, Cox JD. Cutaneous lymphoid hyperplasia: results of radiation therapy. *Radiology.* 1985;155:507–509.

13. Goldschmidt H, Sherwin WK. Dermatologic radiotherapy. In: Moschella SL, Hurley HJ, eds. *Dermatology.* 2nd ed. Philadelphia, Penn: WB Saunders Co; 1985:2074–2075.

14. Borok TL, Bray M, Sinclair I, et al. Role of ionizing irradiation for 393 keloids. *Int J Radiat Oncol Biol Phys.* 1988;15:865–870.

15. Braun-Falco O, Lukacs S, Goldschmidt H. *Dermatologic Radiotherapy.* New York, NY: Springer-Verlag; 1976.

16. Fischer E, Storck H. Zur Röntgentherapie der Keloide. *Schweiz Med Wschr.* 1957;41:1281–1285.

17. Enhamre A, Hammar H. Treatment of keloids with excision and post-operative x-ray irradiation. *Dermatologica.* 1983;167:90–93.

18. Inalsingh CHA. An experience in treating 501 patients with keloids. *Johns Hopkins Med J.* 1974;134:284–290.

19. Ollstein RN, Siegel HW, Gillodey JF, et al. Treatment of keloids by combined surgical excision and immediate postoperative x-ray treatment. *Ann Plast Surg.* 1981;7:281–285.

20. Brown LA, Pierce HE. Keloids: scar revisions. *J Dermatol Surg Oncol.* 1986;12:51–56.

21. Kovalic JJ, Perez CA. Radiation therapy following keloidectomy: a 20-year experience. *Int J Radiat Oncol Biol Phys.* 1989;17:77–80.

22. Edsmyr F, Larsson LG, Onyango J, et al. Radiation therapy in the treatment of keloids in East Africa. *Acta Radiol (Ther).* 1974;13:102–106.

23. Caccialanza M, Dal Pozzo V, Di Pietro A, et al. Radioterapia post-operatioria del cheloidi. *G Ital Dermatol Venereol.* 1987;471–475.

24. Goldschmidt H. Ionizing radiation therapy in dermatology: current use in the United States and Canada. *Arch Dermatol.* 1975;111:1511–1517.

25. Fairris GM, Mack DP, Rowell NR. Superficial x-ray therapy in the treatment of constitutional eczema of the hands. *Br J Dermatol.* 1984;111:445–450.

26. Fairris GM, Jones DH, Mack DP, et al. Conventional superficial x-ray versus grenz ray therapy in the treatment of constitutional eczema of the hands. *Br J Dermatol.* 1985;112:339–341.

27. Goldschmidt H, Yawalkar S, Gruber L, et al. Experimentelle Untersuchungen zur Weichstrahldosierung bei Ekzem und Psoriasis. *Strahlentherapie.* 1962;118:240–249.

28. Groh V, Meyer JC, Panizzon R, et al. Soft x-irradiation influences the integrity of Langerhans cells. *Dermatologica.* 1984;168:53–60.

29. Goldschmidt H. Radiotherapy of benign skin conditions. In: Newcomer VD, Young EM, eds. *Geriatric Dermatology.* New York, NY: Igaku-Shoin; 1989:89–96.

30. Harber LC. Clinical evaluation of radiation therapy in psoriasis. *Arch Dermatol.* 1958;77:554–558.

31. Baer RL, Witten VH. Year Book of Dermatology. Chicago, Ill: Year Book Medical Publishers; 1957.

32. Fairris GM, Jones DH, Mack DP, et al. Superficial x-ray therapy in the treatment of palmoplantar pustulosis. *Br J Dermatol.* 1984c;111:499–500.

33. Lindelöf B. Psoriasis of the nails treated with grenz rays: a double-blind bilateral trial. *Acta Dermatovenereol.* 1989;69:80–82.

34. Gammeltoft M, Wulf HC. Transmission of 12 kV grenz rays and 29 kV x-rays through normal and diseased nails. *Acta Dermatovenereol.* 1980;60:431–432.

35. Wiskemann A. Strahlenbehandlung der Psoriasis und Parapsoriasis. *Z Hautkr.* 1982;57:1317–1324.

36. Finnerty EF. Successful treatment of psoriasis of the nails. *Cutis.* 1979;23:43–44.

37. Kouskousis CE, Scher RK, Lebovits PE. Psoriasis of the nails. *Cutis.* 1983;31:169–174.

38. Caccialanza M, Bonelli M, Rivolta M. I lipidi della superficie cutanea in rapporto alla roentgenterapia dell'acne polimorfa giovanile. *G Ital Dermatol Venereol.* 1980;115:260–262.

39. Jung EG. Die Strahlentherapie der Haemangiome. *Dermatologica.* 1976;153:86–87.

40. Reymann F. The sensitivity of plantar warts to roentgen radiation. *Acta Dermatovenereol.* 1969;49:171–175.

41. Fischer E. Therapeutische Erfahrungen mit Röentgenkleindosen bei akut entzündlichen Prozessen. *Dermatologica.* 1957;114:204–208.

42. Panizzon R. Die Strahlentherapie bei Komplikationen der chronisch-venösen Insuffizienz. *Schweiz Rundsch Med (PRAXIS).* 1980;69:1405–1407.

11

Electron-Beam Therapy

John C. Breneman

Electron-beam radiation represents a significant addition to the armamentarium of the clinician wishing to use ionizing radiation for the treatment of skin lesions. With the introduction of the medical linear accelerator, electron-beam radiation has come into routine clinical use. Electrons have many properties that make them well suited for treating the skin, chief among these being a depth of penetration that can be well controlled with little or no exposure to tissue beyond the targeted depth, as occurs in superficial x rays. However, in contrast to superficial photon irradiation, electron radiation is relatively difficult and expensive to produce.

Although in many situations electrons and superficial photon radiation can be used interchangeably for the treatment of the skin, there are instances where one or the other is preferable (see Table 11.1). Many of these instances are peculiar to the physical and biological properties of electrons, which will be discussed.

Physical and Biologic Interactions

Electrons interact with tissue on a molecular basis in a manner similar to x rays.[1] The ultimate physical effect in both cases is ionization of the molecules with which the radiations interact, leading to loss of reproductive integrity when cellular deoxyribonucleic acid (DNA) is chemically altered. The similarity of the interactions means that the relative biologic effectiveness (RBE) of electrons and x rays are close (electrons have an RBE that is about 90% of x rays),[2] so that a certain absorbed dose of electron radiation will have approximately the same physical and biologic effect in skin as the identical dose of x rays. Although some clinicians increase the prescribed dose of electrons by 10% over the equivalent dose of x rays to compensate for the slightly different RBEs,[3] most prescribe the radiation dose for a given lesion independent of the type of radiation that will be used.

One of the most significant differences between x rays and electron radiation is how the radiation dose is distributed once it enters tissue.[4] Although x rays are attenuated in intensity as they pass through the skin, they are wave-like in nature and have an indefinite range, penetrating subcutaneous tissues to an extent dependent upon their energy. Electrons, being particles, have only a limited range in tissue before coming to a complete stop, so that it is possible to expose the superficial tissues of the body with essentially no penetration of radiation beyond the desired depth (Fig. 11.1). This property has obvious advantages in the treatment of skin lesions, particularly when large areas of the skin are being treated. The depth of penetration of an electron is determined by its energy with typical clinically used beams ranging from 3 to 20 million electron volts (MeV). Approximately 80% of the given dose of an electron beam will penetrate to a depth in centimeters of tissue equal to one-third the energy of the beam in MeV (e.g., 2 cm for a 6-MeV beam, 3 cm for a 9-MeV beam). This depth is often taken as the maximum useful range of a particular energy of electron radiation because the dose falls off very rapidly beyond this point.

Another difference between x rays and electrons is the relationship between the radiation exposure dose (roentgens [R]) and radiation absorbed dose

TABLE 11.1. Comparison of electron radiation to superficial x rays.

Electrons	Superficial x rays
Limited depth of penetration, with no exposure beyond a certain depth	Continued (although diminished) penetration into deep tissues of the body
Edges of radiation field are "blurry"	"Sharp" field edges
More difficult to shape fields due to thickness of blocks	Fields easily shaped with lead foil
Long radiation SSD of accelerator helps create homogeneous radiation doses in tissue	Short SSD may create significant dose inhomogeneities in some situations
Absorbed radiation dose similar in skin and bone	Absorbed radiation dose in bone may be up to 4 times greater than skin
Expensive to use	Relatively inexpensive to use

(cGy) of the two radiations. The photoelectric interaction by which superficial x rays are absorbed depends on the cube of the Z number of the absorbing tissue, with an exposure of 1 R of superficial x rays yielding an absorbed dose of about 1 cGy in skin. However, this same exposure in bone leads to an absorbed dose of almost 4 cGy due to the higher Z number of the bone. Since absorption of electron radiation is not mediated by the photoelectric effect, a given exposure of electrons gives a more similar (approximately 1.5 times) absorbed dose in bone as compared to skin. This is of clinical significance in situations where there is bone closely underlying skin that is to be treated with radiation, such as occurs on the scalp or dorsum of the hand. When treating these areas with superficial x rays, care must be taken because, for any given exposure, the bone may absorb as much as 4 times more radiation compared to the skin. With electrons, absorbed dose in skin and bone is similar.

When prescribing electron-beam radiation to a given skin lesion, three parameters must be specified: dose, energy of the beam, and isodose level to which the dose is being delivered. The first two of these have already been discussed. Prescribing to an isodose level refers to the decision of which point on a graph of radiation intensity versus tissue depth (Fig. 11.1) is to receive the prescribed radiation dose. For example, if 100 cGy of 6-MeV electron radiation is prescribed to the 100% isodose line in tissue, then only a single point in tissue at a

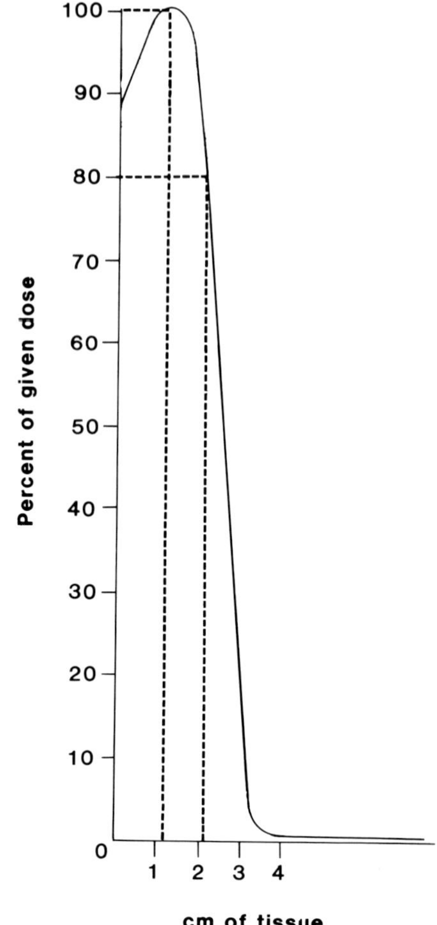

FIGURE 11.1. Penetration of 6-MeV electrons into skin. Note that the radiation intensity increases over the first several mm, reaching its peak (100%) at 1.2 cm. At 2.1 cm its intensity has fallen to 80% of peak, and from there, rapidly falls to 0.

depth of 1.2 cm receives the desired 100 cGy. Tissue both superficial and deep to this point receive less. If 100 cGy is prescribed to the 80% isodose line, then all of the tissue between the surface and 2.1 cm deep receives at least 100 cGy, with some tissue receiving substantially more.

Production of Electron-Beam Radiation

Since clinically useful electron-beam radiation must have energies about 50 times as great as x ray beams, it is much more difficult to produce from a technical standpoint. An x-ray tube cannot be run

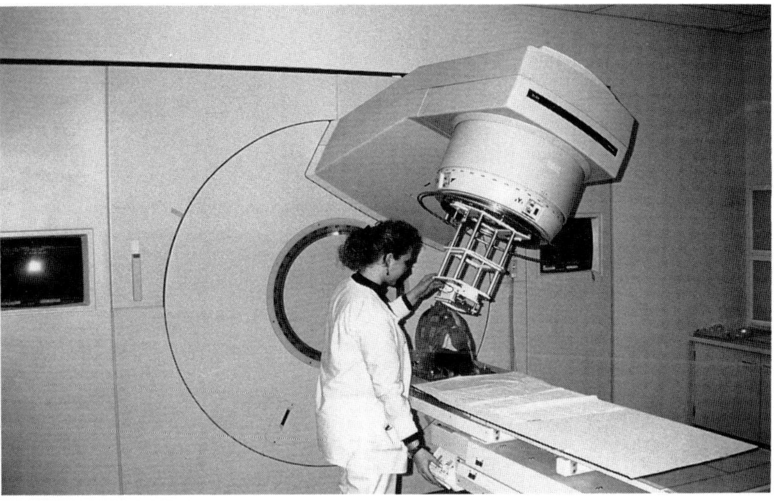

FIGURE 11.2. A medical linear accelerator such as this is capable of producing electron beam radiation with energies of 4–18 MeV. The cost of an accelerator is typically about 1 million dollars.

at these high energies (often 5 million volts or more), so other technologies for making the electron radiation must be employed. Although various types of equipment such as betatrons and Van de Graaf accelerators have been used in the past for this purpose, the most efficient and widely used device is a linear accelerator (Fig. 11.2). In an accelerator, electrons are created by "boiling" them off a cathode element, just as is done in an x-ray tube. However, at this point, instead of using an electric potential to accelerate the beam to the desired energy, the electrons are propelled by a precisely tuned microwave carrier wave. Using this technology, beam energies of more than 20 MeV can be created.

An added benefit of the linear accelerator is that the distance from the source of the electrons in the accelerator to the skin to be treated (source-to-skin distance, or SSD) is relatively long (usually 100 cm) compared to that of a superficial x-ray machine (often less than 30 cm). This long SSD minimizes the influence of the inverse square law on dose intensity in the skin, giving a more homogeneous radiation dose compared to short SSD superficial x rays in areas where the skin surface is irregular, such as the nasolabial region and the pinna.

Total Skin Electron Irradiation

One of the most important applications of electron-beam therapy in dermatology is in the treatment of diseases involving large areas of the skin. For such diseases, treatment with x rays results in an unac-

ceptably high dose of internal radiation exposure. Electron radiation is ideal here because the depth of penetration can be well controlled. Total skin electron irradiation (TSEI) was introduced in 1951 as a method of treating mycosis fungoides[5]; since then, experience with thousands of patients has established it as one of the most effective treatments for this disease.

Treating the entire skin surface with a homogeneous dose of radiation poses a number of technical problems and several different techniques of treatment have been devised to deal with these.[6] All techniques use large field sizes generated by positioning the patient at a great distance from the linear accelerator (usually several meters). The patient is then placed in the radiation field in a number of different positions to spread the radiation evenly over the skin surface. Most techniques use a treatment distance that generates radiation field sizes sufficient to cover approximately half the body length. This permits reasonable treatment times, but necessitates careful, individually planned matching of two electron fields to cover each half (usually upper and lower) of the body without dose perturbations in the region where the fields join. Typically, electron energies of about 4 MeV are used to provide an effective penetration of about 1 cm into the body.

Patient positioning in the beam is done in several ways, ranging from the use of several fixed, discrete positions[7] to rotation of the patient on a platform during the radiation.[8,9] One popular technique devised at Stanford[10] uses six individual

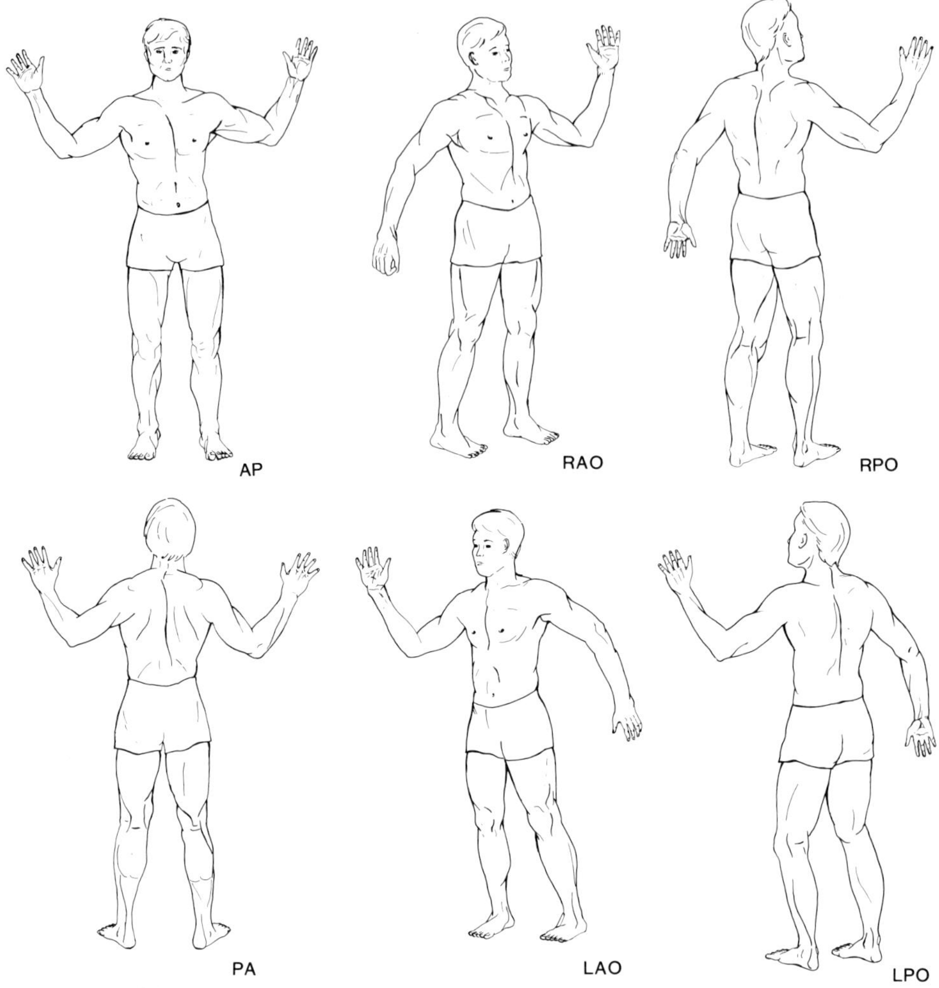

FIGURE 11.3. The Stanford technique of positioning patients for TSEI. The patient must be irradiated in all 6 positions to complete each individual treatment.

positions (Fig. 11.3) designed so that each part of the patient's body is exposed to the radiation beam equally. Since each of the six positions must be exposed twice (once to the upper body and once to the lower body), there are effectively 12 treatment positions necessary to complete each individual treatment. In practice, often only six fields are treated each day to keep the treatment time at 30 minutes or less, therefore taking 2 days to complete each cycle of treatment. During treatment patients may wear a thin hospital gown but are otherwise nude. Leaded goggles are usually worn by the patient to prevent cataracts and supporting straps are provided to help the patient hold his arms in

position. Because of the length of the treatment and the awkward positions the patient must maintain, the treatment is somewhat physically demanding, although most people are able to undergo therapy without significant difficulty. For those patients who cannot tolerate treatment in a standing position, a treatment technique has been described using a reclined patient position.[11]

Despite these carefully conceived TSEI techniques, individual patients will have inhomogeneities in the dose to various areas of their skin. There is always underdosage of the vertex of the scalp, soles of the feet, and dorsum of the penis. Depending on the TSEI technique and body habitus of the patient, other areas may be partially self-shielded during treatment, including under the arms, between the legs, the eyelids (if goggles are used), inframammary areas, and under panniculi. These areas must receive supplemental boost irradiation. On the other hand, some areas may receive more than the prescribed dose of radiation, such as the fingers, tops and sides of the feet, ears, nose, and portions of the arms. This is dealt with by shielding these areas during TSEI using lead sheets or layers of tissue-equivalent "bolus" material. Determination of which areas require shielding or boosting is made by combining clinical observation of the patient's skin during treatment with data obtained from in vivo measurements of radiation dose using thermoluminescent dosimetry chips (TLDs).

Treatment Regimens and Results of Total Skin Electron Irradiation

A variety of different regimens have been used in the treatment of mycosis fungoides. Low-dose (<3000 cGy) TSEI has been used in several hundred patients with excellent remission rates and palliation of symptoms.[12,13] Most patients have been treated with higher dose (3000–4000 cGy) TSEI with complete response of disease reported in about 85% of patients.[14-16] Although most patients with advanced disease relapse after months to years, some patients with early disease have no recurrence of their lesions for long periods of time and are presumed cured.[17,18] Hoppe and colleagues[19] have reported on 140 patients treated with doses of 2000 to 4000 cGy TSEI administered 4 days a week over 5 to 10 weeks. Complete remissions were obtained in 84% of patients, and of those having plaques involving less than 25% of their skin surface, 42% were free of disease after 10 years and presumably cured. For patients with more advanced cutaneous T-cell lymphoma, lower doses of 1500 to 3000 cGy have been shown to give excellent palliation and may permit the use of repeated treatments if necessary.[13,20]

Although TSEI has been used primarily to treat mycosis fungoides, it has also been applied successfully to other cutaneous lymphomas and leukemias,[7,21] as well as generalized Kaposi's sarcoma[22] and cutaneous histiocytosis X.

Toxicity of Total Skin Electron Irradiation

The development of acute and chronic side effects of TSEI depends on a number of factors, which include total dose, fractionation technique, homogeneity of dose over the skin surface, and skin type. For typical courses of TSEI consisting of 3000 to 4000 cGy administered over 8 to 10 weeks, side effects are usually mild and well tolerated.[23] Acutely, most patients experience alopecia with hair re-growth beginning soon after completion of treatment. However, in some patients, hair may return thinner, and sometimes is of a different color or texture. Swelling and tenderness may occur in the fingers and feet and occasionally bullae will form on the dorsum of the feet. Mild dryness and burning of the skin may occur, but is usually easily managed with topical moisturizers. Nail dystrophies are frequent as a result of temporary inhibition of growth of the nail plate, but are usually asymptomatic and self-correcting over a period of a few months. Diminished eccrine gland function has also been described, with function returning to normal within 6 months in most patients.[24]

Chronic effects are usually minimal, with some patients having persistent dry skin and pigmentation.[14] An increased risk of skin cancers is a theoretical concern but has not been widely reported. With high or repeated doses of TSEI, chronic effects may be more severe with telangiectasias, poikiloderma, ulcerations, and subcutaneous fibrosis being reported when cumulative doses approach 6000 cGy.[25]

Localized Skin Lesions, Including Basal and Squamous Cell Skin Carcinomas

For many superficial skin lesions, electron-beam therapy can be interchanged for superficial x rays at identical dosage and fractionation schedules. However, certain considerations when using electron-beam radiation deserve special mention. First, it can be seen by looking at the electron-beam depth dose curves that the peak dose of radiation does not occur at the skin surface, but rather builds to a maximum at a depth that is inversely related to the energy of the beam. One method of dealing with this is to add a layer of tissue-

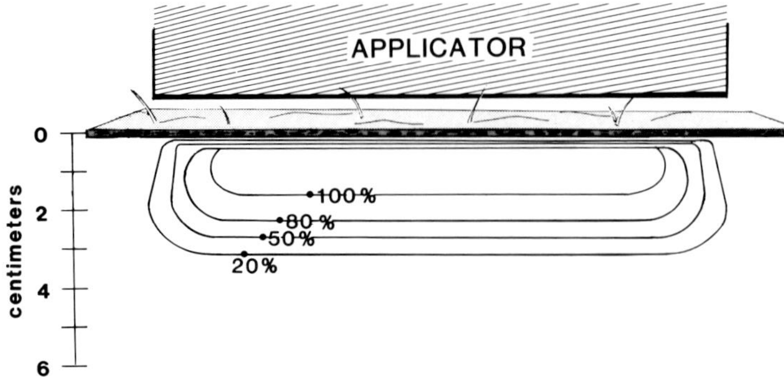

FIGURE 11.4. The profile of a 6-MeV electron beam in skin shows how the area receiving the prescribed dose (i.e., the area contained within the 100% isodose line) is significantly smaller than the area of skin that the applicator cone covers.

equivalent material (called bolus) on top of the skin to absorb this "build-up" area of the beam, and increase the energy of the beam so that the desired depth of penetration into the skin is maintained. Alternatively, one may prescribe to an appropriate isodose line that includes the skin surface and accept the higher peak dose that occurs in the deeper tissues.

Another consideration comes in determining the margins of coverage of the electron beam around the skin lesion. When examining the profile of an electron beam in tissue it can be seen that the area of high dose intensity is constricted inside the borders of the radiation field as marked on the skin surface by as much as 1 cm, creating a "blurred" field edge (Fig. 11.4). This peculiarity of electrons must be kept in mind when shaping the beams to individual lesions.

Finally, when shaping electron beams to lesions, more shielding must be used to block the electron beam than the millimeter of lead that suffices for superficial x rays. The equivalent of 3 to 4 mm of lead will shield >95% of electron radiation in the 4- to 8-MeV energy range usually used for skin tumors.[3] Therefore, electrons may not be the treatment of choice for lesions around the eye. The intraocular eye shields used to protect the lens from superficial x rays may not be sufficient to shield electron radiation, and this combined with the lack of "sharpness" at the edge of the electron field make superficial x rays preferable in this location.

Radiation dose and fractionation for electrons is usually identical to what would be used for superficial x rays. For smaller tumors, common treatment schedules include 3300 cGy in five fractions and 4300 cGy in 10 fractions. Larger lesions may require more prolonged treatment, such as 6600 cGy in 33 fractions, particularly when a good cosmetic outcome is important.

Although little has been reported about the clinical outcome of electron-beam radiation for the treatment of cutaneous basal and squamous cell carcinomas, available data indicate that cure of these tumors should occur about 90% of the time, as is expected with superficial x rays.[26] The choice of treatment modality depends then on individual patient factors and equipment availability. As a rule, superficial x rays will be preferable for most skin cancers because of the ease in shaping the fields and operating the equipment, and the lower costs involved. However, in selected cases electrons may be preferable. These include large lesions where there is concern about radiation exposure to subcutaneous tissues from superficial x rays[27] (especially on the scalp and dorsum of the hand); irregular treatment surfaces such as the pinna and nasolabial fold, where superficial x-ray machines with small SSDs could result in large dose inhomogeneities; and lesions that are too thick to be treated with x rays. These are the same situations that in the past required use of a radium mold for treatment, but with the current availability of electron-beam units, radium molds are seldom used.[28]

Acute and chronic side effects of electron radiation should be similar to those seen with identical schedules of superficial x rays. However, some authors have commented on a low incidence of moist desquamation with electron radiation.[28,29]

References

1. Jackson SM. Clinical application of electron beam therapy with energies up to 10 MeV. *Br J Radiol.* 1979;43(511):431–440.

2. Sinclair WK, Kohn HI. Relative biological effectiveness of high-energy photons and electrons. *Radiology.* 1964;82:800–814.

3. Tapley N. Skin and Lips. In: Tapley N, ed. *Clinical Applications of the Electron Beam.* New York, NY: John Wiley & Sons Inc; 1976:93–121.

4. Tapley N. General Considerations. In: Tapley N, ed. *Clinical Applications of the Electron Beam.* New York, NY: John Wiley & Sons Inc; 1976:81–92.

5. Fromer JL, Johnston DO, Salzman FA, et al. Management of lymphoma cutis with low megavolt electron beam therapy: nine-year follow-up in 200 cases. *South Med J.* 1961;54:769–776.

6. Holt JG, Perry DJ. Some physical considerations in whole skin electron beam therapy. *Med Phys.* 1982;9(5):769–777.

7. Nisce LZ, Chu FCH, Lee HS, et al. Total skin electron beam therapy for cutaneous lymphomas and leukemias. *Int J Radiat Oncol Biol Phys.* 1982;8:1587–1592.

8. Kim TH, Pla C, Pla M, et al. Clinical aspects of a rotational total skin electron irradiation. *Br J Radiol.* 1984;57:501–506.

9. Kumar PP, Good RR, Jones EO, et al. Dual-field rotational (DFR) technique for total-skin electron-beam therapy (TSEBT). *Am J Clin Oncol (CCT).* 1987;10(4):344–354.

10. Hoppe RT, Fuks Z, Bagshaw MA. Radiation therapy in the management of cutaneous T-cell lymphomas. *Cancer Treat Rep.* 1979;63:625–632.

11. Gerbi BJ, Khan FM, Deibel FC, et al. Total skin electron arc irradiation using a reclined patient position. *Int J Radiat Oncol Biol Phys.* 1989;17:397–404.

12. Nisce LZ, Safai B. Once weekly total-skin electron-beam therapy for mycosis fungoides: 7 years' experience. *Cancer Treat Rep.* 1979;63:633–638.

13. Lo TCM, Salzman FA, Moschella SL, et al. Whole body surface electron irradiation in the treatment of mycosis fungoides—an evaluation of 200 patients. *Radiology.* 1979;130:453–457.

14. Hamminga B, Noordijk EM, Van Vloten WA. Treatment of mycosis fungoides: total-skin electron-beam irradiation vs. topical mechlorethamine therapy. *Arch Dermatol.* 1982;118:150–153.

15. Tadros AAM, Tepperman BS, Hryniuk WM, et al. Total skin electron irradiation for mycosis fungoides: failure analysis and prognostic factors. *Int J Radiat Oncol Biol Phys.* 1983;9:1279–1287.

16. VanVloten WA, DeVroome H, Noordijk EM. Total skin electron beam irradiation for cutaneous T-cell lymphoma (mycosis fungoides). *Br J Dermatol.* 1985;112:697–702.

17. Lo TCM, Salzman FA, Costey GE, Wright KA. Megavolt electron irradiation for localized mycosis fungoides. *Acta Radiol Oncol.* 1981;20.

18. Meyler TS, Blumberg AL, Perser P. Total skin electron beam therapy in mycosis fungoides. *Cancer.* 1978;42:1171–1176.

19. Hoppe RT, Cox RS, Fuks Z, et al. Electron-beam therapy for mycosis fungoides: the Stanford University experience. *Cancer Treat Rep.* 1979;63:691–700.

20. Cotter GW, Baglan RJ, Wasserman TH, et al. Palliative radiation treatment of cutaneous mycosis fungoides—a dose response. *Int J Radiat Oncol Biol Phys.* 1983;9:1477–1480.

21. Rubin CM, Arthur DC, Meyers G, et al. Leukemia cutis treated with total skin irradiation. *Cancer.* 1985;55:2649–2652.

22. Nisce LZ, Safai B, Poussin-Rosillo H. Once weekly total and subtotal skin electron beam therapy for Kaposi's sarcoma. *Cancer.* 1981;47:640–644.

23. Desai KR, Penzer RD, Lipsett JA, et al. Total skin electron irradiation for mycosis fungoides: relationship between acute toxicities and measured dose at different anatomic sites. *Int J Radiat Oncol Biol Phys.* 1988;15:641–645.

24. Price NM. Electron beam therapy. *Arch Dermatol.* 1979;115:1068–1070.

25. Grollman JH, Bierman SM, Ottoman RE, et al. Total-skin electron-beam therapy of lymphoma cutis and generalized psoriasis: clinical experiences and adverse reactions. *Radiology.* 1966;87:908–915.

26. Tapley ND, Fletcher GH. Applications of the electron beam in the treatment of cancer of the skin and lips. *Radiology.* 1973;109:423–428.

27. Viravathana T, Prempree T, Sewchand W, et al. Technique and dosimetry in the management of extensive basal-cell carcinomas of the head and neck region by irradiation with electron beams. *J Dermatol Surg Oncol.* 1980;6(4):290–296.

28. Grosch E, Lambert HE. Treatment of difficult cutaneous basal and squamous cell carcinomata with electrons. *Br J Radiol.* 1979;52:472–477.

29. Johnson TS, Garciga CE, Feldman ME, et al. Low-megavoltage electron beam therapy of head and facial skin cancer using a versatile polystyrene collimator system. *Radiology.* 1975;115:695–699.

12

Grenz-Ray Therapy

Bernt Lindelöf

History

The effects of ionizing radiation on the skin became apparent quickly and radiation-induced dermatitis, epilation, and pigmentation first led to recognition of the biological effects of these rays. Some workers early on tried soft x rays in an effort to prevent severe sequelae, but the idea of using soft x rays in treating skin conditions lay dormant until 1923, when Gustav Bucky succeeded in devising an apparatus that produced ultrasoft x rays.[1] Since he believed that the biological effects of these rays resembled those of conventional x rays in some ways and those of ultraviolet rays in others, Bucky called the new rays grenz rays. The name "grenz" means "border" in German.

Physics

A grenz-ray machine is essentially a smaller type of x ray machine that uses electric potentials of 8 to 17 kV for the acceleration of the electrons. The quality of x rays is defined as their penetrating ability. The most frequently used definition for various x ray qualities is the half-value layer (HVL). It is defined as that thickness of a given filter material (in dermatology usually aluminum [Al]) that reduces the intensity to 50% of the original incident radiation. For grenz rays, they will be referred to as soft (HVL up to 0.02 mm Al), medium (HVL 0.023–0.029 mm Al), and hard (HVL 0.030–0.036 mm Al). The HVL is influenced by multiple factors but for practical purposes only two of them are important: kilovoltage and addi-

tional filtration. An x-ray beam produced by higher kilovoltage has shorter wavelengths and greater penetrating power. By placing a filter in the x-ray beam the quality is changed in such a way that the higher the atomic number of the filter, the greater the reduction in beam intensity. The intensity or dose rate of radiation is influenced by kilovoltage (kV), milliamperage (mA), filter, exposure time, and target skin distance (TSD). It increases when the kV and mA are increased. It decreases as the distance is increased, approximately in inverse square proportion, and it is also reduced as the thickness and atomic number of the filter are increased. The radiation dose is directly proportional to the exposure time if all other factors remain constant. The x-ray dose in roentgen (R) specifies the exposure to a certain quantity of radiation, based on its ability to ionize air. It is not identical with the observed dose in the tissue, which is expressed in rads. The unit of the absorbed dose (tissue dose) used today is Gray (Gy): according to the International System of Units (SI) standards, 1 Gy equals 100 rads.

Biologic Effects

Grenz rays are absorbed predominantly through the photoelectric effect. Since their energy is small at the outset, the path of the photoelectron is short, so that its entire quantum of energy is absorbed within one cell. However, thousands of collisions occur along that short path. This produces ions and excited atoms and molecules that are able to enter into chemical combinations with free radicals or other molecules to form new molecules of unpredictable effect on the tissue.[2] Recent research has shown that grenz-ray therapy decreases the number of Langerhans' cells in the epidermis. After a single dose of 400 cGy of 10 kV grenz rays on human epidermis, it was found that the number of Langerhans' cells (OKT-6 positive) was slightly reduced after 30 minutes and markedly reduced 1 and 3 weeks after irradiation.[3] By counting the Langerhans' cells at electron microscopic resolution in human epidermis before and after grenz-ray therapy, it was confirmed that the Langerhans' cells disappeared from the epidermis after treatment. No consistent differences in keratinocyte morphology was observed.[4] By pretreating nickel-sensitive patients with grenz rays and then applying nickel patch tests on the treated area and on untreated control skin, it has been shown that grenz-ray therapy can almost totally suppress allergic contact dermatitis.[5] This suppression lasts for about 3 weeks after treatment and is paralleled by a suppression of the number of Langerhans' cells in the epidermis.[6] The mechanism of action of grenz rays on psoriasis is not known, but an antimitotic effect or an influence on the dermal infiltrate in psoriasis may be an explanation.

Side Effects

Possible effects of grenz-ray therapy are qualitatively identical to those of conventional x rays. The principal adverse effects are erythema and pigmentation. Grenz-ray erythema is relatively asymptomatic, and its latent period is shorter than that of conventional x-ray erythema. It is ordinarily not followed by sequelae other than pigmentation.[2] The intensity of this cutaneovascular reaction varies greatly, not only among different individuals but also among different body regions of the same individual.[7] Pigmentation may result from grenz-ray therapy and close shielding should be avoided in order not to produce a sharp line at the edge of the treated area. Pigmentation so induced varies with race, age, and body region, but is never permanent.[8] Large doses may occasionally give rise to a peculiar pigment displacement, a spotty hyperpigmentation instead of uniform hyperpigmentation.[2]

Cancer Development

In 1959, the first case of squamous cell carcinoma resulting from an extreme overdosage of grenz rays was described.[7] Since then, 40 cases have been reported.[9-11] The carcinogenic effect of grenz rays has also been studied in experimental animals.[12-15] It has been shown that grenz rays can produce metastatic squamous cell carcinoma under certain experimental conditions and that the pattern of tumor development, as in ultraviolet light exposure, was that of carcinogenic summation. The incidence of carcinoma after grenz-ray therapy is small indeed but may follow extremely high doses in persons who are abnormally sensitive to x rays.[9]

Indications

Most inflammatory dermatoses have their pathology in the first millimeter of skin and the rest in the first 3 mm of skin. Grenz-ray therapy may be expected to be beneficial because 50% of grenz radiation administered is absorbed by the first 0.5 mm of the skin. This form of radiation is extremely suitable if one considers the sparing effect on hair roots, sebaceous and sweat glands, eyes, and gonads. The list of conditions for which grenz-ray therapy has been reported to be effective is long, but much of the treatment recorded in the literature is obsolete today. For a full account of grenz-ray therapy the monographs of Bucky and Combes[16] and Hollander[2] should be consulted.

The list of conditions for which grenz-ray therapy today is indicated and effective is as follows:

1. psoriasis
2. lichen simplex chronicus
3. pruritus ani et vulvae
4. seborrheic dermatitis
5. nummular eczema
6. nonspecific, persistent eczematous conditions
7. lichen planus

Psoriasis

Grenz-ray therapy should be considered as one of the most useful agents in psoriasis.[17] Many observers have reported good response to grenz rays but some of them also emphasized the frequency and/or promptness of recurrence and warned against the production of erythema as possibly leading to a Koebner reaction.[18-22] Especially good results have been obtained in the treatment of psoriasis of the scalp,[23-25] which often is difficult to treat successfully. When tar lotions or corticosteroids are unsuccessful, there are fewer alternative treatment modalities left, compared to treatment of psoriasis of other body regions. Ultraviolet B and psoralen-ultraviolet A are ineffective because of the inability of these light qualities to penetrate the hair in sufficient doses. Dithranol cream is often effective but this treatment is messy, time-consuming, and must be carried out with persistence. Grenz-ray therapy should therefore be considered as a useful therapeutic agent in psoriasis of the scalp. Apart from the results obtained, it exceeds other local therapies by its convenience in application. In the treatment of psoriasis of the scalp it is important to remove scales because they and hair absorb an important quantity of the dose. Scales can be removed by pretreating the scalp with topical oils containing salicylic acid a few times before grenz-ray treatment. Hair can be moved by combing in such a way that the cone of the grenz-ray machine lies close to the scalp with a minimum of hair in between. By combining a topical steroid with the grenz-ray therapy in the treatment of psoriasis of the scalp, a faster clearing and a longer remission time has been obtained,[24] but this good result was not reproducible in another study.[25] Overall, about 80% of the patients healed completely after grenz-ray therapy in these studies,[23-25] and 50% to 70% were still healed at 3 months after treatment. At 6 months after treatment up to 50% of the patients were still free of lesions. Grenz-ray therapy (10 kV) could also be useful in nail psoriasis if the nails are of normal thickness. However, no nails healed completely and thick psoriatic nails showed no improvement at all.[26] The penetration of grenz rays was obviously too small, and harder x rays were needed.

Lichen Simplex Chronicus and Eczematous Conditions

In lichenified dermatitis, grenz rays have been uniformly effective.[27] In chronic eczema of the hands, grenz-ray therapy produced superior results compared to nonirradiated controls.[28]

Lichen Planus

Good results have been obtained by many workers in the treatment of lichen planus, but there is a risk of an acute flare-up, possibly because of a Koebner reaction.[29,30]

Other Indications

Darier's Disease

There are several reports of improvement or complete clearing of lesions after grenz-ray therapy for Darier's disease.[2,31,32]

Histiocytosis X

Good results have been reported in one patient with histiocytosis X.[33]

Dosage

The most common radiation quality used for grenz rays is 10 kV; in the United States some dermatologists prefer 15 to 25 kV grenz rays. The interval between treatments recommended by different authors varies from 1 to 3 weeks. In my opinion, an interval of 1 week is suitable, and four to six treatments are usually necessary. The areas of skin vary in their radiosensitivity, which must be taken into account. Palms, soles, and scalp are the least sensitive and 400 cGy for each treatment can be administered safely. The anogenital area is the most sensitive and thus the dose must be reduced to 50 to 200 cGy for each treatment. Light-skinned and/or light-sensitive patients tolerate radiation less well and the dose must be reduced. Scales and hair absorb an important quantity of the dose[34] and in the case of thick hair, the dose must be doubled when treating the scalp. Scales must be removed before treatment by using a salicylic-acid ointment. The maximum cumulative dose for a certain area of skin should not exceed an arbitrary limit of 10,000 cGy. In situations where it seems advisable to go beyond this limit, the patient should be monitored closely and the treated area should be examined for malignant transformations every 10,000 cGy. The only large-scale study of the carcinogenic effect of grenz-ray therapy[11] did not reveal any increased risk of cancer development in 481 patients who had received at least 10,000 cGy on the same body area. In my opinion, palms, soles, and scalp tolerate grenz-ray therapy very well, and can be safely exposed to much more than 10,000 cGy of grenz rays in a lifetime.

Radiation Protection

The exposure to grenz rays of office personnel handling a grenz-ray unit at 10 kV and a dose rate of 100 cGy per 10 seconds has been investigated for different treatment situations. Scattered and leakage radiation and primary radiation at some distance from the grenz-ray unit were measured. Air absorption was found to be most important. Direct exposure of the operator to the primary grenz-ray beam at a distance of 4 m was practically nil. At a distance of 2 m from the unit, the operator was permitted to be exposed 100 hours per year; at a distance of 1 m, the permitted exposure of the direct beam was 3 hours per year. Scattered and leakage radiation from the unit was of no importance and certain clothing was demonstrated to promote absorption.[35]

References

1. Bucky G. Grenz ray therapy. New York, NY: Macmillan Co; 1929.
2. Hollander MB. *Ultrasoft X-rays. An Historical and Critical Review of the World Experience with Grenz Rays and Other X-rays of Long Wave-length.* Baltimore, Md: William & Wilkins; 1968.
3. Lindelöf B, Lidén S, Ros A-M. Effect of grenz rays on Langerhans' cells in human epidermis. *Acta Dermatol Venereol.* 1984;64:436–438.
4. Lindelöf B, Forslind B. Electron microscopic observation of Langerhans' cells in human epidermis irradiated with grenz rays. *Photodermatology.* 1985; 2:367–371.
5. Lindelöf B, Lidén S, Lagerholm B. The effect of grenz rays on the expression of allergic contact dermatitis in man. *Scand J Immunol.* 1985;21:463–469.
6. Ek L, Lindelöf B, Liden S. The duration of grenz ray-induced suppression of allergic contact dermatitis and its correlation to the density of Langerhans' cells in human epidermis. *Clin Exp Dermatol* 1989; 14:206–209.
7. Kalz F. Observations on grenz ray reactions. *Dermatologica.* 1959;118:357–371.
8. Rowell N. Adverse effects of superficial x-ray therapy and recommendations for safe use in benign dermatoses. *J Dermatol Surg Oncol.* 1978;4:630–634.
9. Frentz G. Grenz ray-induced nonmelanoma skin cancer. *J Am Acad Dermatol.* 1989;21:475–478.
10. Mortensen AC, Kjeldsen H. Carcinomas following grenz ray treatment of benign dermatoses. *Acta Dermatol Venereol.* 1987;67:523–525.
11. Lindelöf B, Eklund G. Incidence of malignant skin tumors in 14,140 patients after grenz ray treatment for benign skin disorders. *Arch Dermatol.* 1986;122: 1391–1395.
12. Shapiro EM, Knox JM, Freeman RG. Carcinogenic effect of prolonged exposure to grenz ray. *J Invest Dermatol.* 1961;291–298.
13. Zackheim HS, Kronbock E, Langs L. Cutaneous neoplasms in the rat produced by grenz ray and 80 kV x-ray. *J Invest Dermatol.* 1964;48:519–534.
14. Epstein JH. Carcinogenic and cocarcinogenic effects of grenz radiation. *J Invest Dermatol.* 1970; 54:439–440.
15. Wulf HC, Hou-Jensen K. Metastatic cancer in guinea-pigs irradiated with grenz rays. *Arch Dermatol.* 1979;115:176–178.
16. Bucky G, Combes FC. Grenz ray therapy. New York, NY: Springer-Verlag; 1954.
17. Arouete J. Grenz ray therapy. In: Sidi E, ed. *Psoriasis.* Springfield, Ill: Charles C Thomas; 1968:243–257.
18. Frain-Bell W, Bettley FR. Treatment of psoriasis and eczema with grenz rays. In: *Yearbook of Dermatology.* Chicago, Ill: Year Book Medical Publishers; 1960;61:103–104.
19. Stewart WD. Eczema. In: Maddin S, ed. *Current Medical Management.* 2nd ed. St Louis, Mo: CV Mosby; 1975:144–146.
20. Brodersen J, Reymann F. Effect of grenz rays on psoriasis treated with local corticosteroids. *Dermatologica.* 1981;162:327–329.
21. Wiskemann A. Röntgenbestrahlung von Dermatosen im Genitalbereich. *Hautarzt.* 1977;28:219–223.
22. Wiskemann A. Strahlenbehandlung der Psoriasis und Parapsoriasis. *Z Hautkr.* 1981;57:1317–1324.
23. Johannesson A, Lindelöf B. The effect of grenz rays on psoriasis lesions of the scalp. A double blind trial. *Photodermatology.* 1985;2:388–391.
24. Johannesson A, Lindelöf B. Additional effect of grenz rays on psoriasis lesions of the scalp treated with topical corticosteroids. *Dermatologica.* 1987; 175:290–292.
25. Lindelöf B, Johannesson A. Psoriasis of the scalp treated with grenz rays or topical corticosteroid combined with grenz rays. A comparative randomized trial. *Br J Dermatol.* 1988;119:241–244.
26. Lindelöf B. Psoriasis of the nails treated with grenz rays: a double blind bilateral trial. *Acta Dermatol Venereol.* 1989;69:80–82.
27. Lynne-Davies G. Lichen simplex chronicus. In:

Maddin S, ed. *Current Medical Management.* 2nd ed. St Louis, Mo: CV Mosby; 1975:203.
28. Lindelöf B, Wrangsjö K, Lidén S. A double-blind study of grenz ray therapy in chronic eczema of the hands. *Br J Dermatol.* 1987;117:77–80.
29. Kopp H, Reymann FE. Lichen planus treated with grenz rays. *Acta Dermatol Venereol.* 1956;36:477–481.
30. Brodkin RH, Bleiberg J. Grenz rays and lichen planus: case report of isomorphic phenomenon following grenz-ray therapy. *Arch Dermatol.* 1965;91:149–150.
31. Wiskemann A. Dyskeratosis follicularis Darier. *Dermatol Monatsschr.* 1969;155:200–202.
32. Cipollaro V, Shaps R. The treatment of Darier's disease: a comparison of superficial x-ray and grenz ray therapy. *Int J Dermatol.* 1979;18:580–583.
33. Lindelöf B. Histiocytosis X in an adult: treatment of skin lesions with grenz rays. *J Am Acad Dermatol.* 1988;19:426–427.
34. Wulf HC, Brodthagen H. Transmission of Bucky (grenz) rays through human scalp hair. *Acta Dermatol Venereol.* 1977;57:525–527.
35. Lindelöf B, Karlberg J, Lyckefält S, Gerhardsson A. Grenz ray therapy: practical aspects of protecting office personnel from radiation. *Photodermatology.* 1988;5:248–251.

Index